Urban Design Practice

An International Review

Edited by
Sebastian Loew

RIBA Publishing

© Sebastian Loew, 2012

Published by RIBA Publishing, 15 Bonhill Street,
London EC2P 2EA

ISBN 978 1 85946 449 6

Stock code 77533

Chapters on Argentina and Morocco were translated into
English by Sebastian Loew.

British Library Cataloguing in Publications Data
A catalogue record for this book is available from the
British Library.

Commissioning Editor: Matthew Thompson
Designer: Alex Lazarou
Cover designer: Alex Lazarou
Production: Kate Mackillop

Printed and bound in Great Britain by
Butler Tanner & Dennis Ltd, Frome and London, UK

RIBA Publishing is part of RIBA Enterprises Ltd.
www.ribaenterprises.com

Contents

Foreword

For over 30 years, the Urban Design Group has been promoting excellence in urban design and a better understanding of how to make successful cities. It has done this through its series of lectures, its annual conference, its awards, study tours and educational seminars, and its regular publications, the quarterly magazine, Urban Design, and the biennial Directory. The group was a founder member of the Urban Design Alliance, which brought together the various built environment professions in the UK, and has established contacts with a number of influential organisations, such as the former Commission for Architecture and the Built Environment, now Design Council Cabe, and the Academy of Urbanism. Its membership, open to all those concerned with and interested in the quality of life in cities, includes practitioners from around the world.

The group is pleased to support one of its long-standing members with this new publication, which responds clearly to its objectives. Sebastian Loew's book broadens our perspective, locating the urban design experience in an international context. Reviewing its definition and practice as well as taking on the challenge of looking into the future, Sebastian and his 18 international collaborators contribute to a clearer understanding of the role and potential of urban design at a pivotal moment for our global civilisation.

At a time when many professionals are struggling to respond to the challenges raised by major issues like climate change and economic recession, this book encourages a creative and open view for shaping the future of urban place making, by examining how these problems are tackled in different countries.

Locating the debate in a global context makes a forceful case for the exchange of ideas and design collaboration, working across professions and continents. Crucially, this worldview brings a focus on the civilising imperative of high-quality spaces and places. We trust that this book will become essential reading for urban designers wherever they live or work, and will help promote the aspirations of the Urban Design Group around the world.

Amanda Reynolds
UDG Chair

The Urban Design Group (www.urg.org.uk) is an inter-disciplinary charity with a mission to support and encourage everyone committed to improving life in cities, towns and villages. We work to promote high-quality urban design and collaboration within the design process through our awards, events, research and publications, especially our acclaimed journal Urban Design.

Acknowledgements

First of all I want to thank all the contributors to this book from countries around the world, who put up with my requests and demands, researched the subject, drafted substantial and interesting texts, and managed to meet almost all the deadlines. This book only became possible thanks to their efforts. I am very grateful to all of them, but one in particular has to be singled out: my old colleague from South Bank University, David Truscott, who many years ago first put the idea of a global review of urban design into my head.

Many thanks are due to the Urban Design Group and the Francis Tibbalds Trust for their encouragement and financial support, to David Lock Associates for their sponsorship and to Juan Luis de las Rivas for committing to buy a number of copies for his university library. A long list of people – too long to mention, though I will single out the members of the Urban Design magazine editorial board and my former colleagues at the University of Westminster – helped with contacts, images and ideas. Thank you also to the RIBA Publishing team, Matthew Thompson for believing in the book and James Hutchinson and Kate Mackillop for helping in its production. And thank you to all urban designers around the world!

Sebastian Loew

This book has been generously supported by

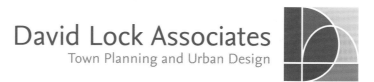

Contributors' biographies

ARGENTINA

Raquel Perahia, Arq. PUR (UBA)

Raquel worked as a consultant in urban and regional planning, advising local and provincial authorities on their local development plans. She has taught on the postgraduate Urban and Regional Planning and Planning and Landscape courses of the architecture faculty of the University of Buenos Aires, where she is also a researcher. Her articles have been published in Argentina and abroad.

Elba Luisa Rodríguez, Arq. PUR (UBA)

Elba was head of urban development at the ministry of housing from 1977 to 2007, having previously held positions as head of planning at municipal and provincial levels. She also taught in the planning department of the faculty of architecture and urbanism of the University of Buenos Aires, and has published a number of articles in Argentina.

AUSTRALIA

Mark Sheppard, BArch DipUD MAUD MPIA

Mark is a practising urban designer, based in Melbourne. He is a principal of urban design and planning consultancy David Lock Associates (Australia), which he established in 1997 after working for David Lock Associates in the UK from 1993. Mark has qualifications in architecture and urban design. He has had numerous articles published on urban design topics, ranging from the design of new town centres to the planning of urban growth areas.

BRAZIL

Vicente del Rio, PhD

Vicente is an architect and urban designer. From 1979 to 2001, he taught at the school of architecture and urbanism of the Federal University of Rio de Janeiro. Since 2001, he has been professor at the city and regional planning department at California Polytechnic university, San Luis Obispo. An experienced planner and urban designer with several projects in Brazil and abroad, he has published extensively and has authored five books in Brazil: Introducao ao Desenho Urbano no Processo de Planejamento (Sao Paulo: Pini, 1990), Percepcao Ambiental (with L. Oliveira; Sao Paulo: Studio Nobel, 1996), Arquitetura: Pesquisa & Projeto (Sao Paulo: Projeto, 1998), Projeto do Lugar (with Rheingantz and Duarte; Rio de Janeiro: Contra Capa, 2001), and the proceedings of the International Conference on Psychology and the Design of the Built Environment (with C. Duarte and N. Iwata; Rio de Janeiro: UFRJ, 2000). In the US, he is the co-editor and co-author of Contemporary Urbanism in Brazil: Beyond Brasilia (with W. Siembieda; Gainesville: University of Florida Press, 2009).

CHINA
Matthias Bauer, Dipl.-Ing. (Arch.)

Matthias has more than eight years of work experience in urban design in China. He is currently leading the urban design team of Atkins in Beijing. Previously, he worked with Scott Wilson, Halcrow and EDAW in China. He graduated from Dresden University with a degree in architecture and subsequently worked in urban regeneration and conservation in Germany and the UK (London and Leeds). His major masterplanning project in Europe has been the Phoenix West in Dortmund, Germany. In China, his extensive work includes masterplans for new towns, residential communities, tourism resorts and science parks, as well as large-scale strategic development frameworks. He has won first prize in numerous planning and design competitions, from high-speed railway station masterplans to logistics parks, and from entire CBDs to artificial islands.

CZECH REPUBLIC
Ing.Arch Veronika Sindlerova

Veronika works in Prague. She graduated in 2006 from the faculty of architecture of the Czech Technical University (CTU). From 2001 to 2003, she worked at the landscape architecture and urban design department of the Bauhaus-University in Weimar, Germany. Currently she practises as an architect and urban designer, and has designed or co-designed several buildings and urban projects in various cities of the Czech Republic. She is enrolled on the doctoral study programme at the Czech Technical University in Prague, faculty of architecture, department of spatial planning. The subject of her doctoral thesis is The System Approach to Urban Public Spaces. At the same time, she collaborates as fellow in the studio Sustainable Cities at CTU in Prague, faculty of architecture.

DUBAI
Tim Catchpole, MA, DipUD, FRTPI

Tim is a development planning consultant with over 35 years' experience in as many countries worldwide. For the past 20 years, he has worked with Halcrow and specialised in masterplanning projects, notably including industrial zones and business parks, major urban developments and transport infrastructure. He has been visiting Dubai regularly since 1991, and has watched it grow rapidly from a provincial town into a major world city.

Manosh De, B. Architecture, MSc Urban Design

Manosh is an urban design and masterplanning professional in Dubai. In 2002, he was selected on the US department of state International Visitors Programme to share ideas with his American contemporaries on historic city regeneration. In 2003, he attended University College London as a Chevening Scholar to study urban design and development. Manosh is currently working with a leading multidisciplinary engineering firm in Dubai. He has worked on a number of complex large-scale city developments across the region for a variety of clients. He has participated in a number of conferences, and has been published extensively.

EGYPT

Dr Noha Nasser

Noha is an architect and academic specialising in culture-led urban design, community development and social cohesion. She holds a PhD in urban design, conservation and regeneration, focusing on Cairo's historic core. Noha has also been a post-doctoral visiting scholar at the University of California, Berkeley. She is a senior lecturer and has held director posts at the Centre for Urban Design Outreach and Skills (CUDOS) at Birmingham City University and the Urban Renaissance Institute (URI) at the University of Greenwich. She is currently researching global influences on British architecture and urbanism.

FRANCE

Thierry Vilmin, Sc. Po. Paris. Dr. IUP

Thierry is a socio-economist by profession. He started his career as an executive in the real-estate branch of a bank. He then studied urbanism, obtained his doctorate and engaged in a career in planning, working for a number of years in local government and other public-sector organisations. He then became a consultant, lecturer and researcher in planning and land policies. This mixture of public- and private-sector work, business economics and development allowed him to discover the multiple facets of the system of 'actors' who create the urban fabric. He has used this wide and varied experience to write a number of books, articles and simulation models, as well as in his teaching at the Institut des Sciences Politiques in Paris and in continuous professional development.

GERMANY

Katja Stille, BSc (Hons) Dip Arch MA (Arch H&T) MA (UD)

Katja is an associate of Tibbalds, a multidisciplinary planning and urban design consultancy. Born in Germany, Katja trained as an architect at the University of East London and has subsequently undertaken the postgraduate course in Urban Design at the University of Westminster. Since 2003, she has worked as an urban designer with the responsibility for a variety of projects. Following an article on the role of plans in German housing development, she undertook further research comparing the German and English planning systems in order to inform a UK government study into the use and practicality of design codes.

Daniel Kräher, Dipl.-Ing. (Arch)

Daniel is currently completing a traineeship in urban planning with the State Government of Hesse. Daniel studied architecture at the Bauhaus University in Weimar and undertook his diploma thesis at the department for spatial planning and spatial research there. As a key member of a research team on urban green space at the University for Applied Science Erfurt (Germany), he explored the impact of demographic, economic and social changes on the use of urban open space, and presented the work to various government organisations and civic societies. Before starting his training with the government in Germany in 2010, Daniel worked as an urban designer for Tibbalds Planning and Urban Design in London. He has also worked as a freelance architect for offices in Vienna and Weimar.

INDIA

Professor Christopher Benninger

Christopher studied urban planning under Kevin Lynch and Herbert Gans, and architecture under Jose Luis Sert – both at the Massachusetts Institute of Technology (MIT), where he later taught. He founded the School of Planning (Ahmedabad) and the Centre for Development Studies and Activities (Pune). He is on the board of editors of CITIES (UK) and is a Distinguished Professor at CEPT University (Centre for Environmental Planning and Technlogy) in Ahmedabad. He is a practising urban planner, whose work includes the Site and Services programme for Chennai, the National Capitol Complex at Thimphu, Bhutan, and numerous university campuses in India.

ITALY

Professor Corinna Morandi

Corinna is professor of Town Planning and Urban Design in the department of Architecture and planning at the School of Architecture and Society of Milan Polytechnic. She is a member of the board of the international PhD in Spatial Planning and Urban Development. Since 1998, she has been the director of Urb&Com – Urbanism and Retail management – a research group in the department (www.webdiap.diap.polimi.it/Lab/UrbeCom). Her main research topics concern planning and urban design in the metropolitan area of Milan, the comparison of urban and regional planning strategies and policies in Europe, urbanism and retail management. Milan. The Great Urban Transformation (Venice: Marsilio, 2007) is one of her numerous publications.

MOROCCO

Gwenaëlle Zunino, Arch DPGL

Gwenaëlle is an architect–urbanist employed by the Institut d'aménagement et d'urbanisme d'Ile-de-France. She works on urban and architectural quality at various scales from the metropolitan to the local, in places as diverse as Casablanca, Tripoli and Paris. Her work also involves thematic studies, such as intensification and the capacity for evolution of urban and peri-urban fabric. She teaches at the school of architecture of Nancy and facilitates workshops on the urban and landscape project for the National Federation of Agences d'Urbanisme of France.

THE NETHERLANDS

ir Martin Aarts

Martin is head of urban planning at the department of urban planning of the City of Rotterdam. Since 1984, he has been involved in the development of Rotterdam's city centre. Recently he has been responsible for the city's Urban Vision, and now for the urban planning agenda. This concerns such themes as climate change, the polycentric city and the implementation of the Urban Vision.

Martin is also a lecturer at the academy of architecture in Rotterdam and the Netherlands Institute of Housing and Planning (Nirov). He has edited and contributed as a co-author to the following publications: Living in the City (1987), 50 Years of Reconstruction (1995), Accelerating Rotterdam, Stad in Versnelling (2000) and Rotterdam, High-Rise City (2001).

Dr Jan van Horne

Jan is an urban and regional planner, working as senior advisor at the department of urban planning of the City of Rotterdam. He has been involved in a large number of urban and regional projects in the city as well as in its greater urban region, and in many research projects in the fields of demography and regional economics. His expertise ranges from small, detailed neighbourhood development, through urban renewal to regional and supra-regional town and country planning level.

NEW ZEALAND

David Truscott, MA BSc DipUD

David is an urban designer, landscape architect and town planner from the United Kingdom, where he was employed in local and central government and worked as a consultant. He taught urban design and landscape planning for several years at South Bank University. Having emigrated to New Zealand in 1997, he now lives in Auckland where he has been involved in a number of development projects. David has a particular interest in the design of the urban public realm.

SOUTH AFRICA

Liezel Kruger

Liezel has an honours degree in Architecture and a master's degree in City Planning and Urban Design. During 10 years as consultant for David Lock Associates, Liezel was involved in a wide range of projects throughout the United Kingdom, at both local and strategic level. She focused on 'visioning', the preparation of structural frameworks, regeneration and masterplanning as well as consultation and participation events. Upon her return to South Africa in April 2010, she joined the City of Cape Town's spatial planning and urban design department where she champions the collaboration of public and private enterprises. Her main aim is to bring her private-sector experience and international expertise to the developing context of South Africa, and specifically Cape Town. Liezel is on the editorial board of the Urban Design Group's magazine as well as being a member of the Academy of Urbanism.

SPAIN

Juan Luis de las Rivas, PhD

Juan Luis is an architect and professor of Planning and Urban Design at the school of architecture in Valladolid. Former director of the Instituto Universitario de Urbanística, he has been visiting professor at the schools of architecture of the Politecnico di Milano; the University of Arizona (Tucson); the University of Texas at Austin; Escola Superior Artística do Porto (ESAP) at Oporto, Portugal; the Instituto de Urbanismo of Caracas, Venezuela; the Iberoamericana University of Puebla, Mexico; and other European and Latin American universities. He is a town planning consultant for regional and local authorities, and leads a team working in several Spanish cities. Juan Luis is currently conducting research related to innovation in planning and urban design. He has published extensively, and his work has been translated into several languages. In 2002, his Directrices de Ordenación Territorial de Valladolid y Entorno – Urban guidelines for a metropolitan area – won the 4th European Urban and Regional Planning Award, from the European Council of Town Planners.

SWEDEN

Mats Johan Lundström

Mats is an urban planner and designer at AQ Architects and a PhD fellow at the KTH Royal Institute of Technology in Stockholm. He is also the editor-in-chief of PLAN, the Swedish Journal of Planning. He has an MSc degree in Physical-Spatial Planning from Blekinge Institute of Technology (BTH), Karlskrona, Sweden, and a licentiate of Engineering in Infrastructure from KTH.

Dr Tigran Haas

Tigran is the assistant professor of Urban Planning and Design and the Director of the Urban Planning and Design Masters Program at KTH Royal Institute of Technology, Stockholm. He has advanced degrees in Architecture, Urban Planning and Design, Environmental Science and Regional Planning. One of his key publications is New Urbanism & Beyond: Designing Cities for the Future (Rizzoli: New York, 2008).

USA

Howard M Blackson III, MAUD, CNU-A

Howard is an award-winning urban designer who teaches at the University of California at San Diego, California, and practises as the Director of Planning for PlaceMakers, LLC. Educated at the University of Texas at Austin and the University of Westminster, London, Howard has worked extensively throughout North America and Asia. Recent projects have included development regulations and plans for the City of Taos, New Mexico; the City of San Marcos, California; and the Form-Based Code Institute's inaugural Driehaus Award winner, City of Leander, Texas.

EDITOR

Sebastian Loew

Sebastian Loew qualified as an architect in Argentina and as a town planner in London. He obtained his PhD from Reading University with a thesis on modern architecture in historic cities in France. After working in architecture and planning in the British public sector he taught planning at the University of the South Bank, and later urban design at the University of Westminster. At various occasions he has been visiting professor at the Institut d'Etudes Politiques (Paris), the University of Paris 4, the Institut d'Urbanisme de Paris, the Ecole des Ponts et Chaussées (Paris), the University of Lille, and Milan Politécnico.

He has collaborated in various European projects and in particular in the development of an urban simulation under the Leonardo programme. He has organised and run a number of urban design workshops for various clients in the private and public sectors. He undertook research for CABE and, together with colleagues from the University of Westminster, organised and ran their Urban Design Summer School for the first three years. At present he is consultant to the eco-cities programme, funded by the French government.

He is the author of four books, including Modern Architecture in Historic Areas (Routledge, 1998). He is co-editor of Urban Design and chair of Ashford Design Review Panel. He has contributed to numerous publications here and abroad.

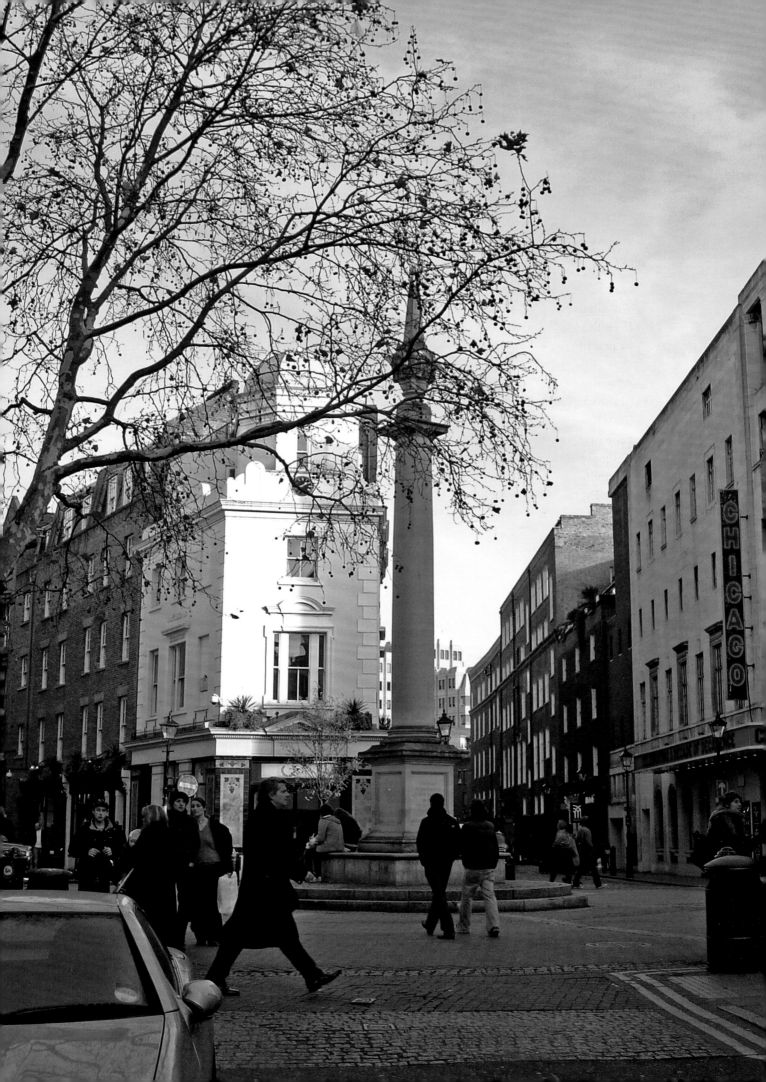

Introduction

What is urban design? The term is widely used among built-environment professionals in English-speaking countries, but even in these contexts its meaning seems to vary. Once translated into other languages, confusion will almost certainly ensue as it will be difficult to find the precise equivalent. That has been the experience from international meetings, whether participants were academics or practitioners.

The tool used by a practitioner may be principally a pencil or more likely nowadays some design software, a calculator or a word-processing package. The scale of the work may encompass the city as a whole, a neighbourhood or a part of a street. The client might be a government organisation, a landowner or a local community. The professional education involved may be based on architecture, engineering, landscape design or town planning, each of which could have a claim to be the dominant discipline.

Even in Britain, the urban design profession has only become recognised in the past 25 years and it does not as yet have the same status as those covered by an official charter. Nevertheless, as it becomes established in Britain it is worth trying to clarify what the position is at the global level, and that is the objective of this book. Is the evolution that has taken place here unique, or have similar changes occurred elsewhere? If the latter is the case, have different countries developed their own individual approaches or is there an international 'school' of urban design?

Other questions follow: who are the urban designers? What do they do and who employs them? What is their training? What are their concerns, and have these evolved over time? Are urban designers trained in one country able to work easily in another, or are the cultural and climatic differences too great? On the other hand, are some countries just replicating ideas, methods or forms from elsewhere, and will this create problems in the future? Is there an 'export trade' in urban designers? Finally, is there a discernible pattern for the future of the profession?

The book's structure

To answer these questions and to try to establish a global view of current urban design practice, 18 professionals working in different countries were asked to describe and analyse what urban design meant in their country. They were all asked the same questions but given the freedom to interpret them, as it was clear that the contexts in which they worked and the meanings of the words varied. The choice of countries, whilst not comprehensive, was meant to be representative of the situation in the wider

(facing page)

Seven Dials, one of the first shared streets in London

region. Admittedly there were omissions, some areas were better covered than others, and the vastness and diversity of a few countries meant that only some aspects could be dealt with. Nevertheless, the rich tapestry that emerged emphasises the fact that there is no international definition of urban design, but that the objective is similar whatever the approach is: to ensure the wellbeing of the population in an economic, ecological and socially sustainable environment.

Each chapter opens with an attempt to define urban design in the specific country. It then assesses the professional place of practitioners of urban design, and whether they are distinct from or part of another profession such as architecture or planning. It also looks at the legal status and the academic position of urban design. The historical development and evolution of urban design then leads to an analysis of current practice and the concerns of the practitioners. A case study (in some cases, more than one) serves to illustrate the position of the profession today. Most contributors conclude by making some kind of comment and by looking into the future. The chapters end with a quick guide which could help a newcomer approach potential work in a particular country.

The book starts with a short summary of the evolution of urban design in Great Britain, as this can act as a benchmark for the global situation. The 18 countries that follow are grouped by continent: Europe, Africa and the Middle East, Asia, the Americas and Oceania. Besides answering the above questions, the conclusion attempts to find patterns of similarities and differences, and to explain their origins.

A note on the European countries

Although each European Union (EU) country has its own legislation, its traditions and its own professional bodies, they all have to follow EU directives and laws. Free movement and open competition are a dominant element of the European treaties. This means for example that professionals qualified in one country are allowed to practise in all other EU countries; it also means that tenders and competitions have to be opened to practices from all member states. The fact that numerous British practices employ graduates from other EU countries, and enter competitions throughout the continent, are a reflection of these policies. Similarly, experts from neighbouring countries are invited to give advice in Britain: Danish urban designer Jan Gehl, for instance, was commissioned to write a report by Transport for London (Towards A Fine City for People), whilst Richard Rogers has been an advisor on the Grand Paris scheme.

The European Union does not have powers over planning, land use or urban design; but it does have environmental policies which are aimed at controlling pollution and greenhouse-gas emissions, reducing waste, encouraging energy efficiency and the development of renewable sources. Article 174 of the Treaty establishing the European Community aims to ensure the sustainable development of the European model of society. These various measures have an effect on urban design, but they seem to have been applied unevenly across the Union.

Great Britain

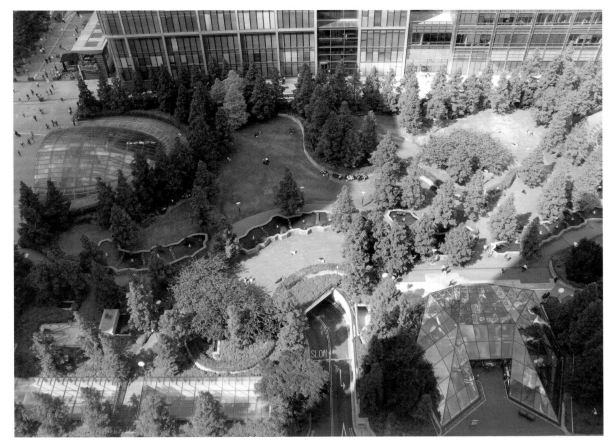

View of Jubilee Park, Canary Wharf, London

U rban design is the art of making places for people. It includes the way places work and matters such as community safety, as well as how they look. It concerns the connections between people and places, movement and urban form, nature and the built fabric and the processes for ensuring successful villages, town and cities.

(By Design, Section 1)

With this definition the term 'urban design' appeared for the first time in an official document in 2000. Soon after, this document was de facto incorporated in the planning legislation through the government's Planning Policy Statement 1, which stated 'Planning authorities should have regard to good practice set out in *By Design*' and 'Good design is indivisible from good planning'.

Early days

Even in 2000, however, the expression 'urban design' was not a new one: it had been in use for about half a century on both sides of the Atlantic. Rob Cowan found it in the Abercrombie and Forshaw 1943 County of London Plan and in various US publications from the 1950s. A more commonly used expression at the time was 'civic design', closely linked to town planning since its inception; the University of Liverpool's School of Civic Design, founded in 1919, was the first to teach town planning as a discipline. However, this latter term gradually became associated with the 'grand' design of civic centres or public buildings rather than the wider urban environment.

The manner in which the expression evolved is significant, in that it reflects the changes in professional practice and the way the disciplines of architecture, town planning and engineering developed. After the second world war, the built-environment professions, dominated by architects, were enthralled by modernist ideas and sought to improve society through the design of cities. On the basis of the horrors seen in Victorian cities, the classic model of the city was considered a failure that had to be replaced by something different. Architectural design ideas that had been developed but not implemented before the war were adopted by the bureaucracies and investors who were in charge of the reconstruction, and later the renewal, of cities, but what was implemented was a debased form of modernism. Helped by new and untested forms of construction, this satisfied a need for mass building and responded to the wishes of the development industry, but did not achieve the societal goals expected. Panel-built housing estates up and down the country are the frequently unloved legacy of these policies. Even though the new dwellings offered greater comfort, their environment and the spaces around them were poorly conceived and created new problems. At the same time, the growth in car use had an unpredicted impact on urban development and urban form.

At least some of Britain's policies were successful: the New Towns in particular achieved international praise and became a model for other countries to follow. Although few people involved in their creation would have called themselves urban designers, that is how we would see them today. Most of them were architects but with a wide view of their task and an understanding of the need to collaborate with a broad range of disciplines. Frederick Gibberd, for instance, architect–planner for Harlow New Town (1974) was also a landscape designer.

Until about the mid-1960s, architect–planners (often trained in both disciplines) were the professionals mostly in charge of urban programmes. But a split gradually evolved, with architects specialising in designing buildings and with planners in charge of policy and the control of development. Architects were seen as the designers, but their concerns were mostly formal and stopped at their client's site boundary. The gap between them widened as town-planning courses increasingly reduced their design input while expanding the social-sciences element. 'Physical' or 'architectural determinism' was seen as an architects' bias that had to be opposed by a more rational, scientific approach to city planning where socio-economic matters predominated. Traffic engineers on the other hand had a clear, though limited, agenda based on ensuring that traffic moved smoothly, safely and quickly; and because of the rise in car use, their role became increasingly important. The Buchanan Report, Traffic in Towns (1963), for instance, had a significant impact on the planning of cities but was not welcomed by all. Gradually the 'design' of cities was split between the professions, each one with its own vocabulary, agenda and objectives, and each fairly intolerant of the views of their competitors (who were not seen as collaborators).

Within this climate, local authority bureaucracies equally divided into separate departments – architects, town planning, parks, valuers, housing, etc – allowed or encouraged developments that destroyed the traditional morphology of cities and created increasingly alienating environments, often dominated by traffic engineering: spaces that had neither function nor meaning, and buildings that did not relate to their context. Rather than reduce social conflicts, these new places exacerbated them. The Thamesmead estate (built from 1967 onwards), with its overhead walkways and concrete system-built blocks, came to symbolise what was wrong.

New beginnings

Gradually, the failures of modernist policies started to become apparent and the excesses of redevelopment caused anxiety among citizens and professionals. In the US, Jane Jacobs was one of the first to write about these emerging issues, but soon a more general and universal debate emerged among academics, practitioners and politicians, about the roles of the various stakeholders in the built environment.

Reactions against modernism originated from different directions. The emerging conservation movement was very influential, as were a number of amenity societies throughout the country aiming at protecting their way of life. Celebrated battles such as the one to save the Euston Arch (which was lost) or to stop the redevelopment of Covent Garden (which was won) brought the issues to a wider public and mobilised professionals and politicians. The effect led on the one hand to a demand for wider public participation in the processes of urban transformation, and on the other to an end to the view that architects had a leading and unique role in these processes.

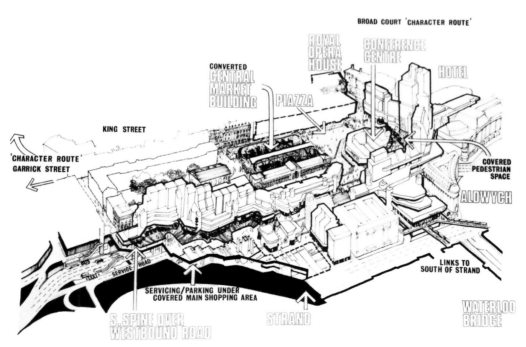

A sketch from the original proposals for major redevelopment in Covent Garden

Outside of London, the impact of suburban development – for which Ian Nairn had coined the expression *subtopia* – led the Essex County Council to produce the Essex Design Guide for Residential Areas (1973), the first of its kind and soon followed or copied by other authorities in the country. The importance of this guide was that it went beyond the design of individual buildings (though it favoured a contemporary response to local vernacular) and encouraged developers and designers to think about the public realm: the streets, the spaces in-between.

It was in this climate that the Urban Design Group was born in 1978 as a forum for people of diverse backgrounds interested in improving the design of the physical environment and the quality of places. One of its objectives was to bring together the various professions that had become isolated in silos and had difficulties in collaborating with each other. The group promoted the idea that the urban environment was too complex and too important to be dealt with piecemeal by separate professionals, and that all stakeholders needed to be involved.

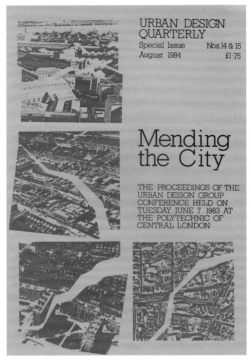

One of the early issues of the Urban Design Quarterly

The late 1970s and 80s were dark days for urban design in Britain, as the government saw any interference with the free market as a block to economic growth. The group's founders realised that they needed to lobby and campaign in order to improve matters. They influenced policy and attitudes by commenting on government documents and by working with other organisations. If the agenda has moved on, if urban design is now a recognised expression used in legislation, in government documents and in development plans, if developers recognise the importance of the public realm, it is to a considerable extent the result of the group's members working towards this – not in isolation, but together with other concerned organisations. One particular high point was reached when in 1988, Francis Tibbalds, one of the founders of the Urban Design Group and its chairman from 1979 to 1985, was elected the President of the Royal Town Planning Institute, thereby being able to bring the message to a much wider constituency.

At the beginning of the 1990s with the appointment of John Gummer as Secretary of State in charge of the Department of the Environment, the profile of urban design started to rise through a number of government publications and initiatives such as the Department of the Environment's Quality in Town and Country. At the same time the media started to show an interest, though not always for the best reasons: iconic buildings and their 'star' architects/authors were often of greater media appeal than more ordinary achievements, and the Prince of Wales' intervention against modern architecture tended to promote both a new kind of civic-design gesture, and pastiche architecture. House builders in particular (but also supermarket chains) decided that covering standard boxes in retro decoration (pseudo-Georgian seemed a favourite) was all that was needed to please the planners and the public. Nevertheless, the fact that the quality of the built environment was a subject of debate was a sign of progress.

Official recognition

In 1997, all the major built-environment institutes came together to create the Urban Design Alliance (UDAL). Two government ministers, Nick Raynsford (Minister for Construction and London) and Mark Fisher (Minister for the Arts), attended the launch and expressed their support for this initiative. Though UDAL has now lost much of its initial dynamism, it marked an important change in attitude as members of the professions understood at last that they needed to work together to achieve the common goal of improving the urban environment.

The establishment of the Urban Task Force in 1998, the publication of its Towards an Urban Renaissance report, and the creation of the Commission for Architecture and the Built Environment (CABE) in 1999 were further landmarks in the acceptance of urban design as a distinct practice and discipline. By Design, mentioned above, was one of CABE's early publications and its impact has been far-reaching. Its indirect incorporation into planning legislation (Planning Policy Statement 1) can be seen as the point at which urban design obtained official recognition.

During the next 12 years, CABE had a significant impact on the acceptance and understanding of urban design through publications and research, education and training, enabling and reviewing panels and lobbying of authorities at all levels. Also encouraging was the contribution of English Partnerships, working mostly with developers and local authorities: its Urban Design Compendium, first published in 2000, was another significant addition to the professional 'toolkit'.

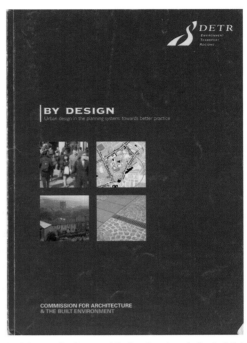

By Design, a landmark publication for urban design in Britain

Education

In parallel with these trends, an academic discipline evolved as a number of universities started offering specialist postgraduate courses in urban design. Oxford Brooks (then, Oxford Polytechnic) was the pioneer, with its Joint Centre for Urban Design (opened in 1972) and the publication of Responsive Environments, now a classic in the literature of urban design. Several universities followed, and today the Urban Design Group lists over a dozen British institutions offering such courses. Most of the students enrolled come from one of the main built-environment professions – architecture, planning, engineering or landscape design – but they see the advantage of obtaining an additional specialisation, and especially one that enables them to collaborate in multidisciplinary teams. Research

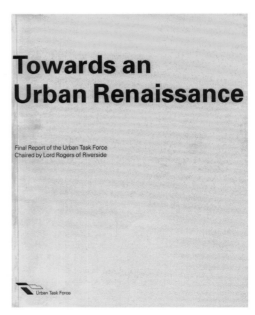

The Urban Task Force's report marked a change in British policy

has evolved at the same time, and is reflected in the increasing number of articles and books that are being published.

During the boom years, graduates from these courses were in great demand as urban design work expanded. Developers and local authorities accepted the importance of urban design and commissioned feasibility studies, masterplans, design codes and other studies for which interdisciplinary teams were required and within which urban designers were seen as key players. An increasing number of architectural and planning practices offered urban design services to their clients, and competition for staff meant that quality improved all around. Short courses and in-house training programmes multiplied as existing staff needed to upgrade their skills and increase their awareness of urban design. Responding to demand, CABE established its very successful Urban Design Summer School (developed for the first three years with the University of Westminster) and the Greater London Authority created Urban Design London.

Current practice

In Britain, urban design work has to a large extent been a reaction to the modernist model and its rejection of the traditional city. People are no longer satisfied with soulless urban spaces and an environment dominated by cars; they want cities that are attractive and humane. A return to traditional urban morphologies seems to be the basis of most urban design schemes: the perimeter block, the shared street, landmarks, mixed uses and walkable neighbourhoods are strongly advocated by most British consultancies.

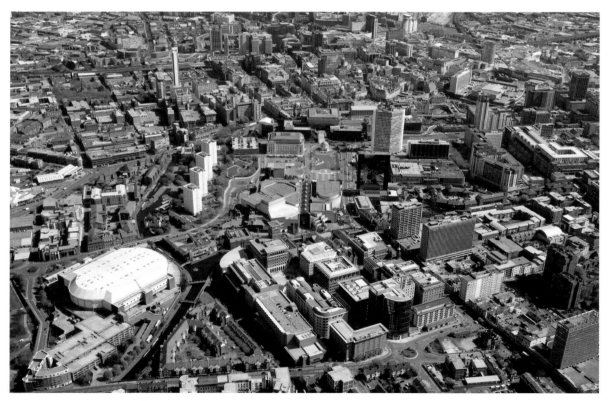

Aerial view of Brindleyplace, a major redevelopment that changed people's perceptions of Birmingham

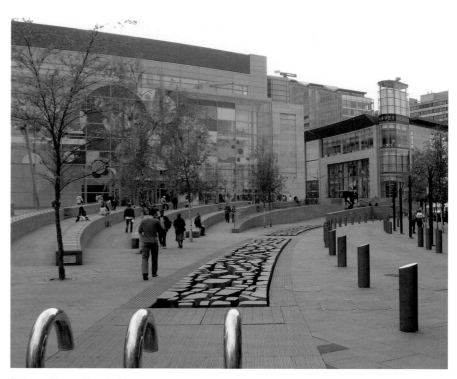

Exchange Square, Manchester

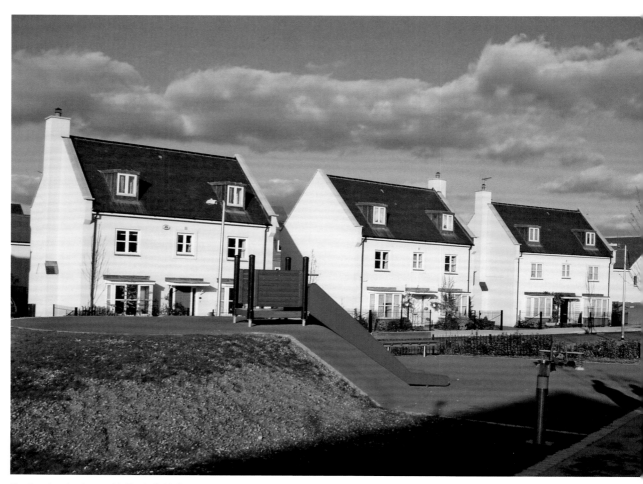

New housing development in Newhall, Harlow,
masterplanned by Studio REAL

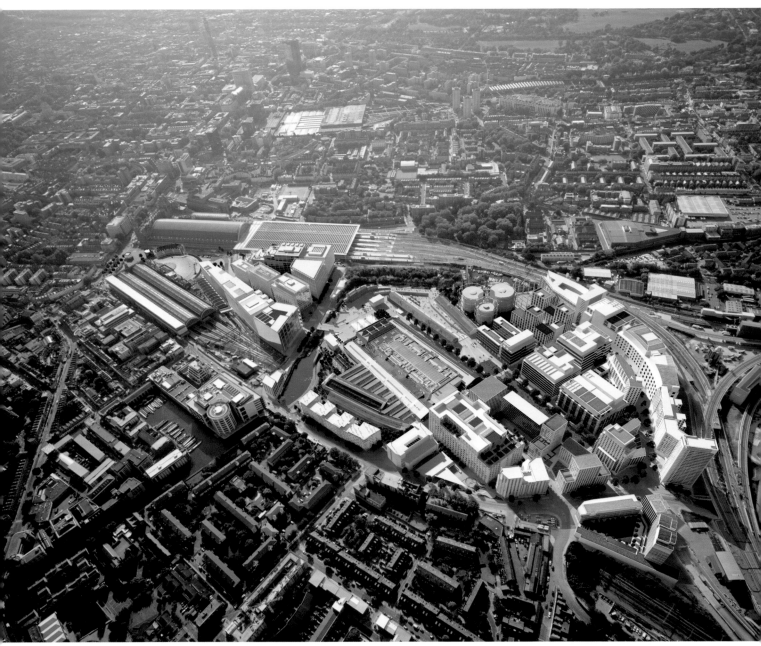

Aerial view of King's Cross redevelopment

It may not have developed into a style, but a common language (reflecting the work of Kevin Lynch, Gordon Cullen and Jane Jacobs) has evolved, with terms such as legibility, permeability and connectivity used ubiquitously, and not just by urban designers. The expression 'urban renaissance' was probably not chosen accidentally by the Task Force team, as many people have also started to understand the disadvantages of suburban living and long commuting times, and to move back to the cities.

The body of work produced by urban designers is impressive as well as diverse in type and in scale: it includes *inter alia* masterplans for whole districts on both greenfield and brownfield sites, the redesign of a square and the total or partial removal of cars from a street. Some important achievements have helped in establishing the profession: the transformation of Birmingham and the creation of Brindleyplace, the renewal of

Hulme, the rebuilding of central Manchester generally and the pedestrianisation of part of Trafalgar Square all made the national news. Some new housing developments, such as Accordia in Cambridge and Newhall in Harlow, won praise and awards. But smaller schemes up and down the country have had at least as much impact on people's everyday lives, and are appreciated by many. This has created a demand for better design, and affected at least part of the development industry. Some of the major players such as the Argent Group, Igloo Regeneration, the Grosvenor Estate and Berkeley Homes are now advocates of good urban design and acknowledge the fact that it makes economic sense.

Since the beginning of the 21st century, a new concern has affected all built-environment professions: climate change and how it will affect the shape of cities. The walkable, dense and mixed neighbourhoods which urban designers have been promoting for a long time are a step in the right direction. As a result, and also because of their interdisciplinary approach, urban designers are ideally positioned to help in the search for solutions that need to go beyond building technology or innovations in transport. New skills and knowledge will have to be acquired and at present the field is wide open, but the design of cities is already reflecting these new concerns.

Conclusion

In Britain, urban design has come a long way in the past 60 years. It is now an established discipline and a profession with an increasing number of practitioners and a substantial body of work. Whilst it would be an exaggeration to claim that everybody understands what an urban designer does, at least people involved in the built environment have a better idea than they did hitherto. Unfortunately the media is still more interested in buildings and star architects, and rarely discusses the quality of the public realm. The war is not won, but advances have been made.

The next decades will be as exciting as the past ones and probably more difficult: how will urban design fare in an economic downturn like the one being experienced at the moment? How will the momentum achieved in the past decade be maintained when developers and local authorities will want to save money, and the government is less keen to defend design quality? How will climate change and limited energy resources affect the work of urban designers?

As mentioned above, certain elements seem to have become ubiquitous in what are considered good British urban design schemes: the perimeter block, the well-connected streets, the active frontage providing 'eyes on the street', the shared street space. Though these appear to be formal elements, they are seen as the basis for places that work and are enjoyed by their users. But are these accepted universally or grounded in culture, tradition and climate?

The experience of other countries may help us answer these questions. In a globalised world, ideas travel in all directions. British urban designers work in other countries and then return to Britain, with positive results for all involved. British practices enter international competitions and participate in tenders all over the world; their success is the result of having developed an expertise and methodologies that are widely recognised. On the other hand, issues that seem to be central here may be peripheral elsewhere, methods of operation are certainly different and lessons can be learned from understanding how colleagues in other contexts operate. It is hoped that the following chapters contribute to this understanding.

SECTION 1

EUROPE

FRANCE

Thierry Vilmin, *economist and consultant*

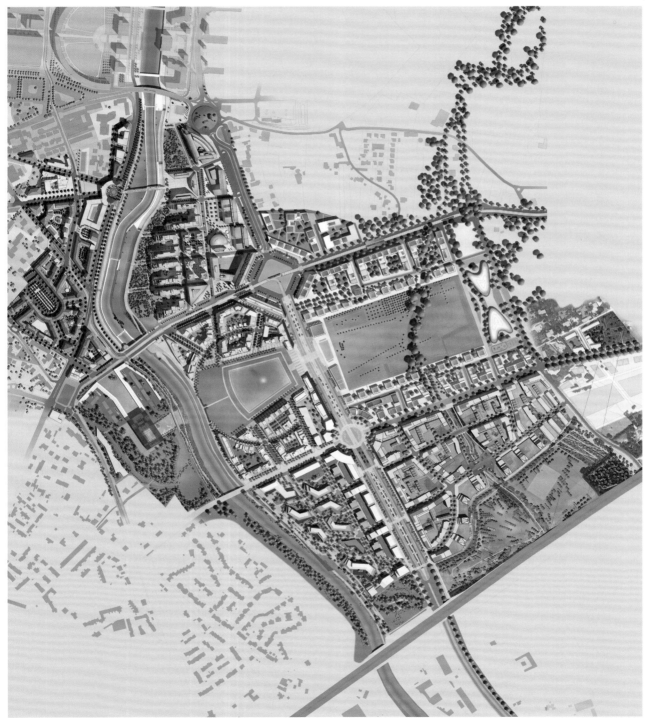

Example of a *projet urbain*: Port Marianne in Montpellier

FRANCE has nearly 65 million inhabitants, but with one of the highest population growth rates in Europe it could reach 72 million in 2050 and overtake Germany. Its population density is lower than that of its neighbours and space is less scarce. The country is divided into 26 regions (four of them overseas), 100 departments and over 36,000 municipalities. Traditionally France has been a centralised country, but since the 1980s planning powers have been decentralised and handed over to the municipal authorities, known as *communes*. These are mostly small, and as a result have limited technical and financial resources with which to fulfil their planning responsibilities. Voluntary groupings of communes take place to reflect changes on the ground resulting from the galloping urbanisation of the past 60 years. The resulting associations of *communes*, which can take various forms, are better suited to respond to these challenges.

According to the International Monetary Fund (IMF), the country has an endemic high level of unemployment (around 9%), a consequence of sluggish growth and the rigidity of the labour market.

Definitions

The English expression 'urban design' is sometimes used in France to mean the formal conception of the city, its physical form. The closest French equivalent is *composition urbaine*, or urban composition, an expression used mostly in an architectural sense of urban form. It is therefore associated with a conservative pre-modernist approach to the city, linked to the Beaux-Arts tradition. The word *urbanisme* is more frequently used, and it relates to both urban form and function; an *urbanist* is mostly an architect who works at a scale larger than that of a building, and the diploma granted to architects is automatically that of *architecte-urbaniste*. But the term can also be translated as planning, and there are urbanists that have not studied architecture. The professional urbanist is probably the closest equivalent to the urban designer.

In between these two terms, *urbanisme* which is too wide, and *composition urbaine*, which is too narrow, the expression *projet urbain*, or urban project, has emerged. This encompasses not just the formal aspects of a scheme but also its social, economic, technical and environmental characteristics. It also assumes a political commitment and a participatory, interactive and iterative process in the preparation of the project which can modify the original brief during its implementation. The expression defines a product and a methodology rather than a profession, but as such indicates what the latter should be capable of.

On the other hand, both practice and history have led to another concept which is more operational than urbanism and fairly unique to France: this is known as *aménagement*, defined by law (Article L.300-1 of the Urbanism Code) as follows:

> The objectives of *aménagement* are to implement an urban project or a local housing policy, to organise the retention, enhancement or reception of economic activities, to encourage the development of tourism or leisure activities, to create community services, research or higher education premises, to eradicate substandard housing, to allow urban renewal, to preserve and enhance the built or non-built heritage and the natural environment.

The law distinguishes general 'actions' that can be localised but have an impact on the whole city (similar to policies in Britain), or 'operations' over a specific area such as an old neighbourhood to be regenerated or an extension of an eco-neighbourhood. In both cases, the public sector is involved in the process, even if it does not necessarily develop the scheme. *Aménagement* is therefore a form of intentional or planned urbanisation – as opposed to spontaneous or uncontrolled development of sprawl. It translates better as planning than as urban design, though it does not correspond precisely to either.

It is therefore difficult to find the exact equivalent to urban design in French: both *urbanisme* and *aménagement* have elements of urban design. And the outcome is mostly the *projet urbain*, which has no legal definition and remains a vague term, particularly in terms of scale (city? neighbourhood? block?), but includes a political commitment. So, *aménagement and projet urbain* are two sides of the same concept: the former is the implementation of the conception of the latter.

Legal status

The above definition of *aménagement* is taken from the Code de l'Urbanisme, a statutory document that regulates the practice of planning in France. It is therefore under this banner that any legal status can be found and although the expression 'urban design' can be found neither in this hefty document nor in the legislation, guidance and constraints on design are set in it and in local planning documents, and must be reflected in applications for permits. These can only be approved if they comply with the regulations, in which case they can also not be refused.

The main planning documents are the *Schéma de cohérence territoriale* (SCOT), equivalent to a British structure plan and covering a large area over the medium to long term, and the *Plan local d'urbanisme* (PLU), equivalent to the British local plan. The latter is normally commissioned by one *commune*, but occasionally by a formally established group of them; it is regulatory, establishes land-use rights and, as a consequence, land values. Planning applications must conform with the PLU to get consent and cannot be refused if they do. Basic requirements of urban design are therefore incorporated in the plans, regulating street alignments, setbacks, building heights in relation to street widths, distances between building, parking, etc. In conservation areas or other sensitive zones, additional requirements may be included.

Contrary to what happens in some other countries, urban development covering an area larger and more complex than that of a single development is mostly initiated by the public sector: these are the urban projects mentioned above. To implement these, local authorities have access to another statutory tool, the *zone d'aménagement concerté* (ZAC) – comprehensive development area – that gives them control of the process. Through this widely used instrument, local authorities have powers to acquire (by expropriation if necessary), masterplan and develop land, within a designated area.

To realise a *projet urbain*, the local authority first commissions a brief from independent or in-house consultant urbanists who may not necessarily have an architecture background. This document translates, mostly in written form, the intentions and the vision of the elected members.

The brief is the basis for a legally regulated tender system (also enshrined in European legislation), through which the local authority chooses a professional who is charged with preparing a masterplan for the area. At this stage, some of the elements of the brief can be questioned: feedback at the design stage may result in a revision and refinement of the initial intentions.

A contract is then signed between the local authority and its designated developer, defining the scheme, the programme and the financial responsibilities of the partners. The masterplan is the basis for the contract between developer and local authority. It therefore acquires legal status and its requirements can be enforced. Urban form is established in advance of any private building taking place, and frequently its armature is laid out by the public authority before it sell the parcels of land to developers. So although urban design as such is not a legally recognised term, the practice is covered by a number of legal documents applying in a variety of contexts.

The professionals

At least three categories of practitioner are involved in the multidisciplinary teams of *aménagement* practice:

- 'spatialists', architects and landscape architects who design the schemes
- civil engineers responsible for the technical aspects of the schemes: roads, networks, transport and traffic
- social sciences professionals: economists, sociologists, lawyers, managers and communication specialists, in charge of the programming of the projects, business plans and contact with the inhabitants.

Nowadays environmental specialists also join the teams and work across disciplines to ensure that sustainability is taken into account in all its facets – ecological, social and economic – and throughout the process from the initial studies, through decision making and implementation, to management after the delivery of the scheme.

All the above professionals may call themselves *urbanistes*. The title has been recognised for a while and an official accrediting organisation – *Office Public de Qualification des Urbanistes* – has been set up. Their status is therefore similar to that of architects or engineers. However, for the general public an urbanist is someone who draws: an architect/urbanist or perhaps a landscape architect. All the other participants in the process of producing an urban project are known by their original discipline: engineer, economist, lawyer, sociologist, etc.

However, although the urban project is the result of a collaboration between various disciplines, the coordinating architect–urbanist remains in most cases the keystone who, through giving form to the scheme, synthesises all constraints and aspirations of the various stakeholders. Architectural 'stars' are often associated with iconic urban projects in the hope that, through their ideological lead, they will manage to transcend the individual visions and interests of the stakeholders. However, this can only happen if the architect–urbanist is backed by a political 'big chief', a mayor or a group of elected representatives.

The discipline

Architect–urbanists study mainly in schools of architecture and follow an integrated curriculum from BA to doctorate. The same is true for landscape architects. The other practitioners have a generalist first degree and specialise during their postgraduate studies. The master's-level courses offer a wide spectrum of subjects that are part of planning and which develop the capacity of collaborating in interdisciplinary teams on one urban project. Architectural students will be involved in large schemes and will learn about traditional urban composition. But with few exceptions, urban design is not part of their curriculum.

It follows from the above that academic research that can be directly attributed to urban design is not easily found. However, analytical and theoretical work on the *projet urbain*, which can be seen as one of the main products of urban design, is undertaken by government and academic institutions. A number of publications also deal with this subject.

Historical development of urban design

France has a long tradition of urban design, in that cities or parts of cities were carefully planned and regulated there from at least the 17th century. Interpreting baroque layouts imported from Italy, France created its own 'classic' layouts, of which Versailles was probably the best-known example. In the 19th century, Baron Haussmann's modernisation of Paris became the model for many other countries, sometimes (as in the United States) under the Beaux-Arts label, reflecting its origins in the Parisian architecture school of the same name. Urban composition and its rules were taught at this school, and for a long time it remained the canonical model for town planning practice in France and abroad.

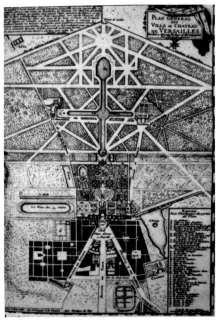

17th-century plan of Versailles' chateau and gardens

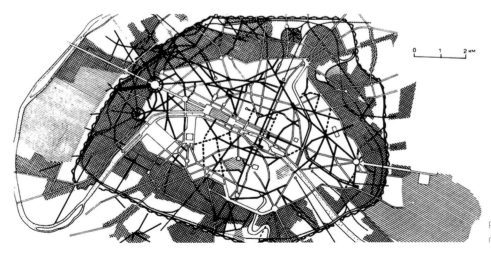

Paris plan with Haussmann's modernisation proposals

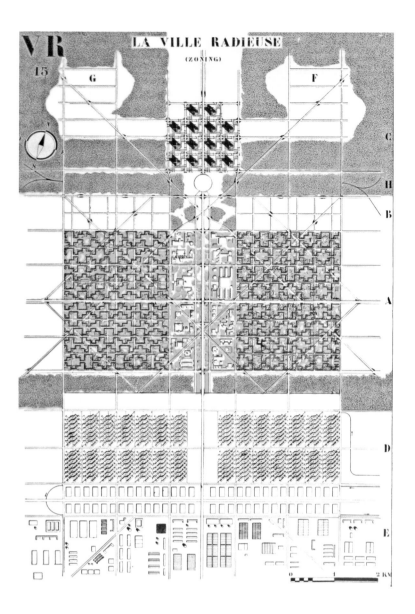

Le Corbusier's diagrammatic proposal for *La Ville Radieuse*, 1929

Perhaps as a reaction to this fairly inflexible model, modernist ideas found fertile ground to develop in France, particularly under the leadership of Le Corbusier. Even though his most radical plans were never implemented, he became a strong propagandist for a new approach to city design and urban form, based on the separation of activities and on the reinvention of the traditional relationship between buildings and the public realm. These ideas influenced the redevelopment of cities after the second world war, and the education of French architect/urbanists. The resulting new paradigm was the basis for the design of reconstructed cities, large housing estates and new towns, which became ubiquitous in France. A new formalist approach to city planning was, to a large extent, possible because of the centralised control of urban development and the dominant position of architects.

In the 1980s, decentralisation handed over much more power to local authorities and in particular their mayors. As quantitative imperatives diminished, the quality of urban environments became more important and appeared on the political agenda. The already-mentioned *projets urbains* are a direct result of this change of direction, as they address all the issues of an area and apply to all kind or urban situations: new centralities where good quality public realm, frequently connected to new forms of public transport, is the key to success; regeneration of former industrial areas; rehabilitation of large 1960s housing estates; conversion of urban motorways into boulevards in order to mend scars in the landscape; restoration and renewal of historic centres, etc. Improvements to the public realm are now frequently seen by mayors as a symbol of the success of their mandate, and have been commissioned during the past few years by small and large *communes* all over the country, frequently in combination with traffic calming or pedestrianisation schemes. When the resources are available, public amenities with an impact that reaches beyond the area are included in the programme as a 'lever' for economic success. And although these schemes are not the only way that cities develop, they represent a good-practice model that others tend to emulate.

Sustainability

Following a national debate on the environment, legislation was voted on to embed sustainability in all aspects of French society. The laws, known as Grenelle 1 and 2, deal with building, energy, transport, waste disposal, health and biodiversity, and have a direct impact on urban development. One of the results of related government-sponsored initiatives are the *EcoQuartiers* or eco-neighbourhoods: these are projects which integrate housing development with its natural, urban and environmental contexts; offer a range of tenures; and involve all stakeholders in their planning and design. The idea behind these is that they will start as models but become the norm for urban development, and the government hopes that by 2012 every city where housing development takes place will have at least one *EcoQuartier*. In the meantime, annual prizes for the best *EcoQuartiers* have been awarded in 2011.

More recently, the government launched a tender for *EcoCités* and selected 13 major cities out of 19 candidates. They are being assisted to expand in a sustainable way, coordinating all policies and actions with this objective in mind. The scale of thinking and the complexity of these projects are much larger than those of the eco-neighbourhoods, but the idea behind them is similar. In the long run, the French government hopes that all urban growth will be planned in a holistic and sustainable manner. One related consequence of these policies has been the construction of tram lines in most large cities, which in turn has led to a redesign of the spaces in the streets they follow. Recently, four new cities have been added to the existing 13 and a network of all of them has been established to exchange good practice.

Most urban projects are now conceived as eco-neighbourhoods, and this affects the design not only of the buildings but also of the urban morphology, the public realm, the landscaping and the movement patterns around them. The *EcoQuartier* and *EcoCité* labels are increasingly seen as an asset, and therefore influence the practice of urban design.

Practice

Practitioners exercise their profession in three main ways: commissioning work, undertaking studies and implementing projects.

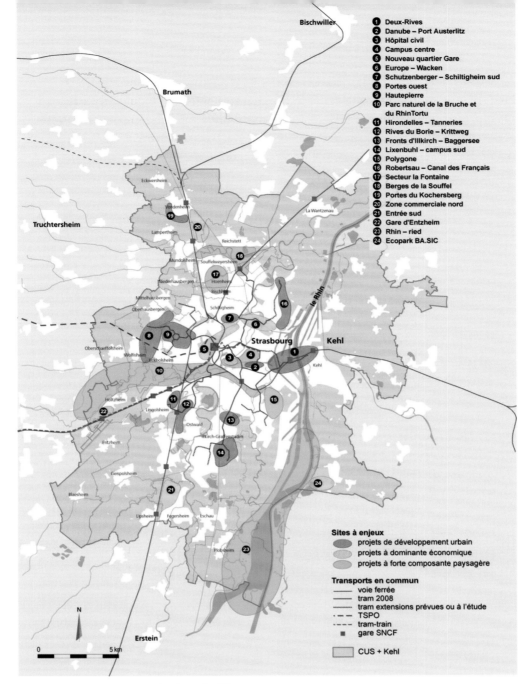

Legend:

1. Deux-Rives
2. Danube – Port Austerlitz
3. Hôpital civil
4. Campus centre
5. Nouveau quartier Gare
6. Europe – Wacken
7. Schutzenberger – Schiltigheim sud
8. Portes ouest
9. Hautepierre
10. Parc naturel de la Bruche et du RhinTortu
11. Hirondelles – Tanneries
12. Rives du Borie – Krittweg
13. Fronts d'Illkirch – Baggersee
14. Lixenbuhl – campus sud
15. Polygone
16. Robertsau – Canal des Français
17. Secteur la Fontaine
18. Berges de la Souffel
19. Portes du Kochersberg
20. Zone commerciale nord
21. Entrée sud
22. Gare d'Entzheim
23. Rhin – ried
24. Ecopark BA.SIC

Sites à enjeux
- projets de développement urbain
- projets à dominante économique
- projets à forte composante paysagère

Transports en commun
- voie ferrée
- tram 2008
- tram extensions prévues ou à l'étude
- TSPO
- tram-train
- gare SNCF

CUS + Kehl

Proposed sites and projects for the Strasbourg *EcoCité*

In France, commissioning urban development projects is done mostly by the public sector, by local authorities either intervening directly or delegating the work to public urban development companies. The latter prepare the land and lay out the infrastructure but do not build; they then sell the land to private developers who undertake the construction. Contrary to what happens in other countries, few private enterprises are willing to take the long-term risk that large urban development schemes imply.

As was already mentioned, local authorities commission preliminary studies from independent consultants, and developers commission pre-operational studies. In practice those preliminary studies, in which the developers are not involved, are often out of phase with economic and technical realities. On the other hand, involving developers in the preliminary studies would risk breaking the competition laws applicable since 2005 (except for those developers which are 100% controlled by the local authority and therefore in-house). This conflict is still to be resolved through case law.

In addition, the relationship between the urban project and the regulatory plan is now being questioned. Practice indicates that large and/or complex schemes often precede the regulatory plan or, when it already exists, lead to its modification. It has shown that to establish rigid regulations first, when the people who will carry the project are not even known, is illusory. Current debate therefore tends towards replacing a regulatory planning system by one based on the project. This attitude also constitutes a recognition that urbanism cannot be purely a top-down activity with the public authority acting independently, but that it must take account of all the stakeholders, private and public, individuals and organisations, that will participate in its implementation.

Furthermore, the implementation of projects raises the question of distribution of responsibilities between the coordinating urbanist (in other words, a masterplanner/ urban designer) and the architects of individual schemes. In the 1960s and 70s, architects designed both the masterplans and the individual buildings in projects such as social-housing estates or tourist resorts. Planning was considered an accessory to architecture and not as a separate entity. In spite of some rare successes most of the resulting schemes are rigid and monotonous, and have aged badly. Therefore these integrated procedures have been abandoned. Nevertheless, the urbanist responsible for the masterplan is generally asked to also design some of the buildings within the overall development so as to test the rules that he/she has established for others, and to give him/her a more substantial financial reward. This is because architecture is better remunerated than urban design.

The future

Even though space is less scarce in France than in other European countries, the country's excessive consumption has become an issue since the beginning of the century. The Solidarity and Urban Renewal Law of December 2000 has given priority to urban renewal (brownfield site development) over peripheral development (greenfield). However as the regeneration of existing areas is cumbersome and takes a long time, development tends to gravitate towards places with fewer economic, political, legal or technical constraints; that means building in the outer suburbs, at low density, in a poorly planned manner and consuming agricultural land at an even faster rate than in the past.

The process of grouping local authorities into larger organisations has not been completed yet, and most small *communes* lack in-house expertise. The link between planning and the implementation of schemes is a weak one, and there are not enough qualified professionals to advise the local authorities on economic, legal or urban design matters.

CLAUSE BOIS BADEAU PROJECT IN BRÉTIGNY

Context

Brétigny, located 30 km south of Paris and well connected to the capital by the regional rail network, the RER, has 23,000 inhabitants. The town is divided in two by the north–south rail track. Urbanisation is more developed on the east side of it, and there are not enough crossings to the west. The new neighbourhood of Clause Bois Badeau has a strategic position next to the station and should rebalance development westward. As it will also provide a transition towards the natural areas further to the west, it has been conceived as an eco-district, and the project includes a park and eco-corridors throughout the neighbourhood to ensure its links to the nearby Orge river valley.

The new district is being built over former agricultural land belonging for the most part to Clause, a local grain enterprise. The scheme's proposals include 1,600 dwellings,[1] 35,000 m² of business activities, 5,000 m² of retail and 10,000 m² of social amenities over an area of 42 ha. Half of this area will be public open space, 50% of which will be green. The average residential density of 90 dwellings per hectare means that dwelling typologies will have to be carefully designed, in a mix of terraced single-family houses and blocks of flats.

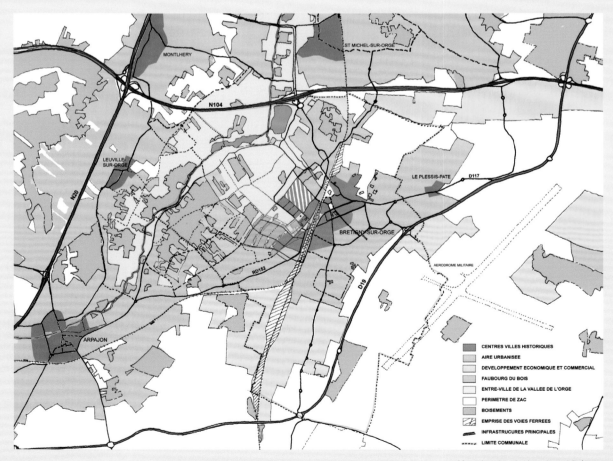

Map showing the location of Brétigny

Case study: Clause Bois Badeau project in Brétigny ~ **FRANCE**

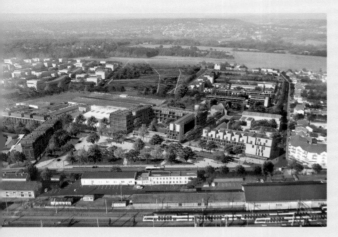

General view of the proposed Clause Bois Badeau project

The actors

The project has been initiated by the local authority, which has used the ZAC – comprehensive development area – tool to maintain control of the process. The ZAC is a widely used instrument that gives a local authorities powers to acquire, masterplan and develop land within a designated area. A contract is signed between the local authority and its designated developer, defining the scheme, the programme and the financial responsibilities of the partners.

The local authority had previously acquired 28 ha from the local enterprise, Clause, using another tool: the right of pre-emption. This allows a public authority to substitute itself for the buyer of a property when a sale between two private parties has been agreed. It is now acquiring the rest of the land required for the project, either by negotiation or through compulsory purchase.

The commune of Brétigny is part of a group of local authorities that has established its own mixed-economy development company, the Société dèconomie mixte du Val d'Orge (SORGEM). Such a company has the legal characteristics of a commercial enterprise, but its majority shareholders are public authorities. As a result the board includes a majority of local councillors, who have a say in the functioning of the company.

SORGEM was first appointed in 2004 to prepare an analysis of the site. Later in 2005, following a tender process in which other private and public candidates participated, it was chosen as the developer for the project. It must buy all the land, reassemble the parcels, commission the masterplan and build the technical and social infrastructure (roads, public spaces, schools, community buildings, etc), but not the housing or the commercial buildings. Land parcels with the right to build are then sold to private operators or investors, who undertake the latter. Within the Brétigny ZAC, some 30 distinct schemes will be developed by different firms, each one with its own project architect but all following the requirements of the masterplan.

In order to finance the project, SORGEM borrowed €9.6 million (£8 million) on the open market, 80% of which is guaranteed by the local authority. Additional finance that may become necessary will not be guaranteed in the same way, and the company is therefore carrying some of the risk.

The project's methodology

To start with, three teams were commissioned to prepare preliminary studies. Analysis of the three different proposals led to a one-year period of debate and consultation, which involved councillors and the local population and engaged the latter in discussions with representatives of the green movement. At the end of this period, one scheme was chosen and the team responsible for it, led by the architect–urbanists Atelier Jam and including landscape architects (Latitude Nord), engineers (Jeol) and lighting specialists (Mission Morel), was appointed as the masterplanner and coordinator for the whole project over the length of the development, predicted to be about ten years. This long-term commitment of the consultant allows the masterplanning team to engage in the details of the scheme, including for instance choosing the materials, in partnership with the architects responsible for the buildings. It also allows it to pursue a pedagogic mission by taking elected representatives on a tour of other good examples of eco-neighbourhoods in Freiburg, Basle or Strasbourg.

As part of their contract, Atelier Jam will also design and build one of the housing areas, restore an old commercial building which is being retained, and be

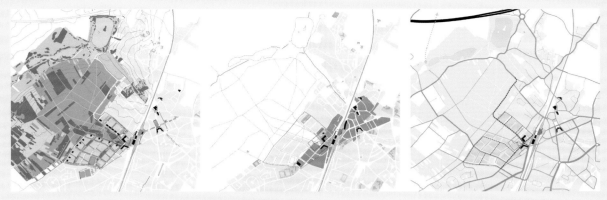

Three studies for the Clause Bois Badeau ZAC

responsible for one public space. One of the other teams that participated in the initial tender will also be responsible for one building operation.

According to Jean-Marc Bichat, one of the partners of Atelier Jam, this is a typical 'urban project'. Formerly traditional 'urban design' was conceived as a rigid blueprint, where parcels were defined in advance and one 'chief architect' imposed his/her regulatory vision on all the other architects who participated in the building operations, or, more often, designed and build them all him- or herself.

Current urban projects such as Brétigny have a much more interactive approach, which involves all stakeholders in a collective conception of the scheme. It also allows monitoring and feedback during the whole period of development, and possible modifications of the initial concept. Instead of a chief architect there is a coordinating architect, a person who will be in constant dialogue with the builders and architects of the different schemes, discussing and reviewing the codes and principles but not imposing them unilaterally. Quoting Mr Bichat: 'a point is reached when the project no

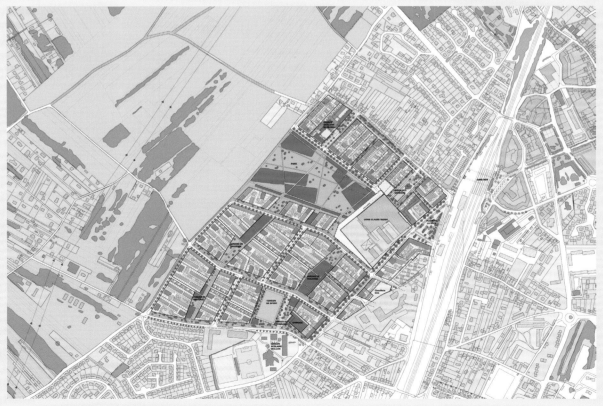

The Clause Bois Badeau ZAC masterplan:
the public spaces and feasibility test

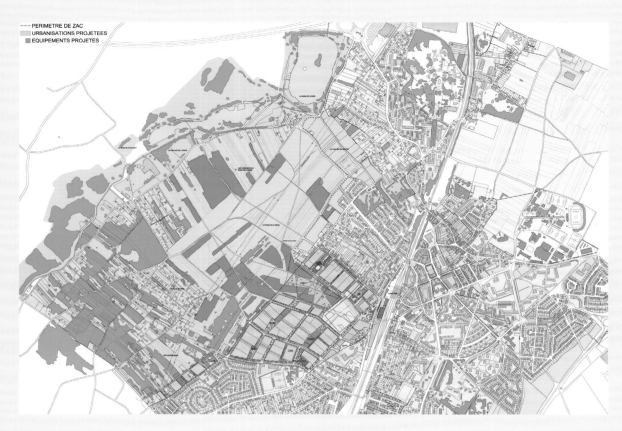

PERIMETRE DE ZAC
URBANISATIONS PROJETEES
EQUIPEMENTS PROJETES

The Clause Bois
Badeau ZAC in its
general context

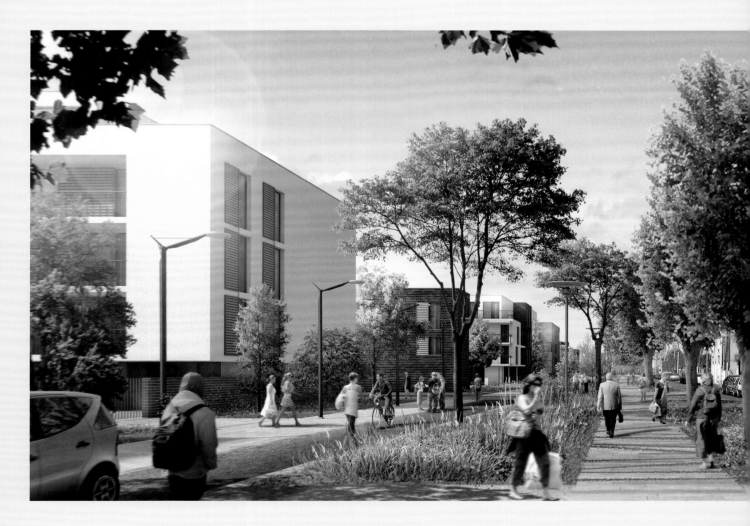

FRANCE ~ *Case study: Clause Bois Badeau project in Brétigny*

longer belongs to you, but to the others; at that point, you've won!'

However, Jean-Marc Bichat observes that some developers and architects in charge of individual parcels tend to follow literally what are only the indicative designs of the masterplanner, thus curbing their own creativity in the hope of more easily obtaining the necessary permits for their scheme. The developers of individual parcels want stable and clear regulations, but the masterplanner wishes to have an open debate about these and the principles behind them before they are formalised. This debate with the architects is particularly important, since at this stage most of them ignore what is going to be built on the neighbouring plot.

The ZAC procedure, which allows for the land parcels to be defined as the development progresses, is well adapted to this interactive method. On the other hand, the masterplanner can only succeed if the project has political support as ultimately the elected representatives evaluate and decide. The political message is transmitted through the mixed economy company (SEM) in charge of the overall development, which is controlled by the politicians.

The scheme

The new district will be an *EcoQuartier*: the buildings and the spaces in between are designed to best respond to climatic conditions and to encourage biodiversity. A range of dwelling typologies and tenures are offered, and all are carbon neutral. A 'green mosaic', occupying a quarter of the total area of the neighbourhood, will link public spaces and private gardens, and two distinct landscape characters will define the urban centre: one around the railway station, and one in the residential areas. Finally, a large park will connect the neighbourhood to the surrounding agricultural land and the Orge river valley.

The scheme is well advanced and a commercial success in spite of the financial crisis of 2008–9, which had the developer fearing the worst. It offers affordable homes in very pleasant surroundings, half an hour by train from the centre of Paris. All the parcels fitted by the overall developer have been sold to individual promoters and some thirty schemes are being built.

The Ile-de-France Regional Council has recognised the quality of the Clause Bois Badeau scheme by giving it the award of best New Urban Neighbourhood; on the basis of established criteria, it had the highest ranking among ten shortlisted schemes.

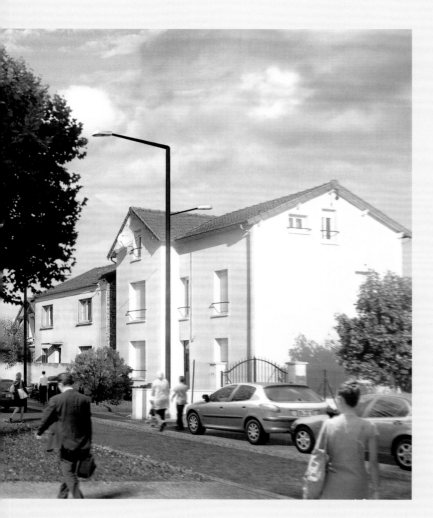

Computer-generated image of the main street of Clause Bois Badeau

Case study: Clause Bois Badeau project in Brétigny ~ **FRANCE**

A quick guide to
France

1 TYPES OF CLIENT

Communes (local authorities), or associations of *communes*

Public developers: *sociétés d'économie mixte, société publique locale, établissement public d'aménagement* (the latter involving the central government, generally for urban regeneration)

Private developers for smaller developments, seldom exceeding 50,000 m² of floor space

....

2 TYPES OF PROJECT/WORK

Masterplan:
- Urban renewal
- Urban extension generally in the form of *EcoQuartiers*

Design guidelines

Architectural coordination when there are several builders, which is generally the case in complex urban schemes

....

3 APPROACH NEEDED TO WORK IN COUNTRY

As most of the work originates in the public sector, the *Code des Marchés Publics* procedures applies. This means open competition according to European Law

Contact with the local mayor is useful

Direct negotiation with client occurs only in small developments by private companies

....

4 LEGISLATION THAT NEEDS TO BE REFERRED TO

Planning laws collected in the *Code de l'Urbanisme*.

Planning documents:
- the *Schéma de Cohérence Territoriale* (SCOT), structure plan for a conurbation
- the *Plan Local d'Urbanisme* (PLU), local plan at the level of the commune, legally binding and compatible with the SCOT

Detailed plans for comprehensive urban development zones (*Zones d'aménagement concerté*, ZAC) embedded in the local plan after being approved by the local authority

....

5 SPECIFIC TIPS FOR SUCCESS

All new developments need to be sustainable (such as *EcoQuartiers*), involving low-energy buildings, a proportion of social housing and activities, public transport, pedestrian and cycling paths, ditches and ponds allowing for absorption of rainwater in the soil, protection from noise, vegetation as a carbon sink, etc

The importance of the image and concept of the new urban development, serving the communication and marketing policy of the mayor, should be emphasised. Foreign urban designers are appreciated inasmuch as they indicate that the city concerned has an international outlook and status

....

6 USEFUL WEBSITES

Certu (publisher): www.certu.fr

Fédération Nationale des Agences d'Urbanisme (FNAU): www.fnau.org

Ministère de l'Écologie, du Developpement Durable, des Transports et du Logement: www.developpement-durable.gouv.fr

Ordre des Architectes: www.architectes.org

Société Française des Urbanistes (SFU): www.urbanistes.com

SELECTED FACTS

1	area	547,030 km^2
2	population	64,876,618
3	annual population growth	0.5%
4	urban population	78%
5	population density	118 p/km^2
6	GDP	$2,560,002,000,000
7	GNI per capita	$42,390

Source: The World Bank (2010)

GERMANY

Katja Stille, *urban design consultant*
Daniel Kräher, *architect and urban designer*

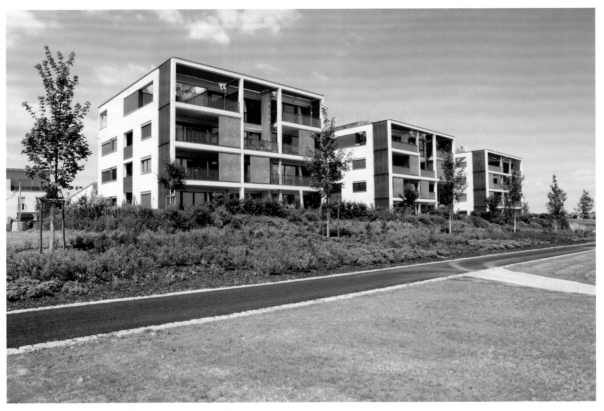

Modern design apartement buildings overlooking one of the
open spaces within the Riedberg development

GERMANY is a federal parliamentary republic of 16 states (*Länder*), three of which are city-states (Berlin, Hamburg and Bremen). The states are divided into 22 counties (*Regierungsbezirke*), 412 districts (*Kreise*) and 11,993 parishes (*Gemeinden*),[1] 0.7% of which have more than 100,000 inhabitants. Compared with other European countries, the number of local authorities is high. About 82% of the German population lives in predominantly urban regions, which cover 60% of the country. In the EU, only the Netherlands, Belgium and the UK have a higher percentage of land characterised as urban. The German population is shrinking and ageing due to decreasing birth rates and increasing percentages of old people; 40% of German households are single-person. The rising number of single-person households leads to an increase in space consumption and a higher demand for smaller flats.

Definitions: dimensions of urban planning

Wherever people choose to live in close proximity to one another, a consensus needs to be found on how to share and to use space. This fundamental requirement of living in settlements can be described as the 'planning of the existing anthroposphere'. Urban planning is a multifaceted activity that can be summarised as the arrangement and programming of void and volumes in relation to one another. As a profession it has two dimensions: to 'create' (design) and to 'manage' (planning) urban forms and functions. In Germany, these two dimensions are brought together under the term *Stadtplanung*, which can be translated as town planning as a statutory activity. It defines regional and place-specific regulations concerning the type, dimension and character of potential development, as well as the land use involved. It establishes the regulatory framework for creating void and volume to design urban space. *Stadtplanung* operates within national, federal and municipal legislation and it sets policies. Together, these two dimensions, urban design and town planning, establish the framework for urban development. Both activities are brought together in one profession called *Stadtplanung*. This can lead to confusion, as the meaning of the term is twofold:

1. *Stadtplanung* as the overall profession, incorporating town planning and urban design. It involves the spatial and architectural planning of the environment; it considers ecological, technical, economical, social and aesthetic issues, including requirements for living and working, culture and recreation. The central purpose of *Stadtplanung* lies in the production of plans and frameworks to control development. All professionals working in this field are generally referred to as *Stadtplanner/in* regardless of their primary background or focus on either town planning or urban design. In the following text the profession and activity of *Stadtplanung* will be referred to as 'urban planning', incorporating both urban design and town planning;
2. *Stadtplanung* is also the term used to refer to the management of urban environments in terms of setting policies for them. The following text will use the term 'town planning' for this.

In addition to the profession of urban planning incorporating activities of urban design and town planning, an academic field called *Städtebau*, which can be translated as 'town creation' (*Stadt* = town [pl. *Städte*], *Bau* = building/creating), corresponds predominantly to urban design. It was introduced into the German language by the Austrian architect Camillo Sitte, who used the expression in the title of his book, Städtebau nach seinen künstlerischen Grundsätzen, translated in English as City Planning According to Artistic Principles. *Städtebau* refers to both the physical manifestation of the built environment and the action of implementing physical planning. It deals with proportion, composition and the relationship between building and space. It is related to the term urban design in Anglo-Saxon countries, but more as a subject field than a profession. *Städtebau* is an identifiable academic discipline, mainly taught within architecture schools.

Basically, the split between urban designer and planner is not that different from its British equivalent. The key differences are as follows:

- Both are called *Stadtplaner*, and only their professional background differentiates them. To clarify this rather confusing situation one German state, Hesse, has invented the particular term *Städtebauarchitekt*, which could be translated as architect/urban designer.

- Architecture is the professional background of urban designers. The opportunity to become an urban designer via a planning degree and a one-year MA does not exist in Germany. Generally, design work is done by professionals trained as architects.

However, as in Britain, the boundaries are fluent and there will always be exceptional people who do not follow the norm, such as architects undertaking policy work and vice versa.

Education and practice

It follows from the above that the education of urban designers is traditionally delivered in graduate courses by architecture faculties of universities and colleges of higher education. Positions in which design work is a necessary and important part of practice are predominately filled by architects, and the design of urban space is an essential element of architectural education at German universities. In pre-Bologna times,[2] most architectural faculties offered programmes leading to an architectural diploma specialising in urban design. The majority of German urban designers therefore have the title of Diplom-Ingenieur in Architecture (Dipl.-Ing.). Some universities also offer postgraduate degrees in urban design, but these depart from the above definition of urban design and from the architecturally based approach. Instead, these new courses focus on the theoretical understanding of urban space and the definition of urban design itself.

Town planning is a separate career taught at universities, mostly combined with higher-level spatial or regional planning (*Raumplanung* or *Regionalplanung*). Although these courses include urban design modules, the extent and depth of design and technical content is not comparable to that of their architectural equivalents. Studies in town planning strongly focus on its legal background and operational processes.

As mentioned above, all practitioners in the wider field of urban planning are called urban planners (*Stadtplaner*), whether they have an architectural degree or a postgraduate one from a planning course. The growing demands on urban planning in terms of economic, demographic and ecological issues led to a broadening of professional backgrounds.

While a century ago urban-planning posts were mostly filled by architects, today the profession is multidisciplinary and urban planners come from a multitude of backgrounds. Their education reflects the current professional challenges in terms of socio-economic issues, history, geography, urban design, building law, construction and landscape architecture. The demands on the profession are changing more rapidly than ever before.

Since Germany has a federal system, planning education differs not only from university to university but also from state to state. Nevertheless, urban design and town planning practitioners are brought together under the professional 'umbrella' of the Chambers of Architecture (*Architektenkammer*). The Federal Chamber of German Architects (*Bundesarchitektenkammer*, BAK) in Berlin, the umbrella organisation for the 16 state chambers, is equivalent to the Royal Institute of British Architects (RIBA) and the Royal Town Planning Institute (RTPI) combined. It represents the interests of more than 124,000 registered architecture professionals (87% building architects, 6% landscape architects, 4% interior designers, 3% urban planners) on a national and international level. The titles 'architect', 'interior designer', 'garden and landscape architect' and 'urban planner' are protected by the chambers' rules and regulations.

Urban designers may work in architectural offices, planning consultancies or local government. However, to be able to progress to higher ranks in the public sector and become a decision maker, architectural graduates would have to go through an internship in local government, focusing on town planning. This takes a further two years and ends with a challenging exam – effectively a second diploma. Urban designers can also work for political parties, universities or research institutions. Although the day-to-day practice of urban design is not very different from that in the UK, the work is predominantly carried out by architecture, planning or urban design offices, contracted by investors/developers or the local municipality. The shrinking workforce in local authorities' planning departments and the growing amount of administrative work in relation to planning applications are generating a need to rely increasingly on external consultants. As a result, technical surveys and urban design work are mainly done by these outside agencies. Masterplans for large or high-profile areas are usually subject to a design competition. More routine plans, at smaller and more detailed scales, or those focusing on conservation or urban renewal, are less often subject to competitions, but may still be outsourced to consultants, especially in the case of smaller authorities.

The planning department's task is to communicate and mediate between politicians and residents, in order to define planning objectives. In line with these, the authorities prepare a brief for an urban design or planning consultant to be appointed. Larger local authorities, such as Frankfurt/Main, have a team of urban designers and planners and draft some of their plans in-house. In all local authorities, the planning department assisted by their legal advisors then use the consultants' work as a basis to prepare legally binding plans for adoption by the council.

As in many other countries, the resources of German planning authorities are being squeezed: they are losing in-house expertise and increasingly relying on external consultants. In addition, the critical economic situation and rationalisation in the public sector is leading to diminishing resources and to a culture of planning-on-demand.

Research

Research is undertaken within the academic institutions, but also extensively on behalf of the federal ministry of transport, building and urban development (BMVBS). The ministry's research covers issues of mobility and transport, spatial and urban development, building, housing and the development of Eastern Germany. The Institute for Research on Building, Urban Affairs and Spatial Development (BBSR) is a departmental research institution that advises the federal ministry. Current topics of the research programmes include: integration and neighbourhood politics, urban strategies for climate change, innovative travel solutions, urban renewal and energy strategies, demonstration projects of spatial planning, building of the future, and more general research on issues such as urban development, building, housing and spatial planning.

Besides these public bodies, a number of nationwide research institutes and academies aim to support spatial planning in theory and practice. These include: the

German Academy for Urban and Regional Spatial Planning (DASL), an association of professionals; the Informationskreis für Raumplanung e.V. (IfR (Forum for Information on Spatial Planning)), a nationwide professional organisation that provides planners with news, discussion forums, facts and contacts; and the Academy for Spatial Research and Planning (ARL), a research institute for 'spatial science' funded by the federal government and states. These organisations facilitate additional research, knowledge transfer and constructive feedback on recent trends in urban planning. With their expert knowledge, they offer a huge contribution to future trends and discussions.

Legislation

The German legal system is based on the Napoleonic code, and on a written constitution which sets out precisely and in detail how it is to be interpreted. As Germany has a federal system, central government shares its powers with the states. The first comprehensive planning legislation, the Federal Building Law (*Bundesbaugesetz*, BauGB), was approved in 1960. It requires each state to set up a series of documents covering issues such as population projections, settlement hierarchies and priority areas, along with regulations to protect the environment. Underneath these, more detailed regional plans are prepared for sub-regions. Within an overall national spatial framework, *Raumordnungsgesetz* (ROG), states develop their own planning policies, resulting in planning practices varying throughout the country.

The BauGB ensures the municipality's independence and responsibility for development control, and makes provisions for two other plans, the Preparatory Land-use Plan (*Flächennutzungsplan*, F-Plan), and the legally binding Land-use Plan (*Bebauungsplan*, B-Plan). The first of these is essentially a zoning plan and it is binding for local authorities but not for private landowners. It defines land use, settlement

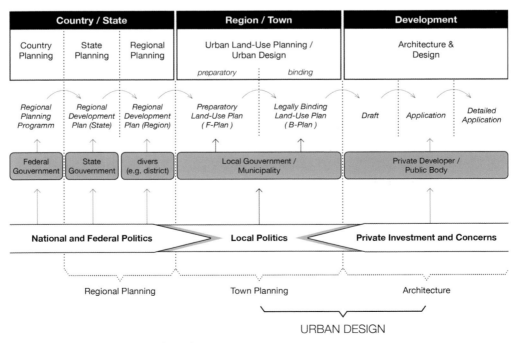

Urban design within the German planning system

boundaries, public facilities, infrastructure, open space, areas of outstanding landscape quality, zones set aside for the production of renewable energies (wind farms or biomass) and land reserved for future infrastructural works. The second plan, the B-Plan, has to conform to the F-Plan and is legally binding for private landowners. It determines the permitted land use of plots and architectural envelope, and makes provision for infrastructure. In some cases, local authorities can attach design guidance (*Gestaltungssatzung*) to the B-Plan in order to control the external design of buildings, their materials, colours, roof forms, proportions and to set environmental targets. However these are sparingly used, for example in conservation areas. The B-Plans' function is to secure an orderly development while leaving as much freedom as possible for specific proposals.

Environmental aspects of planning in Germany

Ever since the adoption of the Federal Building Law (BauGB) in 1960, urban planning has had to consider issues of nature and landscape preservation. This was reinforced by the 1976 Federal Nature Conservation Act (BNatSchG). Additionally, the current BauGB states that 'land-use plans shall safeguard sustainable urban development and a socially equitable utilisation of land for the general good of the community, contribute to secure a more humane environment, and protect and enhance the basic conditions for natural life'.[3] It draws attention to the requirements of environmental protection, the use of renewable energy sources, the preservation of the countryside and 'the ecological balance of nature'.

Issues of nature preservation were made explicit in the revision of the BauGB of 1976, which extended the existing policies to incorporate environmental considerations. In the following ten years, environmental issues were further strengthened by EU legislation.

From 1993 onwards, greenfield development has had to be minimised and, if unavoidable, mitigating preservation measures have to be put in place. For example, if natural ground is to be made impermeable as a result of development or paving, a similar surface area of water run-off has to be provided elsewhere. Except in some inner urban areas, most developments need to determine the amount of impermeable surface and establish a balance between sealed and mitigating areas. Other requirements include the planting of trees within the boundary of the B-Plan, the greening of roofs or the use of water-permeable materials for public spaces and footpaths. Each state has different tools to calculate the balance of what are called *Eingriff* and *Ausgleich:* the former can be translated as the impact of development on the natural environment, and *Ausgleich* is the mitigation of it. If no balance can be achieved on site, compensation must be paid into a local fund that is dedicated to the improvement of the environment elsewhere. Such funds finance, for example, schemes to return streams to their natural state, or the creation of habitats for protected species.

In contrast to the situation in many other countries, environmental protection is defined within German federal law and therefore enshrined in the legal framework at the highest level. In 1998, the BauGB was further revised to include the notion of responsibility to protect the environment for future generations.

The federal government's attempt to reduce the spread of built-up areas shows the level of commitment to protect the environment. According to recent studies, around 100 ha, equivalent to 130–140 football fields, are built over every day in Germany. Suburbanisation and the dream of home ownership are partly to blame for this. To stem the ever-increasing development of greenfield land, the government has set a target of 30 ha per day to be reached by 2020. As a result, the emphasis is now on revitalising brownfield sites such as former railway land, industrial land and army barracks. The principle of mitigation also applies here: investors who propose to develop greenfield land must mitigate the land take by returning other areas to nature or ecologically upgrading them. Thus, the federal government aims to reduce the overall land take and improve the ecological quality of existing areas.

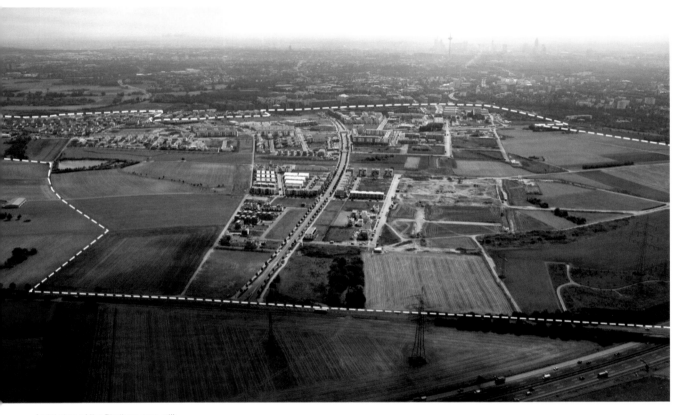

Aerial view of the Riedberg area with
Frankfurt's skyline in the background

RIEDBERG – A NEW URBAN DISTRICT FOR FRANKFURT/MAIN

The most powerful instruments of local planning are based on the special urban planning legislation set out in the second chapter of the Federal Building Code (*Baugesetzbuch*). Among others, the Urban Regeneration Act (URA) (*Sanierungsgebiete*) and the Urban Development Act (UDA) (*Entwicklungsgebiete*)[4] set out essential tools for local planning authorities to directly initiate urban development in the public interest and when comprehensive planning and speedy execution are required.

URAs have been introduced to substantially improve and transform areas with significant shortcomings, either from the physical point of view or because of their location and function.[5] URAs are declared in the interest of public welfare, and conflicting public and private interests are given fair consideration.

UDAs are similar to the above, but are set up to instigate development on greenfield sites. According to the legislation the local authority may formally designate an UDA to meet, for example, an increased demand for housing and employment or to ensure the construction of public facilities.

Both planning instruments are prepared and implemented by the municipality, which therefore acts like a developer. In order to ensure a speedy execution of the measures, the local authority is given increased powers including the rights of 'pre-emption' and expropriation. A local authority can use its expropriation powers on land that is within a formally designated urban development zone. Prior to this, it is required to undertake a number of preparatory studies, for instance to demonstrate that the scheme cannot be achieved through the use of regular contracts or that landowners are not prepared to sell their land. The procedure is comparable to the compulsory purchase order in England, but it can take place early on in the development process. Through these powers the

local authority is in a position to assemble large areas of land, allowing comprehensive development in line with the aims and objectives of the UDA. A UDA is designated by the adoption of a local statute (development statute) that describes the area. It must then be confirmed by higher-level authorities.

To secure long-term planning goals for sites, a common instrument used in combination with the UDAs and URAs is the legally binding Land-use Plan (B-Plan), the closest German equivalent to a development framework in the UK.

Facts and figures for Riedberg

Total area:	266 ha (approx. 1% of the area of Frankfurt/Main)
Net building area:	78 ha (29% of total)
Parks and public green spaces:	94 ha
Social infrastructure:	6 ha
University:	54 ha
Streets and public spaces:	34 ha
Number of dwellings:	6,000
Population expected:	15,000
Jobs created:	3,000
Number of students:	8,000
Total capital investment:	€1.6–2.0 billion (£1.3–1.7 billion)

Riedberg UDA covers 266 ha and is situated about 8 km north of the centre of Frankfurt, surrounded by existing infrastructure, open space and existing neighbourhoods. It is one of the largest UDAs in Germany, more than 100 ha larger than the well-known example of Hamburg's HafenCity. The land, formerly in agricultural use, is on the periphery of, but within, the city's boundaries. The new

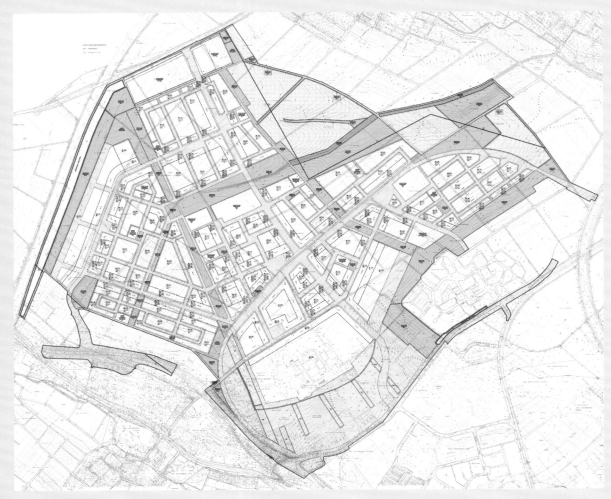

The *Bebauungsplan* for Riedberg

neighbourhood will deliver 6,000 dwellings; new facilities for the University of Frankfurt; technical infrastructure including a light rail system; social infrastructure, with 11 nurseries, two primary schools, a secondary school, a Gymnasium, a Catholic and a Protestant church; two sports facilities; and generous open spaces.

A housing-need assessment found that Frankfurt had a shortage of 6,000 residential units. The development of Riedberg was meant to respond to this need. The area was chosen because of its prominent location, its links to existing neighbourhoods, the proximity to existing public transport and the availability of low-quality agricultural land.

To avoid the mistakes made when building satellite towns in the 1960s and 70s, and to achieve a sustainable and liveable environment, the local authority set a number of key targets:

- a mix of uses to create urban living and work spaces
- the integration of the university campus within the new development to enhance urbanity
- a mix of housing types and tenures to attract a varied population
- a high standard of social facilities
- the best available technologies in terms of heat supply, power generation and storm-water management
- an effective and environmentally friendly public transport system with fast connections to the city centre, leading to a reduction of road infrastructure and parking spaces

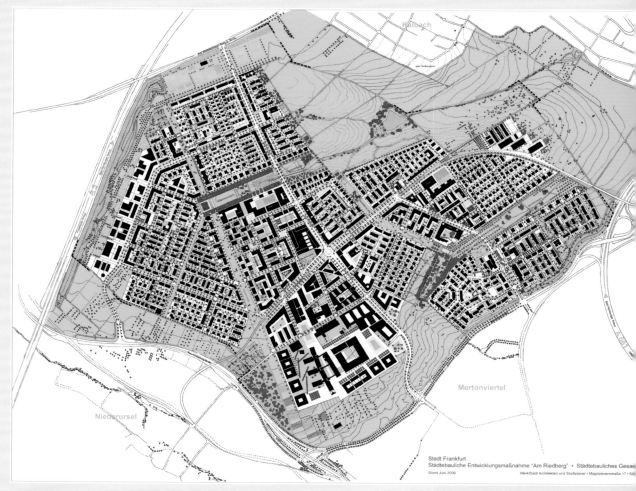

Urban design concept/Riedberg masterplan

- the integration of existing landscape characteristics and features
- the provision of high-quality public open spaces
- the creation of a distinct identity

In 1993, the planning department carried out preliminary studies in accordance with the Federal Building Rule Book, covering topographical, structural and urban parameters as well as the extent, the strategic aims and the feasibility of the UDA. Throughout these studies, the local planning department organised design workshops to establish initial principles. In parallel, it consulted and involved stakeholders and public agencies. In 1994, on the basis of these workshops, consultations and preliminary studies, the planning department commissioned the first masterplan for Riedberg from the urban design consultant

Trojan, Trojan und Neu.[6] This plan formed part of the adoption of the Development Statute in 1996 and was the basis of the ensuing legally binding Land-use Plan (B-Plan) adopted in 2000. The first housing development at Riedberg started in the same year.

The *Forschungs und Entwicklungsgesellschaft Hessen mbH* (FEH), a subsidiary company of the state of Hesse, was appointed as main developer to manage the project, and to prepare and organise the land acquisitions as well as the provision of the initial infrastructure. The UDA designation allows the FEH to buy all land at agricultural value. Through the increase in value of its land assets, the FEH can fund the social and technical infrastructures, and the schools and open spaces, as well as mitigate the environmental impact of the development.

The initial urban design concept was translated by the planning department into the first of several B-Plans, covering the whole 266 ha site. This provides the framework for developers by defining land uses, development blocks and building lines, footprints and heights. During the two decades it would take for the scheme to be implemented, standards for living and working, construction methods and building typologies were likely to change. Because of this, the B-Plan needed to be flexible: it regulated as much as necessary but as little as possible. As the economy and the property markets changed, the planning strategy and the masterplan were amended as well. In 2006, the B-Plan was subdivided into six independent plans, thus allowing further detail to be introduced and changes to be made, for instance in housing density and building heights. These modifications responded to the explicit requirements of the planning department as well as demands from the market. Furthermore, urban design competitions and development contracts were introduced to ensure high-quality development.

The design concept establishes six distinct neighbourhoods, defined by infrastructure and linear open spaces and based on historical and topographical characteristics such as an ancient Roman road, key views and an existing stream. A light railway system that connects the urban extension to Frankfurt's centre in 20 minutes comprises the spine of the development.

A high-density neighbourhood centre of distinct character is situated at the junction of the light railway, the main street and the university campus. Here and in the University Quarter, buildings are generally four storeys high. The main square at the heart of the district is marked and accentuated by a six-storey building, and provides the venue for a variety of activities including a weekly market. A wide range of uses, including housing, a supermarket, shops, a cafe, restaurants, a healthcare centre and other community services, supports the surrounding residential areas of predominately terraced and detached family

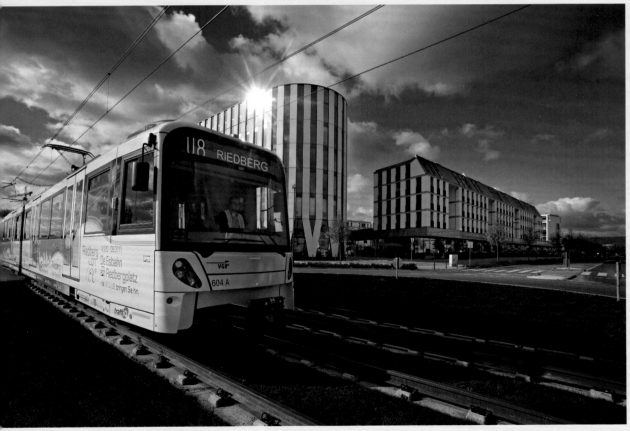

The central area of the Riedberg

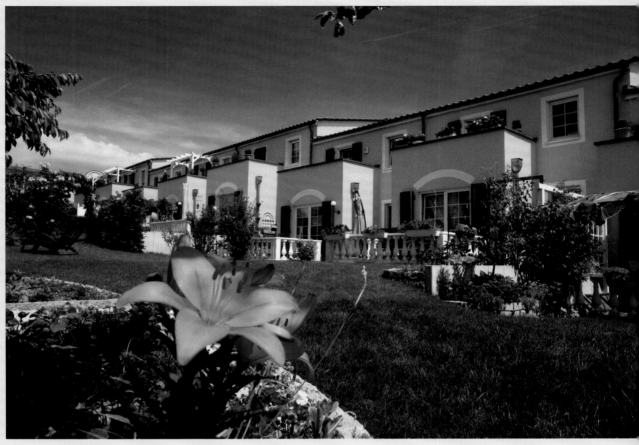

Terraced houses with shared private green space in the backyards

houses, averaging two storeys and of lower density than the neighbourhood centre described above.

Riedberg offers a wide selection of housing types: student accommodation; sheltered housing for the elderly; assisted homes for the less able; smaller flats for younger people; and family houses, either self-build or developer-led. This, together with a wide range of facilities, good transport links to central Frankfurt and easy access to open space, has made Riedberg a success; it is established as a family-friendly and environmentally progressive urban district, attracting a variety of people.

Riedberg has a clearly defined edge and avoids sprawling into the countryside. Two large parks and linear green spaces provide 'green' connections from within the development to the countryside. This green network is an important element that ties the urban extension together and defines the

edges of each neighbourhood. It also provides a good set of pedestrian and cycle routes, leisure spaces and playgrounds for children. In addition, the open spaces offer compensation for the sealing off of large areas of previously open land, and serve other functions. For instance, the parks are designed to form part of a site-wide Sustainable Urban Drainage Strategy (SUDS). Riedberg is connected to a district-wide Combined Heat and Power (CHP) network that is supplied by the local waste-to-energy power plant. In addition, the local authority has made the commitment that all public buildings will achieve *Passivhaus* standard. Since its private housing is also environmentally friendly, Riedberg is set to become a highly sustainable urban extension.

Through the FEH and its planning department, the City can control the quality of proposed developments and the selection of investors and architects, and it decided to make urban design and

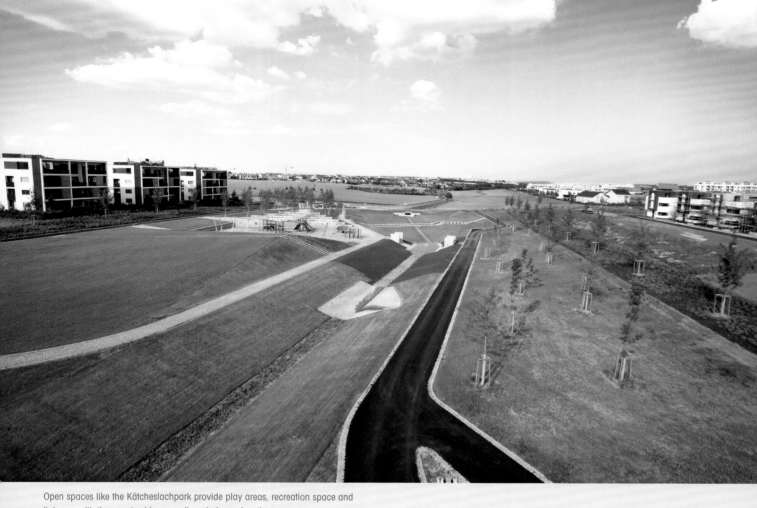

Open spaces like the Kätcheslachpark provide play areas, recreation space and linkages with the countryside, as well as drainage functions

architectural quality a key aspect of Riedberg. For this purpose, it made use of instruments such as:

- architectural and urban design competitions
- urban development contracts with investors
- design guidelines
- involvement of external experts and consultants

In 2011, more than 30% of the site had been developed and the aim is to complete the district by 2017. Because of pressure on the housing market, the City of Frankfurt aims to complete this entire development in less than 20 years.

Riedberg was conceived in the early 90s, and it reflects the planning philosophy of the time: it is a remarkable example of German greenfield development, but the agenda has moved on. Today, the urbanisation of greenfield sites would be avoided, the density would be higher and land would be used more efficiently. Frankfurt's population is projected to increase by 42,000 inhabitants by 2030, leading to a demand of approximately 2,400 additional residential units per year. As a result, the City planning department is searching for new development opportunities and possible areas for growth. A programme called Urban Development Initiative 2030 (*Stadtentwicklunsinitiative 2030*) identifies potential development areas for the coming decades. The main focus of these will be on utilising:

- spaces and gaps between buildings
- existing brownfield land, such as barracks
- land gained from the demolition of oversized infrastructures
- redundant office buildings

Riedberg marked an important change in the way that city expansions were planned and designed in Germany, and it managed to relate well to existing development. But in the future, pressures on urban design are likely to be even higher.

Prospects for the future

Urban design is only one aspect of the urban planning process in Germany. This is not dissimilar to the situation in Britain and other countries, where planning issues have become too complex to be dealt with by one profession only. However, the difference is that in Germany all professionals working within this process are brought together under one umbrella, that of the urban planner. Planning is increasingly legalistic, with laws becoming ever more complicated. Critics argue that it can only be practised with a law degree. Though documents such as the B-Plan have the capacity to be spatial and visionary, the process of turning visions and ideas into a rigid legal framework can water down the original concept. The legal status of plans leaves little room for interpretation, and the development management process is becoming increasingly administrative.

As a result of structural changes and diminishing resources, the design of urban space is increasingly undertaken by the private sector through architectural, planning or urban design consultancies, though it continues to be managed by local authorities. The challenges of urban planning today are characterised by an increasing demand for public participation on the one hand and the need for flexible and time-efficient planning and decision making on the other. It is a conflict between democratic intentions and economic pressures. Limited resources and a shortage of public money, but also the issue of non-renewable raw materials, reinforce this conflict. Small local authorities merge their departments to be more efficient, or reduce the services they provide to a minimum level; larger ones become more dynamic and complex. The varied development pressures and differences in legislation lead to very distinct and place-specific problems. While adhering to the Federal Building Rule Book, the task of urban designers is to find place-specific and sustainable answers to the challenges given. In the future, the focus will lie predominantly with the management and improvement of existing places and less on expansion and new development.

Authorities are being squeezed by a loss of resources and in-house expertise, while issues of demographic and economic change as well as the ongoing scarcity of world resources are challenges that can only be handled by comprehensive planning strategies led by local authorities. Overall, there appears to be a shift from trying to fix everything within the legally binding but very inflexible B-Plan, to regulating urban design issues through contracts and negotiations. This move seems to bring the German system closer to the British one.

In parallel to national laws, European Union legislation is expanding rapidly. The BauGB needs to be continuously amended to incorporate this (environmental impact assessment, legal provisions of the European Union, flood control, brownfield development). The multitude of issues that need to be addressed and the challenges for local planning departments, private practitioners, and planning and urban design consultants are increasing, as are the differences between regions. The next amendment to the urban planning legislation was expected for 2012. However, following Fukushima, the German Government has fast-tracked part of the expected legislation, and in July 2011 it adopted policies with a focus on 'environmentally-friendly urban development' (*Klimagerechte Stadtentwicklung*). The role of renewable energies, especially wind generated, and brownfield development have also been strengthened by the amendment. In the long term, planning may move so far in the direction of legal and administrative practice that a new opportunity will open up for urban design to influence development and urban form.

A quick guide to
Germany

1 TYPES OF CLIENT

Local authorities

Other public bodies such as public corporations, charities, building societies, local and regional development companies

Private developers

....

2 TYPES OF PROJECT/WORK

Legally binding Land-use Plans (B-Plans) and other formal plans

Design guides/codes (*Gestaltungssatzungen*)

Regeneration strategies (*Städtebauliche Entwicklungskonzepte*)

Framework plans (*Städtebaulicher Rahmenplan*)

Masterplans

Feasibility studies

Urban design concepts

Design competitions

....

3 APPROACH NEEDED TO WORK IN COUNTRY

International public tender procedure

International competition

Partnership with local firm

Direct negotiation with client

Urban design competitions are common practice. These are often open to both local and international firms according to European procurement legislation. Any of the formal plans can be based on an open or invited design competition

....

4 LEGISLATION THAT NEEDS TO BE REFERRED TO

Legislation
- Federal Building Code (*Baugesetzbuch*)
- Federal Land Use Ordinance (*Baunutzungsverordnung*)
- Local Planning Policy (*Landesplanungsgesetze*)
- Building Codes/Building Regulations (*Landesbauordnung*)

Regional plans
- County Development Strategy (*Landesentwicklungsplan*) and Regional Development Strategy (*Regionalplan*)

Local plans
- Legally binding Land-use Plans (*Bebauungspläne*), Preparatory Land-use Plans (*Flächennutzungspläne*) and Design Codes (*Kommunale Gestaltungssatzungen*)

Guidelines
- Noise mapping, highway regulations funding guidelines

....

5 SPECIFIC TIPS
FOR SUCCESS

Comply with the federal and local sustainability strategies

Comply with specific federal law

Create viable and realistic projects that can be delivered in an agreed time frame

Create opportunities and potential for projects to adapt to future trends in the long term

Clearly communicate the reasons, aims and objectives of the project to every stakeholder in the planning process

....

6 USEFUL WEBSITES

Federal Chamber of German Architects (BAK): www.bak.de

Federal ministry of transport, building and urban development (BMVBS): www.bmvbs.de

Fraunhofer Information Center for Planning and Building: www.irb.fraunhofer.de

Institute for Research on Building, Urban Affairs and Spatial Development (BBSR): www.bbr.bund.de

....

SELECTED FACTS

1	area	357,112 km^2
2	population	81,702,329
3	annual population growth	–0.2%
4	urban population	74%
5	population density	230 p/km^2
6	GDP	$3,280,529,801,325
7	GNI per capita	$43,110

Source: The World Bank (2010)

ITALY

Corinna Morandi, *professor of town planning and urban design*

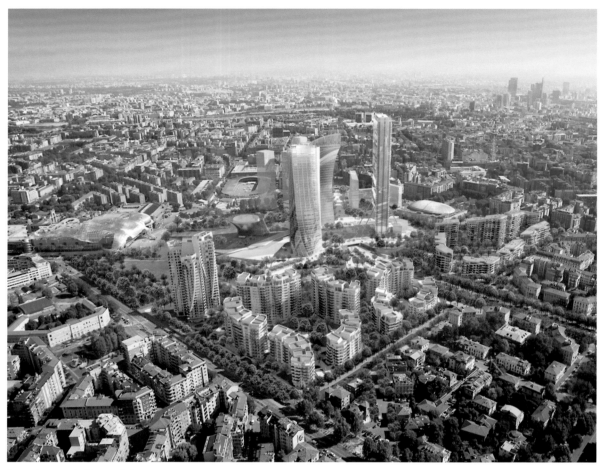

Computer-generated image of skyscrapers,
City Life project by Z Hadid, A Isozaki, D Libeskind, 2004

|TALY has been a democratic republic since 2 June 1946, when the monarchy was abolished. The constitution was promulgated on 1 January 1948. The Italian state is in the process of changing from a centralised to a federal system. The constitution provides for 20 regions with limited but increasing governing powers. The regions were established in 1970, and they elect regional councils. Five regions – Sardinia, Sicily, Trentino-Alto Adige, Valle d'Aosta and Friuli-Venezia Giulia – function with special autonomy statutes. The establishment of regional governments throughout Italy has introduced some decentralisation to the national administration, and recent governments have devolved further powers, among them those related to regional planning. Many regional governments, particularly in the north of Italy, are seeking additional powers.

Definition

A precise definition of urban design does not exist in Italy; instead the expressions *progettazione urbana*, *progetto urbano* and *grande progetto urbano*, translated as 'urban project', or more recently the English 'urban design', are used. This reflects the fact that, as a practice characterised by an empirical approach that addresses the viability of projects and involves both economical and morphological features, urban design is a relatively new discipline in Italy. Its establishment can be traced to the early 1990s, though significant urban schemes had been designed before with an approach that integrated infrastructure networks and public space, destinations and urban form. These, however, should be seen more as 'large-scale architecture'.

Legislation

No specific legislation concerning urban design exists in Italy, as the field itself is not officially recognised. Until the end of the 1980s, tools such as *piani attuativi* (implementation plans) of the *Piano Regolatore Generale* (General Plan), introduced by the first planning act in 1942, were the main regulatory references. A radical change occurred with the approval of a new set of tools (*programmi urbani complessi*, or complex urban programmes), which allowed – with some variations between regions – the spread of an approach to urban design practice similar to that of other countries.

The academic discipline

Until the 1990s, academic teaching addressing large-scale urban projects was known as 'architectural and urban composition'. Only in the last decade have urban design studios been offered at master's level as part of architecture and planning courses. In fact, planning and urbanism are still principally taught in schools of architecture and constitute specialisms in some schools of engineering. The first degree in *urbanistica* was started at the Instituto Universitario di Venezia (IUAV) in 1970 under the direction of Giovanni Astengo. It developed a profile of planners close to the Anglo-Saxon model and removed from the traditional architect's profile. Recently, degrees in *urbanistica* or *pianificazione* have been offered in various Italian universities but they still encounter difficulties in identifying the correct professional profile.

Master's degree and PhD courses in landscape architecture have recently emerged, and a reform of the professional body has transformed the former *Ordine degli Architetti* into *Ordine degli Architetti, Pianificatori, Paesaggisti e Conservatori*, thereby including planners, landscape architects and historic buildings specialists under the umbrella of the architecture profession.

Historical background

As is the case in most European cities, several historical paradigms of this integrated approach to urban development can be mentioned: the baroque transformation of Rome under Pope Sixtus V (introducing the trivium (where three roads meet at one focal point)), which resolved formal and functional issues at the same time as expressing papal power, and 19th-century multifunctional urban schemes such as the opening of an imposing system of public and private spaces in the medieval centre of Milan, all regulated by detailed morphological guidelines (Foro Bonaparte-Via Dante Cordusio). Other examples that show the legacy of an integrated approach applied to a whole new settlement are the 16th-century towns of Sabbioneta near Mantova and Palmanova near Trieste, or the 1930s new towns of Aprilia, Littoria and Sabaudia, developed in a short time to reclaim the marshlands in central Italy. In all these cases a strong power (religious, civic as in Milan, political as in the case of the Renaissance *principi* or of the fascist regime) was the leading driver of the project. Another scheme that can be considered a precursor of urban design is the plan for the Rome E42 World Exhibition, a new urban complex on the former periphery of the city, combining a strong monumental expression of fascist power with architectural projects expressing a rationalist international language.

However, the concern of this chapter is what we understand as urban design today and what is specific to Italy. A first step in this understanding is to look at how the integration of architecture and urbanism (as town planning) has influenced the theoretical and operational work of some key architects, and of movements in the second half of the last century when the Italian approach was an important reference point for international debate.

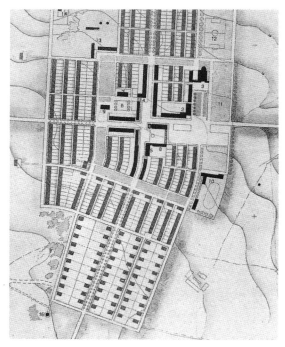

Competition entry for the Plan of Aprilia new town,
L Piccinato (GUR-Gruppo Urbanisti Romani), 1935

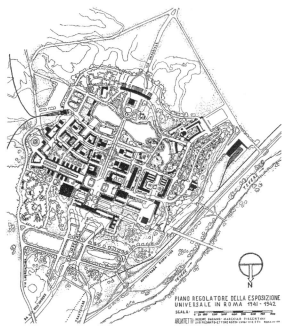

First project of the Rome E42 World Exhibition
by G Pagano, M Piacentini, L Piccinato, E Rossi and L Vietti, 1937

1950s–1970s: Neighbourhood and business districts

The relationship between town planning and architecture found a new and interesting field of development in the concept of the neighbourhood. Postwar reconstruction and the heavy migration of people towards the more economically prosperous regions were at the heart of public housing policies based on a model which was new for Italy at the time. This centred on the role of Ina-Casa (the National Insurance Institute for Housing) and movements such as *Comunità*, led by Adriano Olivetti, which supported experiments in housing typologies and the development of urban neighbourhoods combining functional and morphological issues – defined areas, whose formal organisation is still recognisable. Neighbourhood design became the place for confrontation between two main tendencies: one occurring mainly in the north, representing the inheritance of the modern movement, the other based in Rome (around architect and historian Bruno Zevi) and critical of functionalism and rationalism. Over the course of two decades, a number of schemes showed the effectiveness of these opposing movements; the Quartiere Triennale VIII (QT8) in Milan (1947) and the Quartiere Ina-Casa Tiburtino (1950) in Rome are two representative examples, as is the Quaroni's project for the competition for a large CEP housing estate near Venice.

In 1942, Italy's first town planning act defined the relationship between strategic and comprehensive planning and the design of new neighbourhoods. Different territorial scales of plans (municipal, or *piano regolatore generale*, and regional), as well as zoning, were introduced. The plans for the implementation of the latter were fundamental to the role of urban design; these were the *piani attuativi*, and among them the *piani particolareggiati* (detailed plans), which specified everything from the physical design of an area to the project's budget. Despite the difficulties in enacting

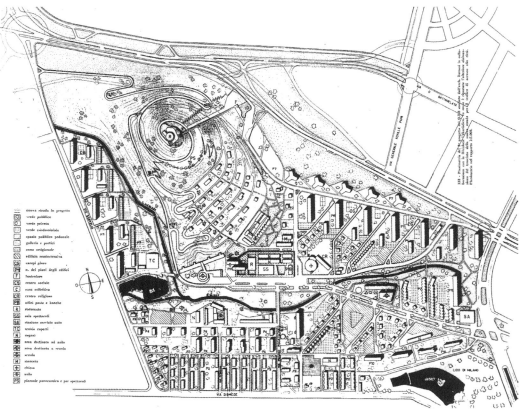

Experimental neighbourhood for the 8th Milano Triennale (QT8) by P Bottoni, 1947

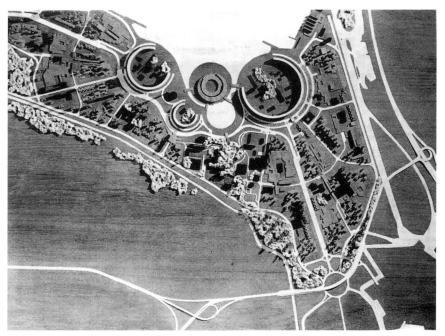

these in practice, they were the tools by which the tradition of integrated design of urban tissues could be updated. This development coincided with the rise of a new preoccupation: the creation of business districts needed to modernise Italian cities such as Milan, Turin and Rome, with the intended introduction of new building typologies and technologies, and the integration of the transport infrastructure.

In mid-sized towns, the backbone of the Italian settlement structure, two examples of the strong, maybe utopian, integration of districts within the overall strategy for a city can be found in Urbino and Assisi. The two architect–urbanists (the term usually employed at the time for lack of urban design definition) were in charge of both the overall plans for the cities and the detailed proposals for their cores. Despite problems of managing both scales, these two very different schemes were successful and influential, particularly as models for the rehabilitation of historic tissues. They were also precursors of the morpho-typological analysis and the pioneering studies of Carlo Aymonino and Aldo Rossi, according to which the results of urban analysis have a direct influence on the design of a neighbourhood.

Other major schemes led to a debate about the relative dimension of architectural projects and town design, and to a questioning of the competence of professionals participating in competitions or assignments at the urban scale. Some key books, published in a short period of time, nourished this debate. Their authors were mostly architects, very few were engineers and none were landscape designers, a profession almost non-existent in Italy at the time.

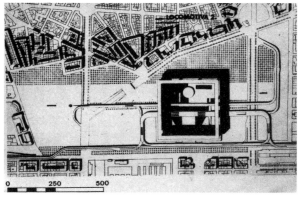

Competition entry for the business district of Turin
by G Polesello and A Rossi, 1962

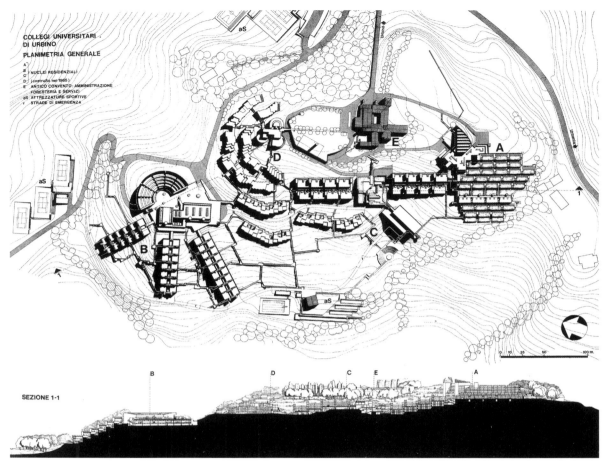

1980s–1990s: Changing scenery

While in the 1950s and 60s a fertile debate had taken place regarding the design of new neighbourhoods and business districts, in the 70s economic and quantitative issues started to become more important. At the same time the economic context was changing, with delocalisation of industry and the modernisation of transport networks, and urban development was moving towards the periphery of cities. As a result, the debate shifted to issues around the transformation of the existing urban fabric and focused on urban morphology. The role of the General Plan was questioned, particularly as projects appeared to be more often in conflict than in agreement with it. Thus, for example, a 1989 issue of the influential magazine Casabella was dedicated to the *progetto urbano* (urban project).

The main concerns of the period were very different from those of previous decades, aiming at reducing the length of time and procedures needed to obtain permits for schemes. At the same time new issues emerged, such as the competition among cities in order to attract urban functions needed for the economic success of countries. In Italy, the use of 'major events' to implement urban projects in a short time often resulted in schemes of questionable quality.

When a General Plan was updated, the opportunity was now taken to give coherence to the various urban projects put forward by local and international investors and developers. In the case of some mid-sized towns, interesting attempts to integrate schemes within the General Plan offered guidelines for decision making rather than a definitive design or a prescriptive code. The General Plan for Turin (1995) was an important reference in that it integrated the planning of the renovation of the city's rail transport system with the location of major urban functions (university, museums, public spaces, offices), and offered guidelines for coordinating autonomous urban design projects.

The case of Milan is different in that after its General Plan's approval in 1980, conditions changed but the plan did not. To overcome this problem, a number of different and specific tools were introduced to adapt to new situations arising, such as the redevelopment of industrial sites or other brownfield land, the coordination of public and private resources and stakeholders, and the integration of planning and urban design approaches. Gradually, this use of new planning instruments spread to other Italian cities where the transformation of the economy opened up opportunities for urban projects.

An additional change affected the planning system when, in 1995, the regions, which had been given powers to draw up their own planning laws, separated in a variety of ways the strategic from the short-term operative plans. Since then, a number of handbooks and texts have been published offering practical information and examples of best practice in the field of urban design. At the same time, academic research and publications have tried to evaluate a decade of urban design theory and practice, and support the development of urban design teaching units.

2000: New scale and new stakeholders
A critical element in the recent debate concerns the effect of urban projects on the deregulation processes and the delegitimisation of the role of the General Plan. However, in the case of plans updated in the last decade, such as those for Rome and Bologna, the role of urban projects is taken into account and accepted.

In Rome, the General Plan states that in the case of new centralities the *progetto urbano* is a compulsory instrument aimed at assessing the sustainability of proposals by various stakeholders, from the planning, environmental, economic and social points of view. In Bologna, the plan identified areas according to their character, suggesting opportunities for spatial and functional changes and combining a strategic vision with morphological patterns for the sites.

In general, the morphological singularity of urban districts is now emphasised. At the same time, new drivers of urban change, often at an international scale, are in charge of major projects such as main shopping centres or the building of large transport infrastructure. A new 'toolbox' of legal frameworks and best-practice for urban designers accompanies these changes. Multidisciplinary teams have now replaced the aforementioned new professional profile, even though major projects continue to be identified by the name of the leading architect (Piano, Gregotti, Valle, Zucchi, and so on). In addition, the change of scale of redevelopment projects that has taken place since the 1990s, helped by the financial stability offered by the Euro, lies at the heart of the establishment of architecture and engineering firms of international size and status, mostly in northern Italy and specifically in Milan.

More recently, the intrusive and widespread presence of international star architects has become the necessary ingredient to obtain financial backing and legitimisation for urban projects. This phenomenon can be viewed in two different ways. On the one hand, the scale and complexity of the schemes require the design and engineering expertise and well-established project-management experience that these firms can guarantee. On the other hand, there is a belief that the complexity of the large schemes can be 'managed by the skill of an "archistar" in dealing with spatial and morphological issues, and designing the solution of the problem' (Palermo 2009, p. 101). This view runs contrary to the real contribution that an architect–urbanist can make to the relationship between context and design. It tends to result in oversized and out-of-scale 'objects', and an urban architecture which ignores both the existing morphology and the ways in which people use urban space.

The government, local authorities or other public sector agencies usually commission projects for infrastructural nodes, such as railway stations or airports, which require a remodelling of whole districts. Most of these major schemes are assigned to architectural and engineering firms in partnership with investors and developers, through competitions launched and supervised by the municipalities.

Apart from such major projects, urban design practice has greatly expanded through local schemes commissioned by municipal authorities concerned with environmental issues and the improvement of public open spaces. Parks, gardens, squares and promenades have been designed by small- and medium-sized firms, still mainly led by architects but increasingly involving landscape architects.

Sustainability

In the last two decades, the importance of issues related to environmental sustainability has also had a significant impact in Italy, both on the updating of legislation and on the attitude of planners and designers. Starting in 1988, laws regulated the procedures needed for the elaboration of environmental impact analysis and the assessment of major projects. This was followed in 1996 by guidelines for regional laws, and other legislation aimed at controlling the environmental impact of urban development and landscape transformations by means of sectoral planning documents. Furthermore, recent surveys of land consumption have underlined the fact that Italy is approaching a very precarious tipping point in its conservation of an acceptable environment for future generations.

Within this legal framework new approaches have become established in planning practice, with consequences for urban and landscape design practices. Environmental standards and parameters have been introduced, for instance those intended to establish the minimum ratio of permeable surface in development schemes (50–70%), aimed at supporting a process of ecological regeneration in urban areas. Equally generalised is the creation of ecological networks and continuous 'green' corridors, obtained free of charge through negotiations between local authorities and private stakeholders in order to compensate for the urbanisation of land.

Sustainable mobility is another issue of concern: the introduction of pedestrian areas and cycle paths within development schemes are seen as integral elements of the design of an area, and not only for functional reasons. The modernisation of railway networks is also seen as a great opportunity to enhance the role of public transport and the importance of interchange nodes; it allows for incorporating drastically reduced car accessibility into the design of the inner city, as in the case, for instance, of the so-called *cura del ferro* (treatment of iron) in the current Rome General Plan.

Finally, regarding energy consumption: national legislation (the most recent batch issued in 2008) is aimed at ensuring that not just buildings but also whole new settlements achieve complete sustainable self-sufficiency.

CASE STUDY

PORTELLO – AN INTEGRATED DEVELOPMENT PROJECT IN MILAN

This case study was chosen for its significance in demonstrating the potential of urban design practice in the recent transformation of former industrial sites. It is also exceptional for its quality of design at all levels, from the masterplan to the detailed landscape and architectural elements. It showcases innovative practice for the size of the scheme and the multifunctional functions of public spaces, for its method of implementation (*Programma integrato di intervento – PII*) and for the success of its negotiations and financial framework. At the same time, it follows the traditional Italian approach analysing the physical features of the urban context: layout, morphology and typologies. Furthermore, the scheme has succeeded in transforming an industrial compound isolated by a fence into a well-connected multifunctional urban district.

The site

The area, defined as Portello Nord, is the northern part of a large former Alfa Romeo industrial plan dismantled in 1982. It is located in Milan's northwestern quadrant, close to the outer ring road. This is one of the most dynamic parts of the region, adjacent to the new Fair District, the site of the 2015 Expo and of City Life, an urban project to redevelop the former Milan Fair site. The 1980 General Plan designated the whole of the former car factory for industrial use, but with the rapid changes in the economic context and the abandonment of urban factories, the projected land-use designation was abandoned. Meanwhile, the need to develop the neighbouring Milan Fair site was at the heart of the process of rethinking the area's land use. After a number of changes, the decision was taken in 1994 by means of a framework agreement (*accordo di programma*) to dedicate the southern

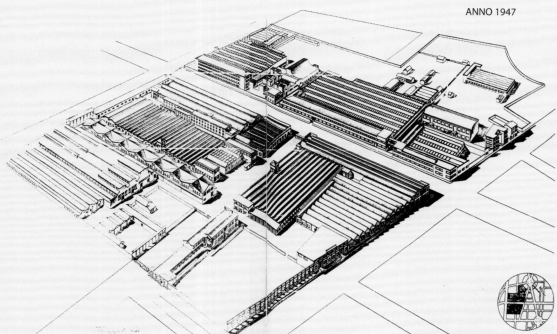

PROSPETTIVA AEREA DELLA FABBRICA ALFA ROMEO

ANNO 1947

The Alfa Romeo factory in 1947

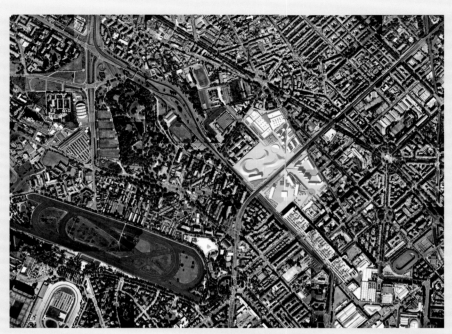

The Portello project in its urban context, between the fair extension and the QT8 neighbourhood

part of the site to new exhibition buildings, and the northern part (about 26.5 ha) to a multifunctional neighbourhood.

The process

The process of transformation started in 1997 when two companies, Auredi and Nuova Portello (both part of the financial holding company Finiper, specialised in commercial development), bought the Alfa Romeo site. In 1998, the Mayor of Milan gave the green light to start redevelopment procedures, subject to approval by the regional authority. This was granted in April 1999, with the establishment of a statutory framework for the comprehensive development programme (*programma integrato di intervento*). In 2000, Milan City Council approved a framework plan and guidelines for the Portello project, which must be submitted for an environmental impact assessment to be undertaken by Metropolitana Milanese s.p.a.

At the end of that year, the city of Milan and the region of Lombardy signed a protocol changing the designated land use of the site to allow a new district with housing, offices, retail and a network of public spaces including an urban park, and to improve its accessibility. The provision of infrastructure was part of the plan, including an underground road link connecting Portello Nord to the City Life site and the northern motorways, funded in part by the Lombardy region. Between 2001 and 2003, other framework agreements were signed; building on site started in 2004 and should be finished by 2012.

In summary, Milan City Council, as overseer of the project, and the Lombardy region – which approves the planning changes and the environmental impact assessment, and funds some of the infrastructure – are the public-sector actors; Metropolitana Milanese s.p.a. is the technical partner; and Finiper (Auredi and Nuova Portello) the private stakeholder.

The masterplan

The site is a rectangle of about 26.5 ha, set along the main northwestern road axis and divided into two more-or-less equal parts by the ring road. It is bordered on two long sides by residential areas: to the west, a regular network of early 20th–century buildings; to the east, modernist parallel blocks. The other sides are bordered by the imposing fair extension pavilion and a large roundabout with heavy traffic.

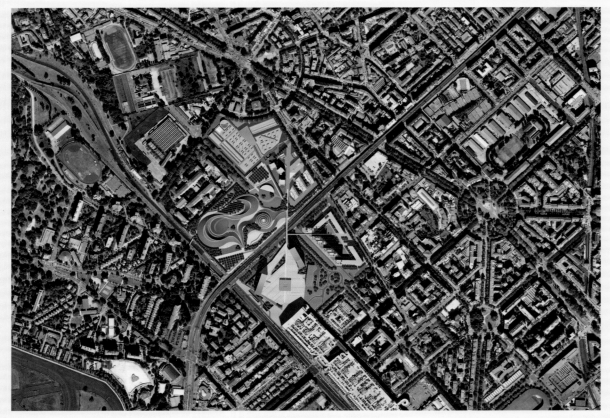

Aerial view of the Portello project

In 1998, Gino Valle, an internationally renowned architect, was commissioned to prepare the masterplan for the area. His studio's approach explicitly refers to the relationship between buildings and location, existing and new settlements, and the integration of urban and architectural design. The general objectives of the Integrated Development Programe for Portello included:

- redeveloping the area where the former Alfa Romeo plants were located
- replacing the monofunctional urban fabric with a new park, complete with public spaces, services, housing and features compatible with the 'flavour' of the surrounding urban context
- establishing a network of paths and of building typologies aimed at reconnecting the existing urban fabric, with its different periods and morphology
- restructuring the road network through the construction of a new underground road
- creating a network of pedestrian and cycle paths

The masterplan concept is very clear: different parts of the site are connected by a sequence of public spaces and paths which allow one to walk or cycle. Moving from south to north these are a large sloping fan-shaped space defined by three office buildings and by the existing Fair pavilion; a footbridge above the ring road leading to two residential areas with different urban patterns, and to the shopping centre made up of several middle-size buildings organised around a piazza, facing the roundabout. Each sector, designed by a different firm, has its own specific characteristics but is well integrated through the sequence of public spaces and the urban park that gives them a morphological focus. The phasing started with the retail park and one housing area, together with earth works to build a hill for the park. The fan-shaped square and offices, and the second residential area, are under construction (2011) and will be finished in 2012, together with the opening of the new underground road and parking.

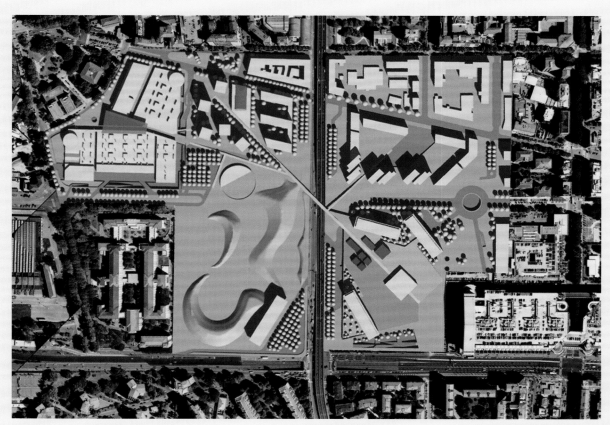

The Portello project's masterplan,
1998–2003

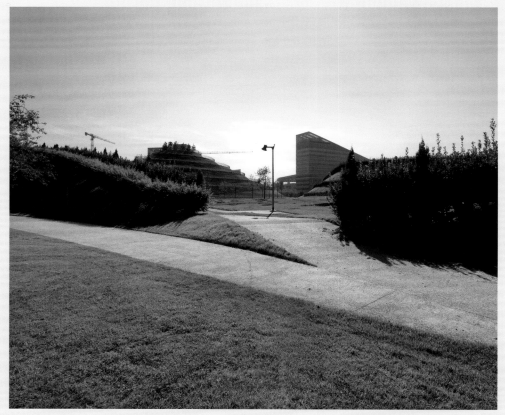

Facts and figures for Portello

Total floor space: 151,725 m², with an overall plot ratio of 0.57.

Land use	Floor space (m²)	%
Housing	75,863	50%
Offices	48,199	32%
Retail	19,600	13%
Production	5,100	3%
Other	2,963	2%
Total	**151,725**	

Public spaces and buildings:
- urban park and open spaces: 166,000 m²
- parking: 47,000 m² (10,000 at surface level and 37,000 below ground)
- nursery school inside the park: 1,000 m²

A population of 2,300 inhabitants and 2,250 jobs are forecast.

The transport network

The local road network and the parking are configured so as to keep the different areas free from through traffic and protect the cycling and pedestrian paths – one crossing the ring road and the other connecting Portello Nord with the 1940s QT8 neighbourhood. As already mentioned, a new underground connection has been built to improve the regional accessibility of the new developments.

As for public transport, accessibility by metro (one existing station, 500 m from the centre of the neighbourhood) will be improved with the opening of a new station, integrating the tram and bus lines.

Architecture

Each part of the new district has its own layout and character, in accordance with the masterplan and with references to the surrounding contexts: the QT8 buildings for the offices, which define the main sloping square; the QT8 artificial hill, a precious legacy of the postwar reconstruction, for the new park and urban landscape; the sequence of piazzas for the shopping mall; and the features of some Milanese residential typologies for the housing.

The sloping square, by Studio Valle in collaboration with Berlin's Studio Topotek 1, has a grid of concentric curves which emphasise the direction of the footbridge; the pedestrianised space is defined by office buildings inspired by the QT8 blocks and has a loggia in the middle, with parking, retail and restaurants underground.

The retail centre by Studio Valle includes five medium-sized buildings, a large supermarket and offices. The design avoided the 'barrier effect' of large box-like developments by setting the buildings with arcades along pedestrian streets and around a

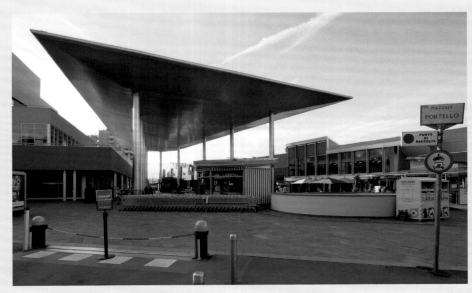

The retail centre with the covered piazza

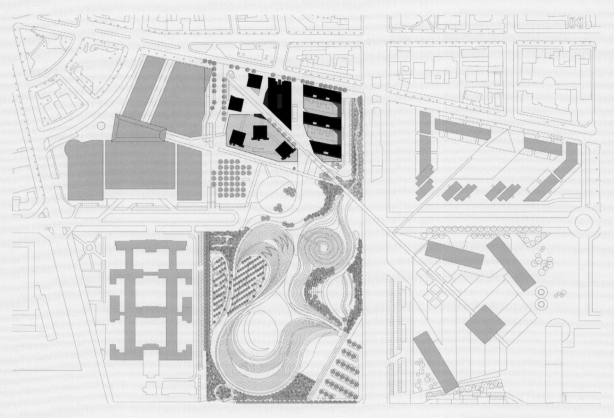

The Cino Zucchi residential area

square covered by a 'sail' at a height of 14 m, which has become a landmark for the neighbourhood.

The northeastern residential area by CZA (Cino Zucchi Architetti) has a porous layout crossed by pedestrian paths leading in different directions and connecting new and existing parts of the urban fabric. The eight buildings are configured so as to create visual connections with focal points in the landscape, and the layout takes into account the former Alfa Romeo canteen, the only building left as a memory of the industrial past of the site, renovated for office and cafe use. The buildings' design, materials and colours are the result of careful research and have created a new landmark.

The southeastern residential area by Canali Associati presents two typologies: a tall building along the perimeter road, and six 15-storey towers facing the pedestrian core and the park. The density is higher than in the other area, and the landscape plays an important role in the design as the buildings are geared to a more upmarket clientele.

The park
Because of its location and design, the park by Charles Jencks and Andreas Kipar represents the functional and morphological focus of Portello Nord. Debris from the old factory and soil removed to make way for new buildings have been used to create a green platform 3 m above the neighbourhood's level, surrounded by a retaining wall which protects the park from road noise and fume pollution. Three hills rise above the platform, the central one 22 m high, and they define a sequence of different, more or less intimate spaces: playgrounds, a garden for old people living in an adjacent home, and a small lake. The idea of a 'vertical park' is a reference to a similar project in the neighbouring QT8, called Monte Stella. The whole scheme, including the land reclamation and the reuse of debris, was funded by private investors and was part of the original agreement between Auredi and the city council, within the Integrated Development Programme. The park is being built in phases and will be completed in 2012.

Conclusion

The project has offered a significant opportunity to enhance the supply of infrastructure and public amenities in the northwestern sector of the city, such as the rehabilitated Alfa Romeo canteen, the underground road and the footbridges. The park is not only an achievement in itself but is also part of a green 'wedge', one of the ecological corridors aimed at improving Milan's environmental performance. Apart from the sloping square of 17,000 m², probably out of scale for the standard Milanese piazza, most of the new urban fabric seems to succeed in creating urban places of quality and character.

To conclude, it is worth mentioning two other large projects, in contrast to Portello Nord and representing different models of urbanism: the Pirelli factories redevelopment, known as Bicocca, by Gregotti Associati (1991–2005) in the northeast of the city; and the aforementioned City Life project (started in 2010) adjacent to Portello Nord.

Bicocca was the result of an agreement between Pirelli, Milan City Council and the Lombardy region: the 1980 General Plan was modified to allow a change of industrial use for an area of 658,000 m². Following an international competition, Gregotti Associati was selected by Pirelli to develop an urban design scheme for a 'technopole'. This was then changed to a mixed-used settlement with the Milan State University and Deutsche Bank as the main stakeholders, in association with various developers for the commercial and residential buildings. One strength of this urban design scheme has been its layout, reminiscent of that of the industrial plant, which was flexible enough to adapt to changes in the scheme but which in time was responsible for its lack of integration with the surrounding neighbourhoods.

City Life aims to transform the 255,000 m² of the former Milan Fair site into a mixed-use area of offices and residential buildings, a park and a contemporary art museum. In 2004, a competition and tender was won by City Life, a partnership of investors and developers, with a scheme designed by star architects Zaha Hadid, Arata Isozaki, Daniel Libeskind and the Italian Pier Paolo Maggiora. In 2005 an integrated development programme was approved by the city council, but several changes were made to modify controversial features, such as the setting of the park, the orientation of the buildings and the resulting shadowing of the surroundings, and, most contentious of all, the building of three skyscrapers, a typology alien to Milan's flat topography.

The park, with the office buildings in the background

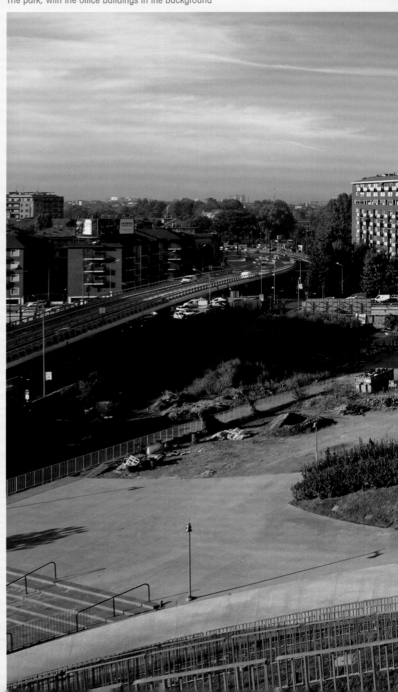

The future

The economic crisis and the population's increasing ecological sensitivity, in parallel with an awareness of the seriousness of the environmental conditions, are once again rapidly changing the context within which urban design projects are conceived and developed. Predictions of the city's population increase from 1.3 to 1.7 million inhabitants, estimated by the General Plan at the beginning of 2011, are already under discussion, together with the contents of several schemes forecasting huge developments. In 2015, the World Expo will take place in Milan, once more along the northwestern road axis. The recent changes in the concept plan for the exhibition site have reoriented the proposal from a traditional sequence of pavilions to an emphasis on the realisation of green open spaces and greenhouses as a major legacy of the event. As a confident vision for the future transformation of Milan, this change in approach could also open up a new vision for urban design projects.

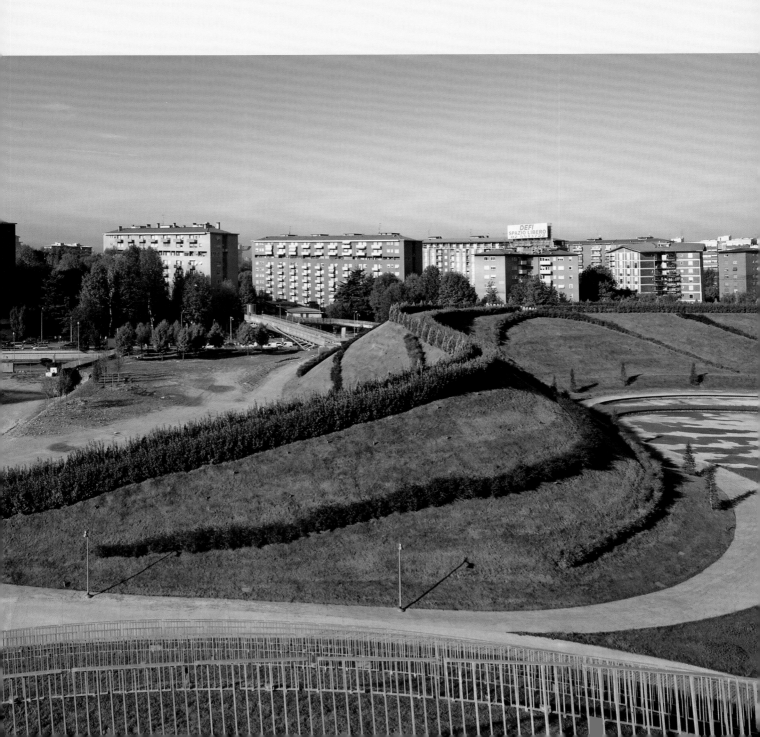

A quick guide to
Italy

1 TYPES OF CLIENT

Local authorities or other public bodies

Public–private partnerships

Railway company

Private developers

....

2 TYPES OF PROJECT/WORK

Masterplans
- Urban renewal
- New community
- Urban extension
- Mixed-use developments
- Sustainable urban renewal
- Modernisation of infrastructure

Design guidelines

Public space design

....

3 APPROACH NEEDED TO WORK IN COUNTRY

Partnership with local firm

International competitions

Direct negotiation with client

....

4 LEGISLATION THAT NEEDS TO BE REFERRED TO

National legislation

Regional legislation

Local plans (detailed plans, integrated development plans and programmes)

Design guidelines and codes

....

5 SPECIFIC TIPS FOR SUCCESS

A percentage of social housing required in all cases

Mixed uses

Quality of architectural design

Multimodal accessibility

....

6 USEFUL WEBSITES

Associazione Nazionale Urbanisti: www.urbanisti.it

Consiglio Nazionale degli Architetti, Pianificatori, Paesaggisti e Conservatori (CNAPPC): www.cnappc.it

Istituto Nazionale di Urbanistica (INU): www.inu.it

Istituto Superiore per la Protezione e la Ricerca Ambientale (ISPRA): www.isprambiente.gov.it

....

1	area	301,230 km^2
2	population	60,483,521
3	annual population growth	0.5%
4	urban population	68%
5	population density	200 p/km^2
6	GDP	$2,051,412,153,370
7	GNI per capita	$35,150

Source: The World Bank (2010)

THE NETHERLANDS

ir Martin Aarts, *urban planning academic*
Dr Jan van Horne, *urban and regional planner*

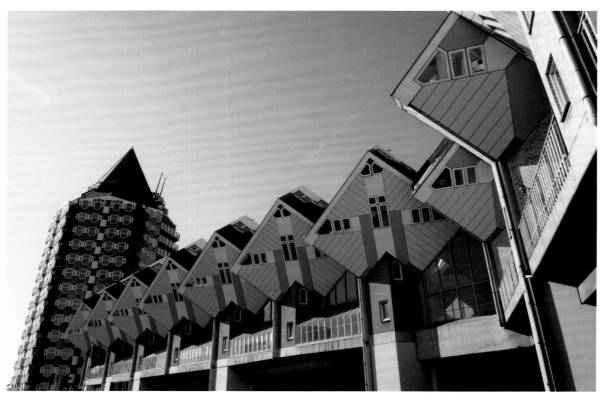

Rotterdam: the 'cubic' housing development on the harbour,
designed by Piet Bloom in 1978–84

THE NETHERLANDS is a constitutional monarchy with a parliamentary democracy. It is divided into 12 provinces and 483 municipalities. The country is highly urbanised, especially the western part known as the *Randstad*. Whether the Netherlands should be regarded as high-density countryside or as a low-density city is a matter for speculation. There are great differences between its urban and rural areas: only 15% of the country is built-up, comprises traffic infrastructure or is used for outdoor recreational amenities. Of the remaining area, 55% is agricultural land, 19% water and 11% woodland and natural countryside.

As a consequence, population density varies greatly: the average density for the country as a whole is 400 inhabitants per km². In the three western provinces that constitute the *Randstad* (Northern-Holland, Southern-Holland, Utrecht), the figure is 825 inhabitants per km². Southern-Holland has the highest density, with 1.025 inhabitants per km², whereas Friesland, in the north of the country, with 1 12 inhabitants per km², is the province with the lowest density.

Definitions

At present the concept of urban design has no clear definition in the Netherlands. However, this was not always so: until the 1980s, when the faith in an 'engineered society' was abandoned, urban design had been a technical discipline with an undisputed and respected status. When it became clear that the engineered society was a fiction, and societal criticism of postwar urban reconstruction became louder, the urban design profession entered a period of identity crisis. As greater evidence and accountability were demanded, other disciplines were asked to collaborate in urban design work. As a result, the profession changed from one of purely technical engineering into multidisciplinary research-based policymaking. From then onwards, all aspects of society played a role in urban design. As a result, a number of similar expressions emerged alongside the concept of urban design: urban planning, urban development, spatial planning, environmental planning and land-use planning.

The concept that best reflects professional practice is now 'spatial planning'. This was defined in the National Planning Act of 1965 and has remained unrevised in subsequent amendments. Spatial planning is defined as:

> directing the spatial development of a region in order to enable the emergence of an entity which is most beneficial to the community as a whole. It should be noted that the concept of spatial planning is broader than the implementation of land use regulations. These give the government specific jurisdiction relating to planning, such as zoning, but on top of these the government and local authorities have ample ways to optimise spatial planning. In particular, they must consider the spatial aspects of all other (non-spatial) activities and the related decision-making.

The professional place of urban design

Professionals from various disciplines are involved in urban design, such as architects, town planners, urban designers, civil engineers, sociologists, spatial economists, lawyers, traffic engineers, landscape architects and real estate experts. Most of these work in private multidisciplinary consultancies. In addition, the national and provincial governments, and the larger municipalities have their own in-house teams that advise politicians on planning and urban design.

The Netherlands has a number of professional organisations in the field of urban and regional planning but none of these has the responsibility of registering professionals or of recognising university courses. The most important institutions are:

- Royal Institute of Dutch Architects (BNA), 3,000 members
- Dutch Association of Urban Designers and Planners (BNSP), nearly 1,000 individual members, approximately 70 consultancies and about 40 institutional members and patrons, such as educational and governmental institutes
- Dutch Society of Horticulture and Landscape Architecture (NVTL)

In addition, there are multidisciplinary professional organisations: the best known is the Netherlands Institute for Planning and Housing (Nirov), an association for professionals in urban and regional development. With more than 10,000 members from various disciplines, Nirov covers the most diverse network of planning and housing professionals in the country.

Education and research

In the Netherlands, universities and technical colleges alike offer education and training for urban planning, urban design and spatial planning. Two of the three technical universities (Delft and Eindhoven) offer a master's in architecture and a master's in urban design. Three of the six Academies of Architecture (Amsterdam, Rotterdam and Tilburg) offer a master's in urban planning and design. Furthermore, urban planning is offered as a non-technical discipline at five Dutch universities (Amsterdam, Groningen, Nijmegen, Utrecht and Wageningen).

In addition, a variety of private educational institutions offer postgraduate courses and seminars. These can either be of a general nature or specifically focused on one or more aspects of urban design, planning and spatial planning. Such courses provide a certificate rather than a master's degree.

Apart from offering education, academic programmes at universities and professional courses at colleges both have a research role. Independent institutes in the private sector and in various government departments also undertake research. The Berlage Institute, for example, is a post-academic laboratory for design-based research in architecture, urbanism and other issues related to the built environment; and the Nicis Institute manages the research programme Knowlegde for Powerful Cities. The research is carried out in collaboration between scientists and professionals from local authorities.

Legal status

A Spatial Planning Act was passed in 1965, supplemented by a decree to implement it. The latest revision dates from 2008. In general terms, the legislation provides for spatial planning regulations at the three government levels: national, provincial and municipal. The decree contains detailed guidelines and requirements concerning analysis, design and legal proceedings. However, since urban design is not a recognised discipline *per se*, the Spatial Planning Act does not mention the term 'urban design'.

In mid-2011, the Dutch ministry of infrastructure and environment announced that a fundamental review of all legislation in the fields of infrastructure, planning and environment was being prepared. This review is taking place in the political context of a move to limit the overall role of government in society, and to broaden the initiative and responsibility of private companies and individuals. The aim is to achieve a smaller, more efficient government, which facilitates services to citizens and social institutions instead of issuing detailed regulations. By 2013, the intention is to replace the present 60 acts, more than 100 council orders and hundreds of ministerial regulations by just one new Environmental Act.

Historical development

The term urban design has actually existed in the Netherlands since the emergence of its trading cities in the middle ages. Commerce emerged at road and waterway intersections, and in the delta region of the western Netherlands, where the rivers Rhine, Meuse and Scheldt flow into the North sea. To enable trade in those cities, it was necessary to negotiate collective agreements on the use and design of the limited space available. Space was at a premium because safe and inhabitable land needed to be defended against the water, then and now a constant threat for the Netherlands. Concerted efforts to build dikes, polders and water-level regulators have always been a condition of Dutch survival. The eternal struggle against the water is concisely revealed in the saying: 'God created the earth but the Dutch created the Netherlands'. Drafting and enforcing usage rules was in everyone's interest and widely accepted. Urban design thus assumed greater significance than the design of buildings. Therefore from the start, the object of urban design involved place making; the development of new neighbourhoods as well as the renewal of existing ones; and even measures to reshape the overall structure of towns, villages and the countryside.

During the Industrial Revolution, a high percentage of the population of the Netherlands moved from rural to urban areas in a very short time, and cities grew rapidly during the second half of the 19th century. Land speculators and builders provided for the almost insatiable demand for housing. This led to the establishment of many new settlements packed with small, crowded dwellings with minimal sanitation, located directly adjacent to the existing cities and within walking distance of industrial and port areas. To this day, some older neighbourhoods are marked by this unplanned urban expansion from the 19th century, and in many cities the original structure of wetlands and ditches is still clearly recognisable through the street pattern.

At the end of the century, living conditions were so bad that industrialists, politicians, and wealthy notables joined forces to end the rampant speculation. As a result the 1901 Housing Act was passed, prescribing minimum standards for housing in terms of light and ventilation, size and sanitation. A separate section regulated land use. The introduction of the Housing Act meant that thereafter urban expansions had to be planned, and therefore urban development plans had to be prepared. At the same time, housing associations were founded with the mission to provide good affordable accommodation for the working population. A number of major industrial entrepreneurs built their own garden cities close to their factories. This was not done just for philanthropic reasons but also for economic motives: since workers lived near the factory and in houses conducive to healthy conditions, their working hours proved more productive.

After the second world war, economic prosperity and mobility grew rapidly. A euphoric faith in the advantages of an engineered society led to strong government intervention. The need for new, larger homes and the diminishing size of the average household made large-scale urban expansion necessary. Planned urban growth was influenced by modernist ideas, in particular the fascination with light, air and space. As a result, isolated blocks of flats and rows of family houses surrounded by spacious green areas became the preferred typologies. In the 1950s and 60s, in order to manage development appropriately, the national government drew up policy documents on spatial planning. Thus in 1965, the aforementioned Spatial Planning Act was approved by parliament.

In the 1970s and 80s, new concepts for urban expansion and development were tested. At the same time, citizens were demanding more involvement in the design of their communities. Urban design and planning were becoming less the exclusive domain of experts and administrators. In response to the criticisms of the anonymous and cheerless housing estates of the 1960s and the dominance of cars, the *woonerf* (home zone) was introduced as a new typology for residential areas: this is a shared public space where pedestrians and cyclists have priority over motorists, giving the residents security in their living environment. This model spread throughout the Netherlands and further afield, but eventually was also found to have limitations.

The search for a more efficient use of land and a reduction in the costs of development, combined with a wish to return to the principles of the garden cities, led the Dutch government to produce the Fourth National Policy of Spatial Planning, known as VINEX. This encouraged designs based on a very rational mix of garden city and modernist ideas, resulting in neighbourhoods with row houses surrounded by open spaces. These typologies, though successful, have, however, not helped to increase urban densities, the issue of which has in the meantime become a major preoccupation. New policies are needed to deal with it.

At present, professionals and administrators have come to realise that the guiding role of government has changed: it should adopt the role of facilitator rather than regulator of citizens' actions. This principle is already reflected in the revised Spatial Planning Act of 2008, but will be fully visible in the future Environmental Act.

Practice and concerns

In the Netherlands, all levels of government – national, provincial and municipal – as well as the water authorities are the main initiators and commissioners of urban planning. The municipal authorities prepare a Structure Plan, which sets out their policies for their city as a whole. For new developments, legally binding detailed project-related plans are required by law, and have to be reviewed every ten years. These plans have to balance the private and public interests, and stakeholders must be involved in their preparation and revisions. The main task of urban designers is to present the policies to all participants in the process through various graphic means: sketches, aerial views, plans, etc. Thereafter, they also have to ensure that individual proposals comply with the approved document.

In the future, the work of urban designers is likely to be more focused on interventions in the existing city than in urban expansion. Concern for history, culture and the character of existing areas will therefore increase in importance for the profession. At the same time, sustainability and financial viability will also become high priorities.

Sustainability is a particularly sensitive issue in the Netherlands. In physical terms, it relates specifically to energy-neutral and climate-change-resilient buildings: a project is energy neutral if its annual energy consumption is equal to the amount of energy produced in a sustainable way. Climate-change-resilient building requires predicting future climate change and adapting to the consequences: temperature rise, precipitation change and sea-level rise. Account must be taken of long periods of drought or rainfall, extreme discharges of river water and sea-level rises of more than one metre. Building on water is also a response to climate change. Moreover, sustainable development is a very broad concept that includes a number of other measures such as green roofs, water plazas, and priority for pedestrians and cyclists.

ROTTERDAM URBAN VISION – SPATIAL DEVELOPMENT STRATEGY 2030

On 29 November 2007, the Rotterdam municipal council ratified the Rotterdam Urban Vision 2030. This document states that as part of the *Randstad*, Rotterdam must follow a strategy focusing on the one hand on the development of the knowledge-based and service economy, and on the other hand on providing an attractive residential and living environment for highly educated, creative workers and middle- and high-income groups. This strategy is necessary to strengthen Rotterdam's prominent position in the 'league table' of international competition between urban regions. The urgency of this matter cannot be stressed enough, as the city's density is too low to accommodate the expansion of its working population. The authorities have decided to build within the municipal boundaries in order to protect the surrounding countryside, encourage sustainable public transport and focus investment on improving the existing city. To achieve these goals, the city needs to make the best use of existing facilities.

The task facing Rotterdam is based on two keystones: a strong economy with growing employment opportunities, and an attractive residential city with a balanced population. These keystones work in tandem: people will be attracted to the city if it offers attractive housing *and* suitable jobs. Conversely, employment opportunities arise only when the city has an inviting environment to attract employees: an environment that provides good housing, related facilities and public space – in other words, complete neighbourhoods that match the requirements of consumers.

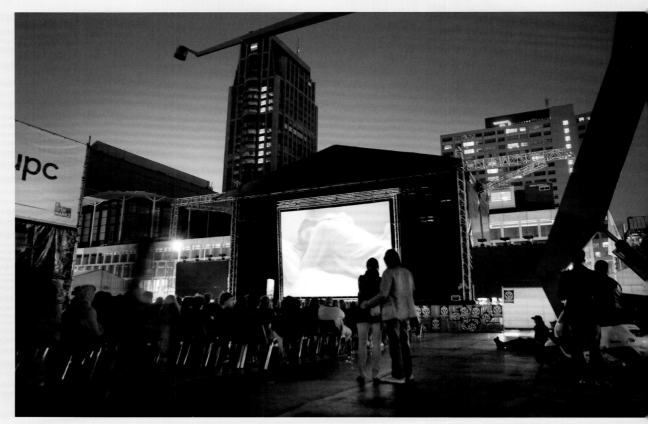

Rotterdam Schouwburgplein, designed by West 8 in the 1990s, has created a vibrant space in the heart of Rotterdam

VIP AREAS

On the basis of an effectiveness assessment, thirteen area developments have been designated that are crucial to achieving the objectives: 'strong economy' and 'attractive residential city', the so-called Very Important Projects, or VIP Projects:

1. Laurenskwartier: mixed urban area
2. Stationskwartier: Rotterdam Central District
3. Coolsingel / Lijnbaan: mixed urban area
4. Ahoy / Zuidplein: southern mall and event area
5. Stadionpark: event area and new football stadium
6. Erasmus MC – Hoboken: medical service area
7. Schieveen Science and Business Park

8. CityPorts: transformation area in synergy between city and port
9. Maasvlakte 2: deep sea terminal and industrial estate
10. Hoeksche Waard: industrial estate
11. Kop van Zuid: quiet metropolitan residential environment
12. Greater Hillegersberg: suburban residential environment:
13. Oud Zuid: tackling the existing housing stock

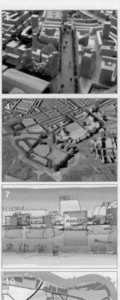

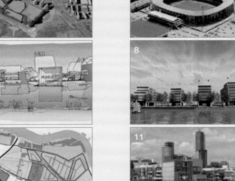

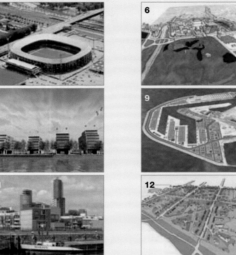

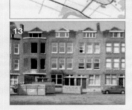

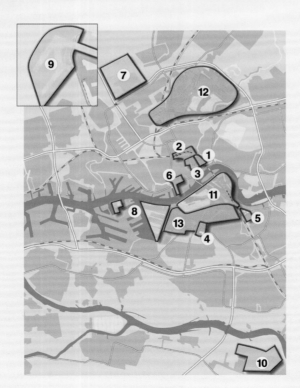

The 13 VIP areas in the Rotterdam Urban Vision 2030

Future perspective

To start implementing these policies, investment has to be directed to the port, the sectors of economic growth (medical, leisure and creative), the small and medium-sized enterprises as sources of urban employment, the extensive range of educational institutions, the popular residential districts and the modern city centre on the river. These assets form the basis for the 'ripple effect strategy', which the city has in mind: what is strong will be expanded, what is weak(er) will derive support from what is strong. This strategy will be applied both to improving the residential quality of the city, and to regenerating the urban and regional economies. Rotterdam's potential is wide-ranging, but analysis of the city's conditions shows some indicators that require immediate care:

- unbalanced composition of the population
- unceasing selective migration
- weak economic growth, leading to insufficient employment

Making Rotterdam more attractive to residents is fundamental and requires urgent action. First of all, the city must take better advantage of its existing assets. Secondly, a number of key decisions must be made in order to define the necessary spatial interventions. The approach to this is outlined in the following paragraphs

Effectiveness of measures

In order to test the feasibility of the measures, plans and projects mentioned in the Rotterdam Urban Vision, the authorities asked private stakeholders to identify the areas in the city where they would want to invest. Next, they checked whether the public sector would be willing to participate through investment in the same locations. The objective was to achieve synergy and get a better return for the city than if initiatives were not coordinated.

Capital investment is the key to achieving the desired positive effects. It is directed to improve and upgrade commercial areas, housing stock (particularly for medium- and high-income groups), various amenities and infrastructure. The hoped-for returns are new businesses, an increase in working population, extra visitors and shorter travelling

times. An evaluation was made of the economic returns on different investments, and these were then prioritised. The outcome was a list of 13 large-scale developments which would get the 'Very Important Project' (VIP) label over the next ten years. These are grouped into four area types.

City centre: the challenge is to achieve densification, mostly with residential development, and to strengthen functional and spatial underutilised potential. Laurenskwartier (1), Stationskwartier (2), Coolsingel/Lijnbaan (3), Erasmus MC – Hoboken (6), Kop van Zuid (11) belong to this category.

Southbank: the aim is to upgrade a large area through housing and community regeneration, and to achieve a better integration of existing facilities. Ahoy/Zuidplein (4), Stadionpark (5), Oud Zuid (13) are the corresponding VIP areas.

Port area: more space is needed for port activities; at the same time, areas no longer needed for these can provide space for large-scale city-related business and ancillary facilities. City Ports (8), Maasvlakte 2 (9), Hoeksche Waard (10) are in this category.

Airport area: airport-related enterprises and research institutions connected to the Technical University of Delft are to be located in these VIP areas: Schieveen Science and Business Park (7), Greater Hillegersberg (12).

Within the designated VIP areas, the role of public–private partnerships will be particularly significant. In addition to the 13 VIPs, a number of other important projects will also receive the necessary resources. An overall implementation programme, including an investment and monitoring plan, has been drawn up.

The role of the urban designer in the VIP process

Focusing on the regeneration of the existing city, and especially on areas attractive to investors, demands new methods of working for the urban planners and designers. It is no longer appropriate to draw masterplans and let the city council approve and implement them. Nowadays stakeholders, including residents, participate in the process from the beginning and establish its objectives together with the city authorities. This means that they are involved with, and become advocates of, the plans instead of protesting against published proposals after the city has worked on them for years.

The process has thus changed from blueprint to 'green print'. The task of the urban designer in this process is to draw together the different ideas, and present scenarios for discussion. Although this may sound easy, it makes it imperative for the professional concerned to listen and translate the emerging ideas into robust and sustainable proposals that benefit the city as a whole. The investors also realise that through collaboration with the city and other stakeholders, results will be more than the sum of their parts and their investment will be more sustainable.

Three examples

The Central Station

At the central station the authorities wanted not only to build a new station, but to create a destination so that it would become a part of the inner city. To start with, the car-based environment had to be transformed into a bike-based one, and the monofunctional office district around the station had to be transformed into a mixed-used area. That meant adding buildings with dwellings above ground and amenities such as cafes at street level. A partnership with companies already present in the area was created for this purpose.

The urban designers' job was to show the opportunities for transforming vacant as well as occupied land, and most importantly convince the stakeholders that the qualities already existing in the area could be exploited in a better way. Therefore they produced a plan of 'potentialities', not a traditional blueprint but a flexible document that could become a contract of common interest for the stakeholders.

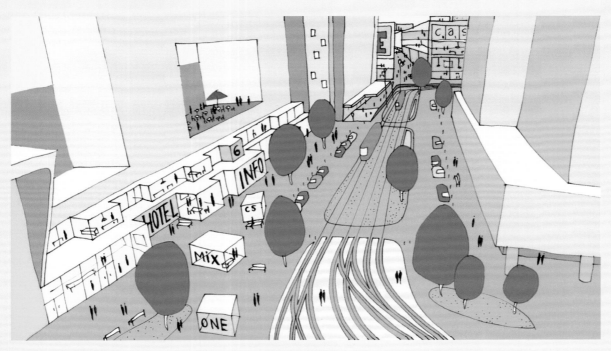

Future streetscape near the central station

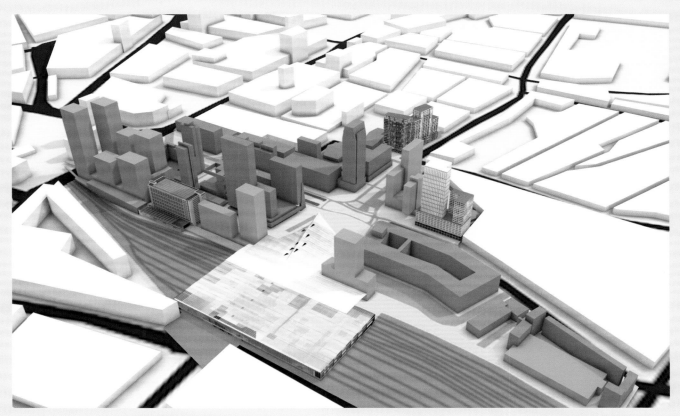

3D model of the plan of possibilities for the
central station area

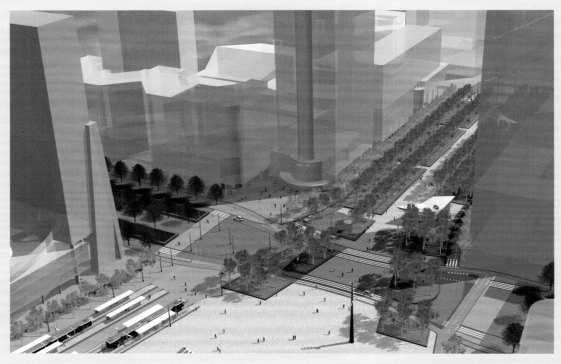

Esplanade with the new gateway
to the inner city

Case study: Rotterdam Urban Vision – spatial development strategy 2030 ~ **THE NETHERLANDS**

Hoboken

In the Hoboken area, where the university hospital and the Museumpark are located, major construction activity will take place in the next few years to build a high-quality centre for culture and science. An intensive process with stakeholders, residents and professionals was established in order to ensure that their various goals were realised. Urban designers presented the ways in which they proposed to do so, and the stakeholders accepted them as professionals who could deliver quality.

A good example of the resulting synergy is the way a solution was found for parking for both the hospital and the museums: a large underground car park was built under the Museumpark, and this in turn made it possible for the municipality to achieve its long-standing ambition to renew the park in accordance with Rem Koolhaas/OMA designs.

Heart of the South (Ahoy/Zuidplein)

The third example concerns the competition held to redevelop a part of the centre of Rotterdam South. Although some regional and national facilities are already established there, they are not contributing to city life. The challenge is therefore to create a 'heart' for the southern part of the city, a pleasant urban environment that will attract people to the area.

Here, the approach has been to prepare an inspiring brief with a predetermined maximum investment. Potential investors were then invited to compete by presenting their best scheme within the brief's framework and budget. The role of the city's urban designers was to show, through the brief, the possibilities for a spatial solution to the problems of the Heart of the South, and to challenge developers to come with schemes that achieved real urbanity.

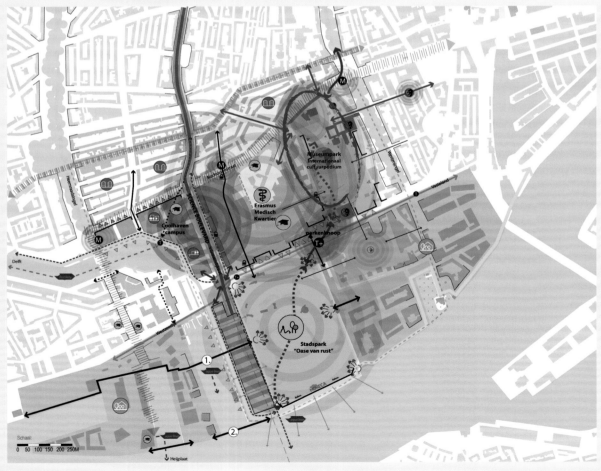

Hoboken masterplan for stakeholders

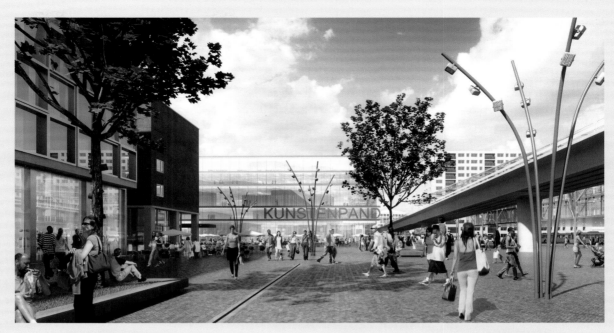

Computer-generated image of the
proposed Heart of the South

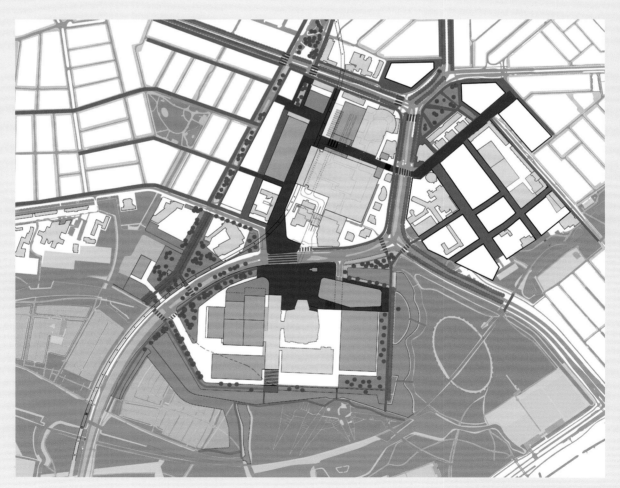

Framework design for the Heart of the South area

Conclusions and the future of the profession

In western society, faith in endless growth has come to an end – mainly as a result of a large number of negative consequences. The new paradigm no longer deals in grand economic models, but in a local economic reality and a safe government context (Europe, the Netherlands) that facilitates it. Saskia Sassen (2008) calls it 'the Importance of Place', adding that 'Cities are no longer part of a national arena, but part of a world economy. But cities can easily become less relevant if they do not continue developing'. Richard Florida (2010) examines the social consequences when he writes that 'The places that ultimately emerge from the crisis as the strongest and most resilient will be those that recognize the need to build economic and social systems, can harness the full creative capacities of a much broader range of their workforce, and stoke the creative furnace that lies within everyone'.

But people want more. Once the preconditions of safety and employment are met, they subsequently expect more from their environment: 'physical beauty and the level of maintenance of the place itself – great open spaces and parks, historic buildings, and attention to neighbourhood aesthetics. In the city it must be easy to meet others, make friends, and plug into social networks. And last but not least is the level of diversity, open-mindedness, and acceptance' (Florida 2010, p. 86). This does not mean that people will be less footloose in the future, as a flexible lifestyle will prove even more important than comfort. It is less about possession ('my home is my castle') and more about investing in personal development (education, travel, business).

Unfortunately, the European Union has no planning policy. This task has been voluntarily retained by the member states. It is therefore still possible for infrastructure not to continue beyond national boundaries, and for railway engines to have to be repeatedly replaced at the borders. However, Europe has indeed recognised metropolitan regions as engines of the economy. The Netherlands comprises several such metropolitan areas, Rotterdam–The Hague, Amsterdam and Eindhoven. And it is clear that as they grow increasingly important, they also must perform better. Powerful city-regions offer excellent opportunities for social cohesion because they reinvest in the existing community rather than in expanding it. Urban areas also make a more efficient and sustainable use of public transport systems, and offer more opportunities for protecting the environmental quality around cities. This is partly achieved by taking a different approach to the management of agricultural land, and by directing food production towards the urban population.

Thus the Dutch metropolitan regions are permanent 'team players' in the European cities' competition. And as is the case with all European cities, the Netherlands will continue to invest in its existing urban centres. Likewise, businesses follow the preferences of their employees who choose those cities that offer excellent residential and leisure opportunities. The most appealing Dutch cities have a historic town centre, an attractive nightlife with a variety of cafes and culinary offerings, and a generous cultural programme; they are safe, surrounded by beautiful natural landscape and offer a good choice of housing, high levels of employment and reasonable commuting times. Most of all, Dutch cities are known for their historic centres whose strong heartbeat is deemed exemplary for offering these preferred qualities.

Therefore, a number of significant developments can be observed in Dutch cities:

- A legitimate focus on investing in the existing urban fabric as a key opportunity for the country's socio-economic future. This calls for the involvement of all disciplines, because the existing city reflects the complexity of issues affecting contemporary society: social, economic, physical, cultural, transport, ecological, etc.
- A stronger intervention in steering (urban) programmes. It is important to focus on the major challenges and aspirations of the community; to select, in partnership with stakeholders, the actions required; and to determine which partners are most suitable in each case. Increasingly, urban development will be produced with the participation of all stakeholders.
- A transition from development to maintenance. The previous model – 'design, build, maintain' – which suited the expansion areas, is not working for interventions in the existing city. Here, maintenance is already in place and it must be linked to development from the start. In the future, there will be no such thing as a temporary situation as there will be no finished situations either. Quality will have to be delivered at every stage,
- The current focus on sustainable development is vital for a successful future. The city and urban life need to be sustainable; their design and redesign are to be based on sustainable principles.

These current developments will make urban design more complex, but also more realistic and challenging. More disciplines and networks will have to collaborate. A new approach, more 'actor-oriented', will be needed, based on complex networks of government, research institutes and business. Short- and long-term measures alternate on different spatial scales; each requires lucid decision making derived from a common shared vision. The knowledge and skills inherent to entrepreneurs and consumers (residents) must be correctly aligned with urban policy frameworks and the budgets of the city as a financial entity. Neighbourhood and district councils have a stronger position as managers of their neighbourhoods than the city government. At the same time, citizens, housing associations, entrepreneurs and developers call for a government that supports them.

This changing role of designers and planners involves a different way of working. It is no longer about predicting the future; it is about anticipating the relevant developments and exploiting the existing energy already apparent in the city. This requires a more entrepreneurial attitude and a better knowledge of the socio-economic and physical realities. The unique value of local creativity will guide urban designers to operate at diverse spatial scales: strategic developments that are relevant at a more local level, as well as small-scale initiatives that can be of the utmost importance for the city as a whole.

The masterplanner no longer has an overarching role but instead has become a team player who, using his/her professional skills, provides, together with other stakeholders, a vision for an area. The urban designer operating in this way can present a rich world of ideas that will yield the best results for the cities concerned.

A quick guide to
the Netherlands

1 TYPES OF CLIENT

National government (ministry of infrastructure and environment)

Provincial and regional authorities

Municipalities

Semi-governmetnal corporations

Developers and other private companies

Housing associations

....

2 TYPES OF
PROJECT/WORK

Spatial development strategy (national, regional, municipal, thematic)

Land-use plan (urban expansion, urban densification, urban renewal, business areas, port areas, shopping centres, recreational and green areas)

Subdivision plans

Visual-quality plans

....

3 APPROACH NEEDED
TO WORK IN COUNTRY

Contact head of department of urban planning

Contact director of a private town planning consultancy

Participate in a competition

Contacts at conferences on urban and regional planning

Apply directly in writing to a public administration, other public institution, private organisation or potential client

Consult professional journals

....

4 LEGISLATION
THAT NEEDS TO BE
REFERRED TO

Spatial Planning Act (Wro)

Environmental Act (Wm)

Building Decree

Land-use plans

Spatial development strategies (national government, provinces and municipalities)

Other policy documents (without legal status)

....

5	SPECIFIC TIPS FOR SUCCESS	Sustainable designs
		Innovative sustainability measures

6	USEFUL WEBSITES	Berlage Institute: www.berlage-institute.nl/institute/mission
		Dutch Association of Urban Designers and Planners (BNSP): www.bnsp.nl
		Dutch Society of Horticulture and Landscape Architecture (NVTL): www.nvtl.nl
		Netherlands Institute for Planning and Housing (Nirov): www.nirov.nl
		Nicis Institute: www.nicis.nl
		Royal Institute of Dutch Architects (BNA): www.bna.nl

SELECTED FACTS

1	area	41,453 km^2
2	population	16,612,213
3	annual population growth	0.5%
4	urban population	83%
5	population density	400 p/km^2
6	GDP	$779,356,291,391
7	GNI per capita	$49,050

Source: The World Bank (2010)

SPAIN

Professor Juan Luis de las Rivas, *architect and town planning consultant*

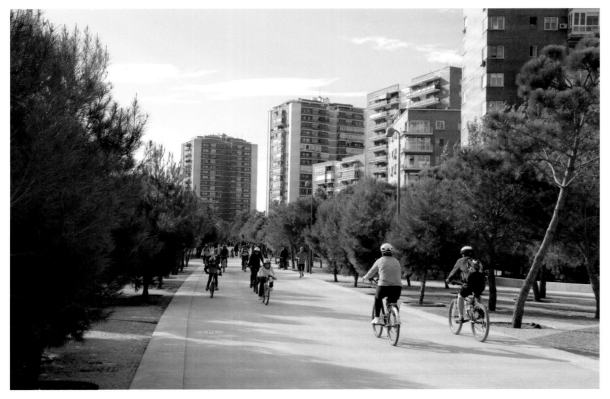

The Salon de los Pinos in Madrid is a recent example of urban design based on landscape, and an invaluable addition to the public spaces of the city

THE KINGDOM OF SPAIN, located on the Iberian peninsula between the Atlantic ocean and the Mediterranean, is characterised by its climatic diversity. The Balearic islands in the Mediterranean and the Canary islands in the Atlantic are also part of Spain. These geographical factors have influenced the country's history whilst the complexity of its topography and climate produces its varied landscapes. These range from mountains to fertile valleys, and from the wide inland plateau – the *Meseta Central* – to the coasts, with the humid north governed by the Atlantic and other regions influenced by the Mediterranean. These regional variations are reflected in the forms of Spanish cities and their architecture, as can be seen by comparing the northern cities of Galicia and the Basque country, such as Santiago or San Sebastian, with those of Andalucía, such as Granada or Seville. Furthermore, it is in the countryside where these differences are most relevant: seen in the diversity of Spanish vernacular architecture and in thousands of villages where the variations of the buildings' adaptation to landscape can be observed.

Since the approval of its Constitutional Charter in 1978, Spain has had a quasi-federal structure with a clear administrative organisation at three levels: national, the state (a parliamentary monarchy); regional, the 17 *comunidades autónomas* (autonomous regions); and local, 8,116 municipalities plus two autonomous cities in North Africa. A national land use law, the 1956 *Ley del Suelo* (last amended in 2007), establishes the national framework, which each region adapts to its own territory. The responsibility for urban issues such as town planning is deeply rooted in a tradition of local autonomy and therefore the main planning documents are drawn up by the municipalities, although these have to respect regional legislation.

Urbanism in contemporary Spain: designing cities in an outstanding context of urban growth

Over the past 30 years a positive economic evolution founded on constant growth, averaging 2.7% per year in the GNP index between 1985 and 2005, has been the most important factor in the changes experienced by Spanish society. As a result of this growth, the expansion of Spain's cities has been extraordinary and has been accompanied by steady investment in infrastructure and great improvements in urban spaces and public facilities. Undoubtedly, these decades of economic growth have transformed urban Spain. The increase in urbanisation has been widespread throughout the country, in every city or town: the proportion of urban land has grown during this period by approximately 100% in comparison to that existing before 1978.[1] However, this Spanish 'growth machine', created in the second half of the last century, has shown its weakness in its relationship with the construction industry: the breakdown of the Spanish economy in 2008 is deeply related to the slowdown in building activity in a country where the housing production level was once the largest in the European Union.

Growth has modified the shape of Spanish cities, expanding their traditional compact structure, splintering their edges and creating new models of urban space. In the outskirts of the main cities, urban sprawl emerges with its usual sequence of individual homes, commercial malls and industry or business parks. However, this process of urban expansion has been balanced by the progressive recuperation of inner-city areas, starting with the rehabilitation of historic centres from the 1980 onwards, and moving from the mid-1990s to include the regeneration of 'social neighbourhoods' created after the civil war.

Urban design in contemporary Spain must be placed in this context of large schemes, and it presents many stark contrasts. The international success of urban creativity in cities such as Barcelona, connected to the 1992 Olympic games, or Bilbao, with its urban regeneration symbolised by the Guggenheim, is probably the main contributor to Spanish prestige in the design of new public spaces. But on the other side of the coin are the numerous anonymous new neighbourhoods in urban peripheries, and the banal and immense built frontages along the Mediterranean coast. Not surprisingly, the role of architects and the quality of Spanish architecture are central to understanding the meaning and significance of urban design in Spain.

Architecture as the dominant discipline:
the lack of specialisation in urban issues

A specific urban design culture has not really developed in Spain. Although everybody can understand the generic meaning of urban design – translated as *diseño urbano* – and the relationship of this concept to urban development, it is not clear whether the term refers to a specific discipline.

Every Spanish architect is potentially an urban designer, even without specialised training. This is a consequence of the lack of specialisation in urban studies[2] and the peculiar Spanish control of professional practice. Only architects and civil engineers – and of these, only those belonging to the *pont et chausses* (highways and bridges) tradition – can sign urban plans. They are considered competent as a result of a generic town planning knowledge gained at university (as part of the architecture curriculum) and because of the official support of professional organisations – *colegios profesionales* – which regulate practice. As a result, Spain does not have a separate professional body for town planners, let alone one for urban design professionals.

The situation of urban design as a discipline is very similar: only architects have an education relevant to urbanism, but even this is generic. In graduate programmes, urbanism represents about 10% of the whole course. Within the context of the Bologna directive, some schools of architecture – such as Valladolid – have developed a new specific subject of urban design. The same is true for postgraduate planning education: the main programmes, specialist or master's courses, are oriented towards urban legislation and management or towards town and regional planning, with no specific units in urban design. Furthermore, no Spanish legislation relates specifically to urban design, and when this concept appears in official documents it is only as a colloquial reference.

For architects and engineers, urbanism is more an area of practice than a structured field of knowledge, as is evidenced by the paucity of urban design publications in Spain – even allowing for a short list of classic translations.[3] Geographers are perhaps the ones that have generated the largest body of knowledge on urban issues. In contrast, the design practitioners' culture demands publications that describe cases or have a selection of good examples but little analysis.

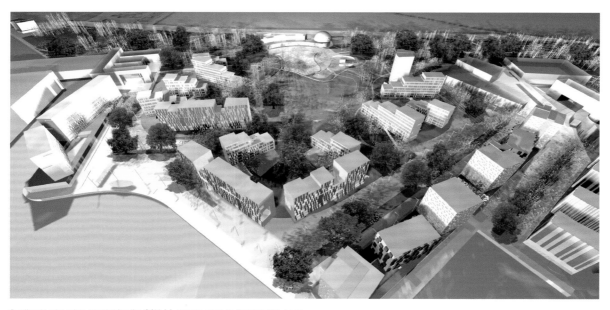

Synthesis of a *plan parcial* for the SSU 11 growth area in Ponferrada, Leon

The clear difference in practice established by law between the two main tools of Spanish urban planning is an additional factor: the *Plan General*, equivalent to a city's framework plan, hardly deals with urban design issues; its aims are regulatory, establishing property rights and land uses, with a programmatic perspective for controlling urban growth or change. The *Plan Parcial*, equivalent to the development plan or urban project (and to a masterplan in the British context) has a clear urban design content as it establishes the conditions for buildings and spaces. However for the majority of architects, apart from its normative contents, the *Plan Parcial* is only about architecture and the urban project is seen as architecture at a large scale.

With this in mind, the exceptional cases where local culture and the excellence of projects have created relevant examples of urban design must be distinguished from routine urban practice. And to understand this reality, the opportunities created by the aforementioned period of urban growth must not be forgotten. After 1979, with the return of democratically elected municipalities, Spanish cities were highly motivated to initiate a process of change with a unique convergence of issues to be dealt with: historic urban landscapes, abandoned industrial areas, old neighbourhoods needing regeneration, a lack of new urban facilities, etc. Some Spanish cities led the way, creating their own particular 'images' which have gradually achieved worldwide renown.

The experience accumulated in this way constitutes a valuable store of urban design ideas, although such a heterogeneous ensemble is not easy to classify. The consequences of the architects' dominance of urban design is twofold: the lack of rules or specific knowledge on the one hand, and the independence of design, which relies only on the architect's talent, on the other. However, some issues permit the introduction of an element of order into the field of Spanish urban design.

Spanish culture and urban public spaces

Contemporary Spanish urban design cannot be understood without reference to the country's urban history, and not just to the physical diversity and quality of its built heritage. In the second half of the last century, and after centuries of neglect, Spain's historic urban areas went through a particular drama of destruction and recovery. Since the beginning of the 1970s, historic city centres have had a marked influence on the evolution of urban design in Spain. Indeed the rediscovery of this urban heritage, its preservation and enhancement paved the way for a full-scale reassessment of quality in urban projects. In turn, this approach gradually focused interest in the city as a whole, and laid the foundation for better urban development in Spanish cities.

Historic city spaces offer a potential for experimentation in urban design which contrasts with the developers' approach in urban extensions. In the case of unique historic centres like Santiago de Compostela, Salamanca, Seville or Toledo conservation is the logical strategy to achieve urban quality.

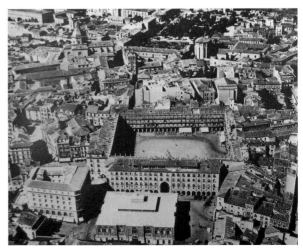

Historical view of the Plaza Mayor in Salamanca

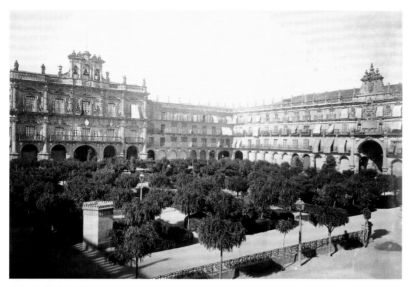

At the end of the 19th century, the introduction of trees changed the plaza into a garden

Conservation plans were also part of the initial phases of the best-known examples of urban regeneration: the pioneering plan for the *Ciutat Viella* in Barcelona, or the old-city reconstruction plan of Bilbao following the 1983 floods. As a result, the rehabilitation of existing urban spaces and historical buildings (an incredible number of such projects achieved in only two decades) has grown into an industry in which Spanish architects have found a new role and developed a particular talent for relating the old and the new in existing urban areas.[4] As this work was going on two decades of economic growth started, making it possible for dynamic cities to make a leap to more ambitious programmes and enabling the experiments of Barcelona and Seville in 1992.

In this process, public spaces and urban facilities offer the most significant urban design achievements, far more interesting than the new coastal and suburban developments where, as already mentioned on page 81, the logic of real estate imposed different rules. The importance of the public realm is in tune with one of the characteristics of the Spanish and Mediterranean lifestyles: urban life is lived 'on the streets' and there is a popular link between everyday life and public spaces, not just in city centres but also in other neighbourhoods. This has an impact on all urban design projects, though success is more evident in the reworking of existing spaces than in the creation of new ones. Spanish urban designers can show many good examples of *plazas* and *paseos* (promenades), and an amazing number of renewed streets in every historic town or village. The high density of urban areas, and of their housing in particular, can also be related to this urban tradition: this level of density is needed for urban life, but its management is a constant issue for debate in urban design circles.

In this context, the prominence of architects engaged in urban design work generates a particular approach to the design of public spaces, which has become obvious in the last few decades. Its main feature is the independence of ideas and skills applied, which rely on the architect's own experience and talent. The second most notable feature, directly related to the first, is a purely aesthetic approach to the layouts of both new and existing public spaces. Environmental psychology and other environmental sciences, including consideration of the point of view of inhabitants/users, are either nonexistent or purely intuitive in Spain's urban design methodology.

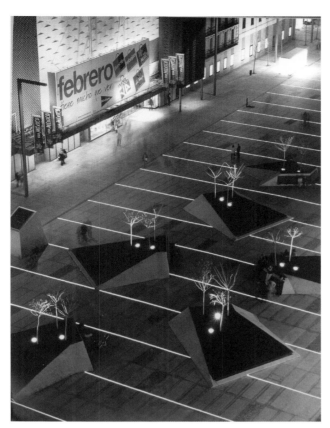

The emergence of landscape and sustainable urban design

Currently, three factors influence urban design practice in Spain: a new interest in
landscape architecture, the search for more sustainable urbanism and the constraints
created by the economic crisis that ended decades of urban growth.

Work on waterfronts is probably the source of many Spanish architects' interest
in urban landscape. Two seminal schemes are worth mentioning: the first is the Wind
Comb, at the edge of the bay of San Sebastian, created in 1976 by sculptor Eduardo
Chillida and architect Luis Peña Ganchegui. Here, urban design becomes a work of
civic art, a place which is in deep dialogue with the genius loci. The second is the *Moll
de la Fusta*, the old wharf at the edge of Barcelona's medieval city where in 1986 Manuel
de Solá Morales began the reinvention of that city's seafront with a smart mixed
'corridor' of development. The 1992 Olympic games would subsequently offer the
conditions to complete the seafront's transformation. In those early days, landscape was
not really mentioned; urban art and function were the aims at the time. However, the
promenades along the urbanised seafront as well as the urban integration of riverbanks
in cities of the interior, generated the need for new approaches.

Two Catalan professors, Manuel Ribas Piera and Rosa Barba, were the pioneers
of landscape architecture in postwar Spain. As architects, their strong concern with
landscape converged with urban issues and in particular with the improvement of design
in urban projects. Works like the *Fossar de la Predera* by Beth Galí, the Botanical Gardens
of Barcelona and the new Benidorm waterfront by C. Ferrater, or the parks by Batlle and
Roig, are good examples of how these initial ideas were consolidated. Furthermore, the

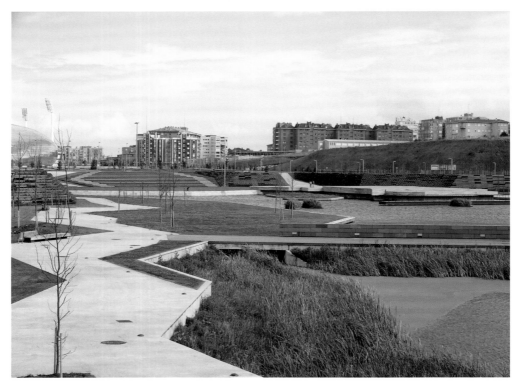

Cabecera Park on the old Turia riverbed in Valencia.
Eduardo de Miguel, Arancha Muñoz and others, 2001

series of European Landscape Biennials celebrated in Barcelona offered a good overview of this new landscape culture. The catalogues that have accompanied all five such events thus far are one of the best resources for understanding the evolution of landscape architecture in Europe and its deep relationship with urban design.[5]

The increasing interest in landscape as part of urbanism happened at the same time as sustainability emerged as a new urban philosophy. The concern for sustainable urban design is no different in Spain from that in other European countries, but Spanish architects are not leading the research in this field and their commitment to sustainable urban design remains generic. Nevertheless, the work of research groups such as *BCN Ecología* led by Salvador Rueda[6] and several recent schemes show the relevance of sustainability in the current Spanish urban perspective. The urban regeneration of old social housing estates; the introduction of modern public transport systems in medium-sized cities like Victoria, Bilbao or Seville; and the creation of new park systems are the more evident results of sustainable urban design in Spain.[7] However, the sustainable urbanism debate has provided more theoretical reflections than concrete proposals, and few connections between theory and practice – although some improvements in urban legislation have also been achieved.

Within the field of new urban development, the urban design debate is evolving around the creation of eco-neighbourhoods. However for the time being, only the case of Sarriguren in Navarre offers an example of real accomplishment based on integrated sustainable urban design concepts.

Finally, the seriousness of the Spanish economic crisis and its specific characteristics could lead to a new scenario in which changes in legislation would promote a more integrated approach to urban regeneration. This could provide the stimulus for developing a more sustainable urbanism.

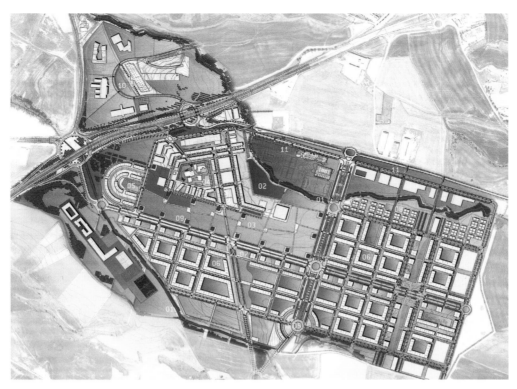

Sarriguren Eco-City plan (Pamplona).
Alfonso Vegara and others, since 1998

Urban design in practice:
echoes and *chiaroscuros* in the Spanish *Ensanche* tradition

The status of urban design in Spain is not a high one: as already mentioned, architects are in charge of urban design schemes without having specific training other than that of accumulated experience. This weakness is reflected in how urban design is perceived; people cannot understand the value of the concept itself. The corresponding lack of theoretical work on urban design is also symptomatic of this low status.

The dominance of the field by architects is the clear result for the lack of specialisation in urban issues. The organisations that regulate the design professions – *colegios profesionales* – are not interested in specialisation. In addition, a new type of consultant, engineering firms, now offer all the services related to urbanism. However, they are more interested in winning big commissions and in the application of technologies than in integrating urban designers into multidisciplinary teams. In important competitions for large urban projects, these firms call on recognised architects to join their team, hoping that this will guarantee their success.

In spite of these circumstances, urban design still has a role in Spain. The more responsible professionals involved in the built environment retain a particular interest in urban design and understand its close relationship with quality. But the field is a narrow one: since the 1980s, some architects have defended the 'intermediate scale', the urban project, but these practitioners have had a limited impact. Almost all the new neighbourhoods created since then have displayed generic layouts, typologies and land uses.

The sequential process of Spanish urban planning nevertheless allows a place for urban design practice. The hierarchy and interdependence of planning documents is

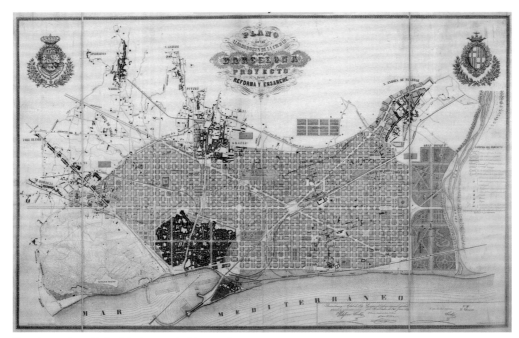

Though a precise grid, Cerdà's plan was flexible enough
to adapt to the topography and the pre-existing layouts
of Barcelona

described as a 'cascade', which runs from the *Plan General* down to the *Plan Parcial* and others. As already mentioned urban design is the key for defining urban development (*Plan Parcial*), but it is also needed to define the urban structure, to allocate land uses and urban facilities, and to measure their scale (*Plan General*). Furthermore, urban design is present in the large new urban projects related to transportation, urban regeneration or environmental improvements. It is here, both in the middle of dense and compact cities and in their banal peripheries with uncontrolled growth that the real challenges lie.

It is worth remembering that, as stated by Françoise Choay, Ildefonso Cerdà was the first modern town planner, not only because of his memorable *Ensanche* of Barcelona, but for his seminal *Teoría General de la Urbanización* (General Theory of Urbanization) published in 1867. Although Cerdà did not establish a school and had no disciples, only followers or imitators, his teachings remain in his plans. The genius of his urban block (the Spanish word is *manzana*, apple) and the precision and practicality of its dimensions for creating extraordinary urban structure are even more evident in the ways in which the pattern has been adapted to the existing topography, deforming the blocks if necessary, as is the case on the *Paseo de Gracia* in Barcelona. It may be that this ability to adapt – taking adaptation as the norm, in fact – is the most important characteristic of what is best in Spanish contemporary urban design.

The *Plan Parcial* for Ponferrada forms the basis for this case study. The *Plan Parcial* is the planning tool most closely related to urban design, and it is similar to a sector plan, an action area or an urban project.

Ponferrada is a medium-sized city with a population of about 60,000 people, located in the province of Leon on the route to Santiago de Compostela. At the beginning of the 20th century, it became an industrial centre as a result of successful coal mining in the nearby mountains.

As already mentioned, Spanish local planning operates at three levels with documents adapted to each of these: *Plan General* (urban structure, regulations and framework for every planned area), *Plan Parcial or Plan Especial* (masterplan for a specific area, detailed lands uses, design of public spaces, building regulations and typologies, envisioning) and *Proyecto de Urbanización* (construction project for urban infrastructures and public open spaces).

The new *Plan General de Ordenación Urbana* (PGOU) of Ponferrada was approved in 2007. The district of Ponferrada comprises nearly 30 villages around the historic town. One of the main planning objectives was to connect these dispersed urban areas in order to create a more continuous and structured urban framework. Over the past few decades, urban development had been very heterogeneous with polycentric growth spreading along the principal roads or around small existing villages. The city is now trying to fill the gaps between settlements. To this end, the *Plan General* has established some strategic design decisions crucial for the future of the city: closing of some roads and avenues to cars, in order to improve urban connectivity; creating a green 'ring' based on a new park system; and redefining local centralities with new or existing public facilities.

The *Sector de Suelo Urbanizable Delimitado* No 11 (area designated for urban development), with 32 ha, is one of the new development sectors defined by the *Plan General* as crucial to the completion of the green ring. In order to develop it, the municipality has put forward a *Plan Parcial* for the youth park. The area, very close to populous neighbourhoods, was in the past occupied by a 400 m high slagheap, but as coal mining declined it was abandoned. At the end of the last century the municipality decided to buy the area and to incorporate this brownfield site into the city. The coal waste was removed and the *Plan General* proposed the creation of a 16.5 ha urban green space, the youth park, thus completing the northern section of the green ring and connecting this area to the city with a new bridge across the river. The cost of this scheme will be partially paid for by the development of a new neighbourhood of 850 dwellings, half of which will be public housing.

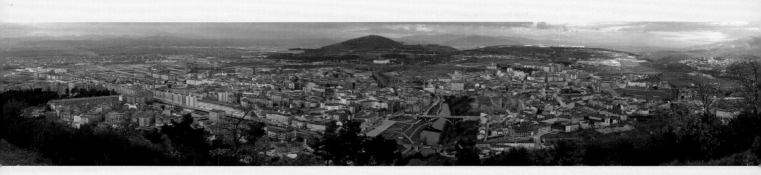

The urban centre of Ponferrada from the Pajariel hillside

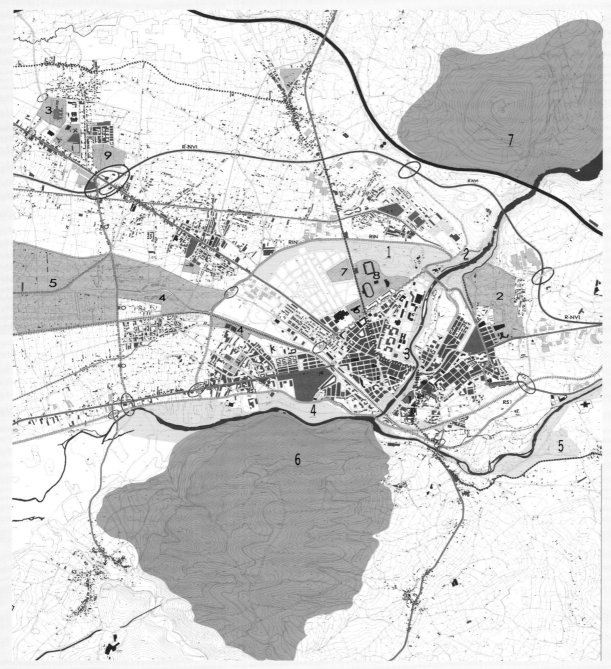

Detail of the *Plan General* charts defining the
new development areas

In addition, the municipality wanted to develop a
new local centre with public and private services.

Once the *Plan General* had established the
framework, the *Plan Parcial* could develop the
design for the area.[8] The first step was to define
the character of the new neighbourhood. Usually
the municipality manages this process, but the
developers and their consultants are relatively
free to decide on the design while respecting the
overall planning legislation and the *Plan General*.
In this case, however, the municipality was both the
landowner and the developer. All design decisions
therefore involved the mayor and his team, and they
wanted to create a unique urban space, attractive
to young families and professionals and with a
percentage of housing for students and for seniors.
An additional planning objective was to include as
much landscaping as possible, in order to obliterate
the neglect of the past.

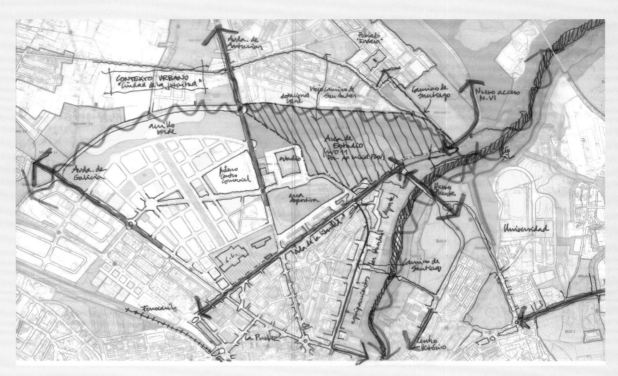

Initial analysis of the SSUD

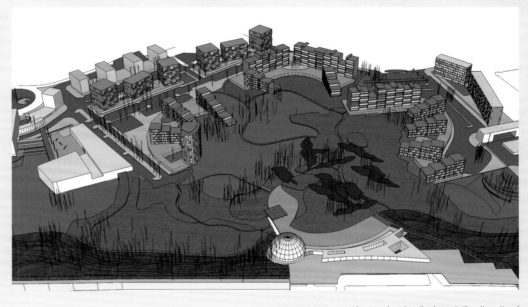

Image showing the layout, the diversity of typologies and solar efficiency

Initially the urban design concept aimed at establishing a visual order, connecting the dwellings with the new park and resolving the articulation between new and existing urban spaces. The second objective was to generate life at the ground level. Two well-defined public areas were proposed: the park and a commercial area along the new streets, as an extension of the existing avenue.

Working in close collaboration with the local planning committee led by the councillor in charge of urbanism, the urban design team (architects assisted by a firm of civil engineering consultants) put forward three alternative proposals, variations on the same theme but with different building typologies. The objective was to define the local constraints and to establish a design concept. After

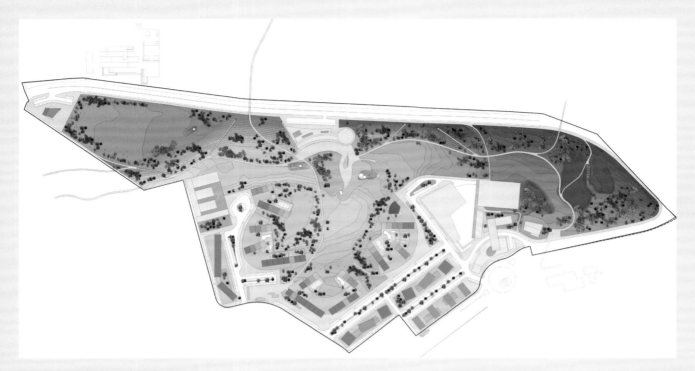

The *Plan Parcial* for the youth park:
dwellings in brown, public and private buildings in blue

discussions between the committee and the officers, the selected option was to be reworked and developed into an urban project.

The choice of building typologies was probably one of the most important decisions, particularly with respect to their diversity and their relationship to the two public spaces. The creation of the main 'spine', with urban spaces at either end, allows continuity and synergy between the new urban activities: public buildings, commercial buildings and public transport. From this active urban frontage, it is possible to access the park through the buildings. The design of the park gives priority to natural features, and is inspired by the local landscape: the tree corridor at the north edge, the arboretum in the east and the meadow acting as a water reservoir in the middle – a large open green area, visible from most of the dwellings.

Other important concerns of the plan were the solar efficiency of the buildings based on their orientation, the future function of the public buildings (youth centre, conference hall, children's museum with planetarium, and seniors' centre) and the quality of private services (small hotel and pilgrims' reception centre).

At first, the local committee was puzzled by the scheme's apparent discontinuity with the existing urban fabric, and the lack of the usual regular urban blocks. But it soon realised that the area was beyond the city limits, separated from it by a large urban avenue and virtually inserted in the green ring. There was therefore an opportunity to create a new kind of neighbourhood, in which quality of design was present throughout the developing process, from the masterplan down to the building details.

The masterplan shows a regular pattern close to the existing urban fabric and a different geometry around the open space that takes advantage of the contact with nature. The latter, more irregular, design also adapts the position of the buildings to views and solar conditions.

For the purpose of public participation a video was prepared, emphasising street life and the relationship between the buildings and the park. Computer technology helped people to understand the design proposals and participate in the decision-making process. This kind of tool is developing into a basic necessity for urban design work, allowing

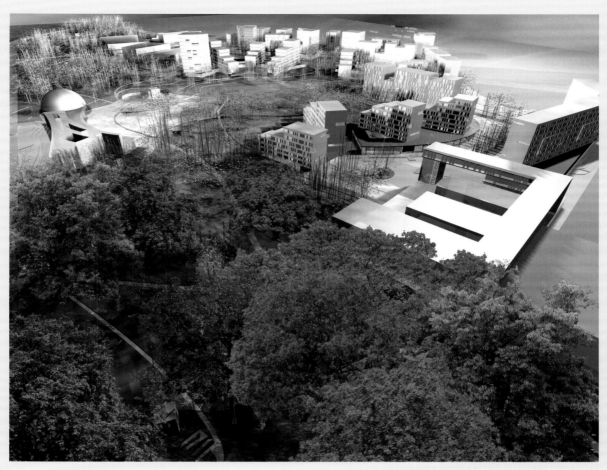

General aerial view of the proposed urban design

people to envision and evaluate the future of their urban environment.

The *Plan Parcial* also includes its own regulations, which develop those of the planning legislation and the *Plan General*. These are mainly detailed standards for buildings, streets, public spaces and urban infrastructure. Sustainability standards are also included: solar energy for dwellings, energy savings in the buildings, mixed-uses recommendations, etc. The municipality is now considering the creation of a district heating biomass plant for the youth park, though for the time being it is only an idea.

In effect, the *Plan Parcial* establishes the detailed conditions for the design of the whole development. To facilitate the implementation of the scheme, the area has been subdivided into several units or urban plots, better adapted to the possibilities of local developers. Therefore, the plan must specify through various documents how each

of these units is to be developed. The *Proyecto de Urbanización* is now in the hands of a firm of engineers that collaborates with the design team. The local authority, as landowner, will offer each plot to developers through a tender process, and its planning committee will ensure that the planning and urban design conditions, the regulations and the timings set down in the plan are respected.

At present (2012) all the planning documents for the area have been approved and the project is progressing. The final economic evaluation of the youth-park area is being undertaken before starting with work on the infrastructure.

A quick guide to
Spain

1 TYPES OF CLIENT

Municipalities (local authorities)

Regional government (*comunidades autónomas*)

Public-sector developers (public enterprises linked with local or regional authorities)

Private developers (local or national)

....

2 TYPES OF PROJECT/WORK

Masterplans and urban projects:
- Urban renewal (*Planes Especiales* and *Estudios de Detalle* in urban regeneration areas)
- Urban extensions (*Planes Parciales* and Planes *Especiales*): these are the more frequent types of urban design commissions.
- Urban preservation, including rehabilitation and urban design guidelines

Landscape plans and projects

....

3 APPROACH NEEDED TO WORK IN COUNTRY

Contact with regional authorities

Contact with mayors and their advisers

Partnership with local firm

International competition

Direct negotiation with client

....

4 LEGISLATION THAT NEEDS TO BE REFERRED TO

Regional plans: regional laws of urbanism and/or of regional planning

Local plans: Spanish Urban Law, local urban plans (*Planes Generales de Ordenación Urbana*), municipal and other local ordinances

Other requirements: sectorial laws (water, environment, roads, etc)

Public competitions and procurement legislation

In certain cases, regulations from the professional organisations (*colegios profesionales*)

Building regulations (*Código Técnico de la Edificación*)

....

5 SPECIFIC TIPS FOR SUCCESS

Sustainable development, including orientation of buildings

Public–private partnerships in regeneration schemes

Percentage of social housing required in all cases

....

6 USEFUL WEBSITES

Asociación Española de Técnicos Urbanistas (AETU): www.aetu.es

Consejo Superior de Colegios de Arquitectos de España: www.cscae.com

Ministerio de Fomento: www.fomento.gob.es

....

1	area	504,645 km²
2	population	46,081,574
3	annual population growth	0.4%
4	urban population	77%
5	population density	91 p/km²
6	GDP	$1,407,405,298,013
7	GNI per capita	$31,750

Source: The World Bank (2010)

SWEDEN

Mats Johan Lundström, *planner and urban designer*

Dr Tigran Haas, *architect and urban designer*

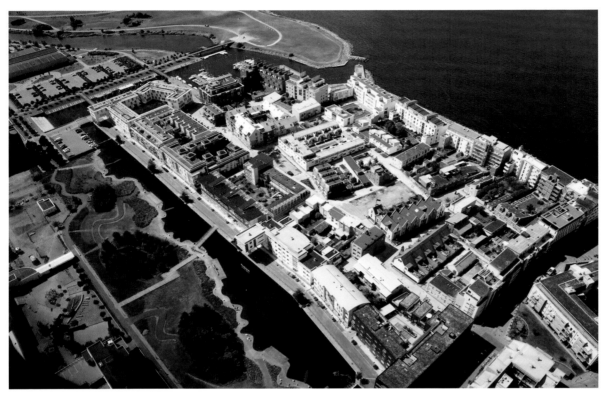

Aerial view of part of the Bo01 area

SWEDEN is a constitutional monarchy with an elected parliament. The country is divided into 21 counties and 290 municipalities. All levels of government have planning responsibilities corresponding to their scale, but most planning documents are prepared and implemented by the municipalities. The 1947 Planning and Building Act was the main piece of legislation until 1987 when it was replaced by a new one. Additionally the Environment Code was introduced in 1999, covering a wider range of subjects than the latter act.

Definitions

From a Swedish point of view, the concept of urban design and its relationship to architecture and town planning is hard to grasp. Does it operate at the level of streets, parks, squares and buildings, or at that of the structure of urban districts and towns? Is it only concerned with the physical form of land and built structures, or does it include mental images and perceptions of the city? Is it just an expert's exercise or does it involve the general public and decision makers? The answer to these questions will probably differ according to who is being asked. There is no Swedish term or concept corresponding to urban design. The closest equivalent is *stadsbyggnad* (city building or town planning), or in older texts *stadsbyggnadskonst* (the art of building cities), related to the German word *städtebau*. There is no widely accepted clear definition of the concept of *stadsbyggnad*: architects, landscape architects, planners and engineers may all say they are involved in its practice, although the meaning given by each of them may vary. The National Encyclopaedia defines *stadsbyggnad* as 'the methodology of ordering and shaping, composing, designing buildings, streets and public spaces in their entirety'. This is therefore the definition of urban design in a Swedish context that will be adopted here.

The professional place of urban design

There is no officially recognised urban design profession in Sweden, and no special certificate or licence is needed to work in urban design. Historically, most people working in urban design were architects, with sometimes some engineers too. In the past few decades, the urban design field has also incorporated landscape architects and various kinds of urban and physical planners. There is no special body or association for urban designers but most professionals are members of the *Sveriges Arkitekter* (the Swedish Association of Architects), which was created in 2002 by the merger of the four associations of architects, landscape architects, interior designers and spatial planners. Among other activities, the association publishes the magazine Arkitekten and administers architectural and urban design competitions, as well as the annual Siena prize for landscape architecture and a biannual prize for planning.

The academic discipline

The academic discipline of *stadsbyggnad* has existed in Swedish schools of architecture since Uno Åhrén was appointed to the first professorship of *stadsbyggnad* at Stockholm's Royal Institute of Technology (KTH) in 1947; other schools of architecture, at Chalmers University of Technology (Gothenburg) and Lund University, followed a few years later.

Landscape architecture education was introduced in the early 70s as the agronomy education at the Swedish University of Agriculture (SLU) in Alnarp and Ultuna was split into two disciplines. At first mainly involved in garden and park design, landscape architects have gradually become more involved in urban planning and design.

The number of architecture students interested in urban planning and design declined during the 1980s and the municipal planning departments had problems attracting architects to the planning sector. As a result, a new course in physical–spatial planning (*fysisk planering*) was launched in Karlskrona's Blekinge Institute of Technology (BTH) in 1989, combining the disciplines of urban planning and urban design.

Today, urban design courses are offered mainly by the schools of architecture in Stockholm, Gothenborg, Lund and Umeå, at SLU in Alnarp and Ultuna, and BTH in Karlskrona. No full academic programme focuses exclusively on urban design. The Master of Science programmes in Urban Planning and Design at KTH (involving collaboration between the departments of architecture and urban planning) and the physical–spatial planning at BTH are probably the nearest to what might be considered urban design in international terms. Since the introduction of the European Bologna higher education system, there has been a rapid increase in the number of programmes in urban planning/development/management offered by Swedish universities. Most of them, however, do not focus on the design aspects of planning.

Research on urban design (such as urban morphology or space syntax) is mainly conducted at the schools of architecture, although not very extensively. Urban planning researchers mostly focus on the process aspects of urban planning and the built environment.

Legal status

Neither national legislation nor guidelines deal specifically with urban design. Construction and planning are regulated by the Planning and Building Act (PBA), which mostly controls the processes rather than the content of these disciplines. The PBA states what kind of issues must be regulated in a detailed plan, but the content issues are formulated in very imprecise terms, such as

> With due regard to natural and cultural values, planning shall promote a purposeful layout and an aesthetically pleasing design of built-up areas, green belts, routes of communication and other constructions. It shall also aim at promoting good living conditions from a social point of view, good environmental conditions and a long-lasting and effective management of land and water areas, energy resources and raw materials.
>
> (PBA: Chapter 2, section 2)

or

> Sites used for development shall be arranged in a way that is suitable with regard to the townscape or the landscape and the existing natural and cultural assets.
>
> (PBA Chapter 3, Section 15).

In addition, the National Board of Housing, Building and Planning (*Boverket*) has issued national regulations and general recommendations on the accessibility and usability of indoor and outdoor public spaces for people with limited mobility or orientation capacity.

Historical development

Swedish politicians and planners of the early 20th century were heavily influenced by socially conscious German architects such as Peter Behrens, Heinrich Tessenow and Walter Gropius. Political movements advocated housing policies to provide good and affordable dwellings for all, and the development of cities in a more planned manner. The 1930 Stockholm exhibition had a considerable impact, as it introduced modernist design and architecture to a broad Swedish audience. Thereafter, modernist ideas of light, air and sun were reflected in new housing developments in the suburbs: narrow buildings were aligned to get as much light as possible; local shops such as dairies, bakeries and butchers were placed on the ground floors.

After more than a decade of investigation, the social housing commission presented a new social housing policy to parliament in 1947. In the same year, a new Planning and Building Act was approved by parliament, giving local authorities the power to decide where and how new buildings were to be developed. The social-democratic postwar period was characterised by new housing developments in the suburbs and much urban renewal in the inner cities – clearing the old and dirty urban reminders of the previous class-bound society. New ideas about urban planning were imported from the UK and the US as books by Stein, Mumford, and Geddes were introduced at the end of the second world war. The first area in Sweden to be planned as a neighbourhood unit was Norra Guldheden in Gothenburg (1946), followed by

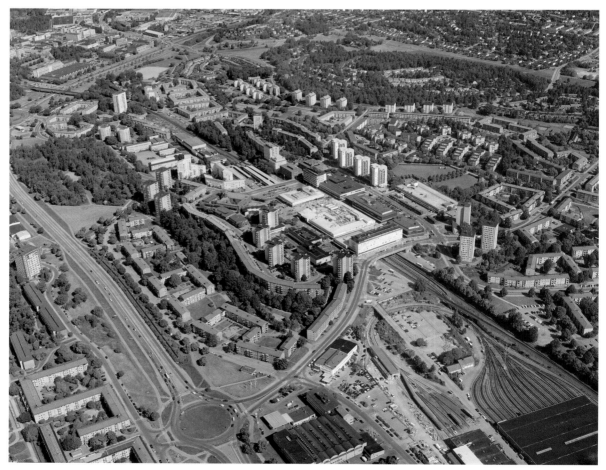

Aerial view of Vallingby

districts in Stockholm like Årsta (1951) and Hökarängen (1954). Their neighbourhood centres offered both commercial and cultural services. The aim of the new welfare society was to foster good democratic citizens in a small-scale social environment.

In the 1950s, these ideas were developed into a planning concept called the ABC city (*Arbete-Bostad-Centrum* = Work-Housing-Centre), meaning that people were to live, work and have access to important social, cultural and commercial facilities within a short distance. In Stockholm, this suburban planning model was closely linked to the development of the underground system: the neighbourhood centre and high-rise apartments were close to the underground T-station, and less dense housing in the periphery of the suburb. Vällingby and Farsta are the most famous examples of the ABC city, attracting visiting architects and planners from around the entire world.

In the 1960s, the ABC model was developed further at a much larger scale, mainly due to the retail industry requiring fewer and bigger stores and thus larger catchment areas. The 'million house programme' launched by the Swedish government in 1965 aimed at producing 100,000 new apartments a year for ten years. This, in combination with a weakness for rational architecture among Swedish architects, increased the scale, the monotony and the industrialisation of the building process. The adaptation to the landscape of the modernist urban design of the 30s, 40s and 50s was now replaced by an orthogonal grid, which also made economic sense for the large construction cranes lifting prefabricated concrete slabs. Most multi-family housing

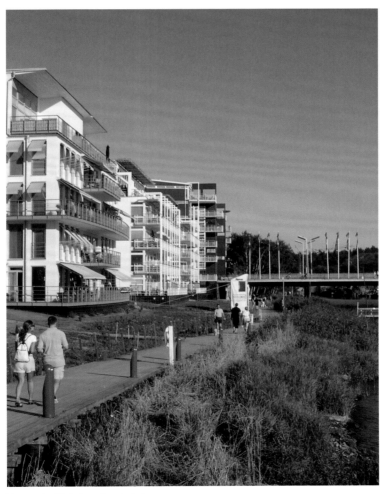

Hammarby Sjöstaden attempts to be an environmenally friendly development

built during this period is on three stories with no lift, or eight stories with only one lift. Towards the end of the programme, in the early 70s, most new dwellings were single-family houses, since the large scale multi-family developments had (and still have) a bad reputation.

In the 1970s and 80s, the reaction against the large-scale developments was strong. The Danish planning concept of 'low-and-dense' inspired many architects and planners, especially in the southern parts of Sweden. The anti-modernist reaction also spurred a renaissance of the traditional city, similar to that of the American New Urbanism movement, although less organised and structured. The term *stadsmässig* (urban-like) has been a buzzword ever since, expressing the will to create more lively and less car-dominated urban environments that promote social encounters.

Since the 1992 Rio conference, sustainability has been addressed in various ways. The self-sufficient eco-village, isolated and separated from existing urban systems, was the first expression of sustainable living in the 1980s and early 90s. The second phase of sustainable development and planning developed in the late 1990s – through eco-districts such as Hammarby Sjöstad/Waterfront in Stockholm and Bo01 in Malmö. These focused on 'smart' growth within the urban system: closing resource loops; finding synergies in urban functions; building energy-efficient buildings; using renewable energy sources; and promoting biking, walking and public transit – at the same time creating inspiring and attractive architecture and urban design.

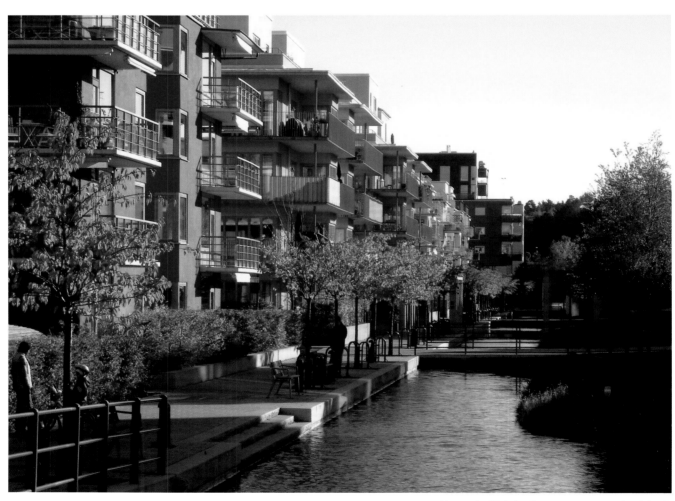

Hammarby Sjöstaden linear green spaces and sustainable drainage systems run through the development

Practice and concerns

The Swedish distribution of legal, fiscal and administrative powers is such that the national and local levels are strong and the regional level is weak. This, in turn, influences the planning system. The Planning and Building Acts dictate that the municipalities are responsible for land-use planning (the so-called municipal planning monopoly). Regional land-use planning is only mandatory in the County of Stockholm, but due to the municipal planning monopoly the Stockholm Regional Plan has no legal power or mandate. The county administrative boards' planning units, run by the national government, mainly monitor the municipal plans, making sure that national interests (such as heritage, environmental and military issues) are being taken care of, and that the procedural regulations of the PBA are obeyed. There is no national plan to steer spatial development in Sweden. However, the National Board of Housing, Building and Planning (*Boverket*) has recently been asked to prepare a 'Vision of Sweden 2025' in cooperation with other authorities and organisations.

The Planning and Building Act states that all municipalities are to have an up-to-date comprehensive plan (*översiktsplan*): a masterplan showing the municipality's intentions for the spatial development of the area. Since many Swedish municipalities cover large areas, these plans only show the general outlines of development; they are not legally binding documents. In order to give more detailed indications on the development of a specific part of the district, an in-depth and detailed district masterplan can be drawn up. A detailed plan regulating land use, amount of building (heights, number of floors, plot ratio, etc), elevations, materials, parking standards, roads, noise reduction, etc, must be prepared before a developer can build, and the ensuing permit must conform with those regulations.

Designs for new urban developments are usually commissioned by the landowner, be it a private development company, municipality or the National Road Authority (which owns some arterial roads in towns and cities). Municipalities usually prefer to prepare plans in-house, especially the comprehensive plans. However, an increasing number of them bring in consultants to prepare parts of, or entire, plans – especially detailed plans covering streets, roads, parks and other public spaces. Therefore consultants may be commissioned to prepare detailed plans by either a municipality or a developer. All documents must always be approved by the planning committee and the local council, as the municipal planners have to ensure that the public interest is taken care of.

When external consultants are involved, the allocation of contracts is usually based on standard procurement agreements or the result of a competition. During the last 10–15 years, the commissioning of private planning and design consultancies has increased considerably. This is either due to the fact that local authorities have fewer financial or professional resources, or the result of downsizing which started during the early 90s' crisis and has increased sharply in the new millennium.

Bo01 AND THE WESTERN HARBOUR (VÄSTRA HAMNEN), MALMÖ

Malmö is the third largest city in Sweden: its population has recently (2011) exceeded 300,000 inhabitants. It is the regional capital of the Skåne (Scania) region in the extreme south of Sweden. Malmö is also an important node on the cross-national link of the Öresund, connecting it to the east of Denmark and its capital, Copenhagen.

Historical background

Malmö was founded in the 13th century. Strategically located on the Öresund strait and the Baltic sea, it was an important trade city in the eastern part of the Kingdom of Denmark. After the 1658 Roskilde peace treaty, Skåne and Malmö became Swedish.

During the 19th century, rapid industrialisation and urbanisation contributed to the fast growth of Malmö. In 1870 it was the third largest city in Sweden with 25,000 inhabitants, and its population increased to 100,000 in 1920 and to 200,000 in 1950. The development of modern transport infrastructure such as harbours, railways and roads was an important factor in the expansion of Malmö as a leading commercial and industrial city. The construction of the Western harbour started in the late 18th century and, as a result of growing activity, a larger South-eastern harbour was built in the mid-19th century. During the first half of the 20th century, shipbuilding became the dominant industry as a result of the growth of the Kockums Company. As Kockums expanded, so did the harbour by filling out more land in the Öresund strait.

However in the late 1970s, industrial decline – especially in the shipbuilding industry – struck Malmö a hard blow, and thousands of workers lost their jobs. Since then, Kockums' industrial production in Malmö has diminished, although research and development activities still take place in the Western harbour. In order to alleviate the impact of high unemployment, the government invested heavily in new infrastructure for other industries; in the late 1980s, the last landfill of Western harbour was carried out and a large SAAB car manufacturing plant was built. It closed down after only a few years, and was then converted into Malmö Expo.

New developments in Western harbour: Malmö University and Bo01

In the mid-90s, after an envisioning exercise, the authorities took the strategic decision to transform the image and economic base of Malmö from an industrial city to a 'knowledge city'. Malmö University was opened in 1998, strategically located on an artificial island now named University island, in between the Western harbour and Malmö central station. This new strategy, combined with the purchase by the city of large areas of land in Western harbour, led to the decision to postpone the housing exhibition Bo2000, planned to take place in Limhamn on the outskirts of Malmö. Instead, the exhibition was held in 2001 in the western part of the Western harbour, marking another important step in the transformation of Malmö.

Bo01

The Bo01 international housing exhibition was an opportunity for the City of Malmö to change its image from a harsh industrial city with social and economic problems to something more positive and contemporary. Furthermore, the exhibition was a way to attract new higher-income inhabitants in order to redress the socio-economic profile of the Malmö region and to increase the tax revenue of the city. The Malmö metropolitan area had a socio-economic structure similar to that of the North American 'doughnut' city: a poor population in the centre (Malmö city), and a wealthy one in the surrounding suburban low-tax municipalities, benefiting from the activities (jobs, leisure, culture, etc) and infrastructure of Malmö, without paying for them.

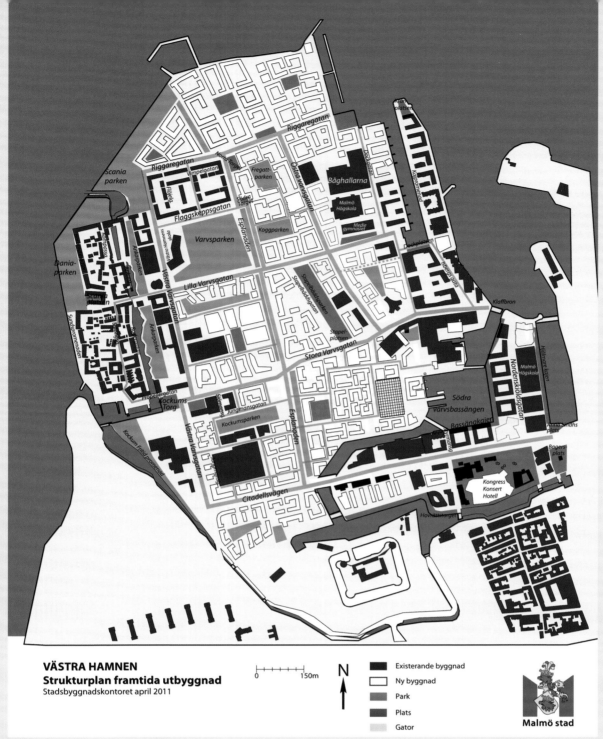

VÄSTRA HAMNEN
Strukturplan framtida utbyggnad
Stadsbyggnadskontoret april 2011

0   150m

N ↑

- Existerande byggnad
- Ny byggnad
- Park
- Plats
- Gator

Malmö stad

The Western Harbour masterplan

One of the main objectives of the development of Bo01 and the Western harbour was to establish a sustainable urban district with closed eco-cycles. The environmental agenda had been established in the mid-90s for the Bo2000 millennium exhibition; it was a development of so-called eco-villages for ecologically aware people, which had started in the urban periphery in the 1980s and 90s.

With the move to the Western harbour – a larger and more centrally located area where the city had a large stake in land – the idea of closed eco-loops was discarded. Instead, the vision of a large compact district with sustainable systems connected to the rest of the city was developed. Its inhabitants would not need to be aware of the resource efficiency of their lifestyles. In the spring of 1998, the planning administration presented a comprehensive plan for the Western harbour area. The masterplan for the Bo01 area, the first stage of the development, was prepared by the head architect of the Bo01 exhibition, Professor Klas Tham, in October of the same year. The legally binding detailed plan and the quality schedule that followed it were prepared by the City of Malmö planning office, following Tham's layout and design guidelines.

The fact that the City of Malmö owned the entire Bo01 area, and that the high profile of the project attracted developers, ensured that high standards of design and environmental quality could be achieved. The municipality was able to choose ambitious developers with good architects, and to place higher demands in the sales contracts of individual parcels of land than they could have done in a regular city plan.

The design and scale of Bo01 is inspired by older towns in northern Europe: low, dense, intimate and space efficient. Tham wanted to create an urban district with a traditional scale, narrow streets, varied heights of buildings, a mixture of private and public gardens, and an atmosphere inspired by Camilo Sitte. The variety of building types, colours, sizes and designs is the result of Tham's scheme and the performance of many architects and developers, giving the area an interesting and unique character. The zigzag-shaped western edge of Bo01 is fronted by five- to six-storey apartment buildings, like a medieval city wall. But instead of protecting its citizens from evil intruders, this high wall protects the inner parts of the area from the mighty winds of the Öresund strait. Narrow, crooked lanes connect the boardwalk with the lower and calmer inner area, buffering the wind from the sea – an urban design concept borrowed from old fishing villages. The internal distorted-grid street network also slows down the wind and the traffic. Terraced dwellings and town houses of two to three storeys are mixed with larger apartment buildings. Some 1,450 apartments were designed by 24 different architecture studios and built by 26 developers.

As required in the quality schedule, the materials and design of the public spaces in the Bo01 area are of a very high quality. The inner streets paved with red or yellow bricks are edged by mini-canals, part of a beautifully designed open storm-water system connecting three 'pocket parks', biotopes imitating nature, with granite and wooden detailing, ponds and mini-waterfalls, and plants.

The western boardwalk along the Öresund strait, with a wonderful sunset view of the recently built bridge connecting Sweden and Denmark, has become a popular place for leisure activities. The planners wanted the ground floors of the buildings to have public facilities (cafes, shops and restaurants) facing the boardwalk, but the developers were hesitant. Hence this was only achieved in the southern blocks, making the private– public relation of ground floor apartments along the boardwalk somewhat awkward. In order to improve this relationship, a wooden stair-shaped structure, used both for sitting and walking, divides the boardwalk into two linear zones. The one closest to the buildings is surfaced with granite paving stones, followed a little further away from the buildings by asphalt pavement for pedestrians and cyclists. The zone on the other side of the wooden stairs has a timber pavement, making it suitable for walking at a slower pace.

The promenade ends at Scandiaplatsen (designed by 13.3 landscape architects, Norway), an open plaza with a lower terrace by the sea with stairs to sit on or to walk down. Further on is Daniaparken (designed by Torbjörn Andersson, Sweco FFNS Architects), a public park with a wonderful view over the Öresund strait. The design is rather austere, reminiscent of those of the Inca and ancient Egyptian cultures. The main part is a sunken lawn protected from the wind, suitable for sunbathing, picnics and play as well as musical events. Pedestrians can continue their promenade along the shore, and stop at one of the panorama points.

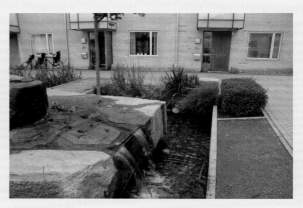

'Pocket park' with storm-water treatment

Both Sundspromenaden and Daniaparken became popular places for diving and swimming. In 2005, the city built an official bathing place with beach facilities such as a diving tower and volley courts in the older park, Scaniaparken (1990, Jörgen Carlsson), north of Daniaparken. Besides its bathing element, Scaniaparken is an open park with formal lawns and only a few trees. In 2005, a few years after Bo01 was completed, a public bathing place (Scaniabadet) with large jetties for sunbathing and diving was opened as a new feature of the park.

The northern part of Bo01, east of Daniaparken, was mostly built after the exhibition. The blocks facing Daniaparken and the Öresund strait are large and rather monotonous. The design of the two white rental blocks at the north-western corner seems to be influenced by New York architect Richard Meier, while the following block resembles an Ibiza hotel complex from the 1970s. However, the inner part retains the small scale, character and details of the exhibition area, although the overall quality is not as high.

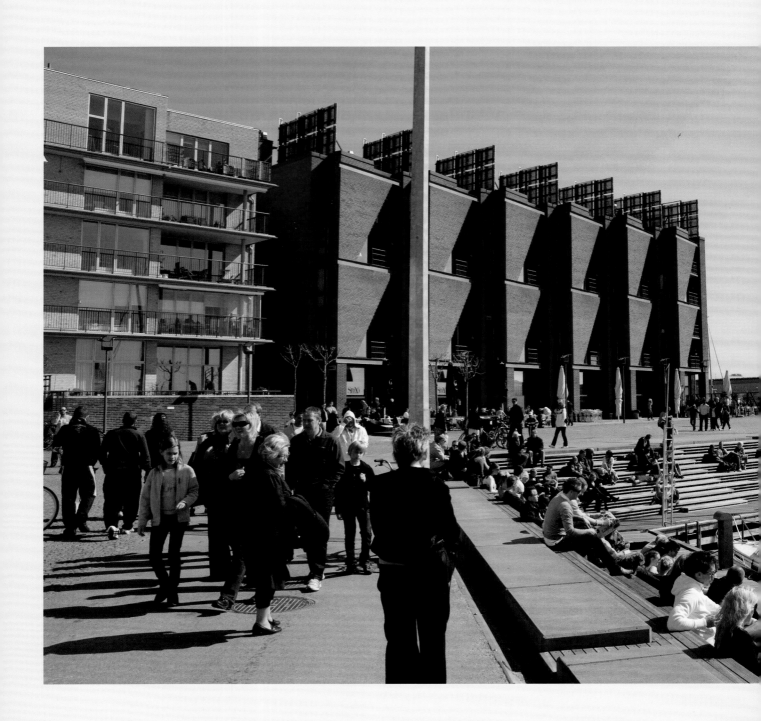

The European Village is part of this section of the area. As a part of the Bo01 exhibition, the Swedish government invited all the member states of the EU to take part in the European Village project, demonstrating small-scale building within various traditions of architecture and indigenous materials. Nine countries participated, building detached houses with their national characteristics, construction methods and approaches to sustainable development. The remaining 14 lots of the village were developed by a Swedish–German company after the exhibition. The result is an urban village within the village, with a varied yet calm character, established around a blue and green corridor.

The eastern edge of the Bo01 exhibition area also has a city-wall character, although with a more rational, rectilinear form. The buildings face a street and a saltwater canal which continues north, passing the European Village and ends in a pond in the Scaniaparken, before going out to the sea. On the opposite side of the canal, the form is curvilinear and more playful, being part of the Ankarparken (designed by Stig L Andersson, APS Landscape architects, Denmark). This is a park with its own ecosystem, composed of a variety of Swedish biotopes distributed like islands in a 'sea' of grass. Apart from being popular among the people living and visiting the area, this park is used for environmental and educational purposes.

As the density of Bo01 is high (the average plot ratio is approximately 1.1), the city wanted to enhance the 'blue–green' network and make an attractive ecological habitat for both humans and fauna. One way of securing this was to apply the 'green surface factor', inspired by the German compensation system for green areas. This is used to create high-quality vegetation and deal with storm water in densely built-up areas with limited land by using green walls, green roofs, ponds, trees, shrubs, etc. The factor is a mean value showing the relationship between areas of vegetation and storm-water treatment on one hand and built-up area on the other.

Apartments facing the sun on the Öresund strait

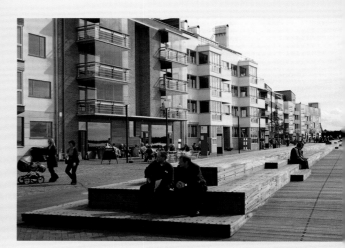

View of the Sundspromenaden facing the Öresund strait

Case study: Bo01 and the Western Harbour (Västra Hamnen), Malmö ~ SWEDEN

The Turning Torso: high-rise urban design

The twisting high-rise building in the north-eastern corner of the Bo01 area, the Turning Torso by Santiago Calatrava, is the most internationally recognised building in Malmö. Inspired by Calatrava's sculpture Twisting Torso, the CEO of the Malmö cooperative housing company HSB Malmö commissioned him to design a building based on the same concept. The idea of a landmark building designed by a 'starchitect', and the highest housing tower in Europe at that, acting as a symbol of the new Malmö was tempting for the city leaders. The City sold the land to HSB, building started in February 2001 and the first tenants moved in almost five years later. It is 190 m tall and has 54 floors grouped in nine cubes. The first ten storeys contain offices and the top two floors a conference venue; in between there are 147 apartments. Though not part of the original scheme for Bo01 or the Western harbour, the sculptural Turning Torso has become a much-appreciated landmark, replacing the disassembled Kockums industrial crane as the symbol of Malmö.

North of the Turning Torso is a multistorey car park combined with housing and a shopping galleria on the ground floor, serving the adjacent buildings. With its long block structure and 'dead' street front, this creates a barrier and it is a less attractive environment for pedestrians than the rest of the Bo01 area.

Energy and environment

The entire Western harbour is supplied by 100% renewable energy (transport not included). The main source for heating buildings and water is a central heat pump using heat from the sea and an aquifer system. The 1,400 m^2 of solar collectors integrated in the buildings provide the rest. The electricity used for the heat pump, ventilation, pumps and household appliances is produced in a 2 MW windmill called Boel, a 78 m high tower located in the Northern harbour which also exports surplus electricity to the grid. The 120 m^2 of building-integrated solar cells also contribute to renewable electricity production. Waste is separated in a sorting room close to each home: solid food waste is collected in a vacuum system,

then composted; food waste from grinders in the kitchen sinks is collected and anaerobically digested into biogas. The waste water is connected to the citywide waste-water system.

The City's aim was to have buildings with low energy consumption. However, hardly any building reached the maximum target of 105 kWh/m^2 a year (considered good ten years ago), mainly because of very large window areas and faulty energy-use models. Some building even had energy consumption over 200 kWh/m^2. In recent developments in the city, however, energy performance has been a top priority.

Later developments in the Western harbour

Bo01 was a way to show that creating sustainable and attractive neighbourhoods was possible, albeit with heavy subsidies from national environmental funds. It was a flagship project with expensive apartments and public spaces. In the newer projects in the Western harbour, such as Flagghusen and Fullriggaren, the City wants to mainstream sustainability, showing the possibilities of creating sustainable housing that doesn't cost a fortune: 'Everyday planning under ordinary market conditions'. To accomplish this, the City has developed a communication planning process with regular seminars and workshops, in which city officials and developers learn together and create consensus on visions and sustainability, and on how to implement them. This process has been well received and has led to higher sustainability standards. However, compared with the Bo01 area, the resulting architecture and urban design are more traditional, larger in scale and with a lower quality of detail in their public spaces.

On the former SAAB factory site, the Masthusen blocks will be the first Swedish district certified according to the BREEAM Communities system of sustainable development. For some years to come, the Western harbour will be the principal sustainable urban development tested in Scandinavia.

Critique of practice and suggestions about the future of the profession

At present, architecture, landscape architecture and urban design remain both theoretically and professionally very much isolated from each other in Sweden. Although there is an understanding that one profession alone cannot solve the problems of cities and urban development, a real integration of disciplines has never happened. Architecture remains definitely the strongest profession, most prominent in the media and politically involved, while urban design is arguably worst off since it has no real professional identity or stable theoretical and practical basis of its own.

The question remains of whether academia (the schools of architecture and planning) will bring about changes and encourage the professions to work in harmony instead of isolating them. The situation could change if professional degrees in urban design were fully recognised and if certification emerged. Within the Swedish system, the lack of a certification of Masters in Urban Design may not be a problem but it could be one for those hoping for an international career.

The fact that most leading architectural practices have urban design sections and projects, and that ecological urbanism and sustainable architecture are expanding to respond to climate change and the energy crisis, means that positive changes are appearing on the horizon. But the most important and positive factor is the growing interest in urban design from young academics and students; this will give legitimacy to urban design, still a very young and fragile discipline in Sweden.

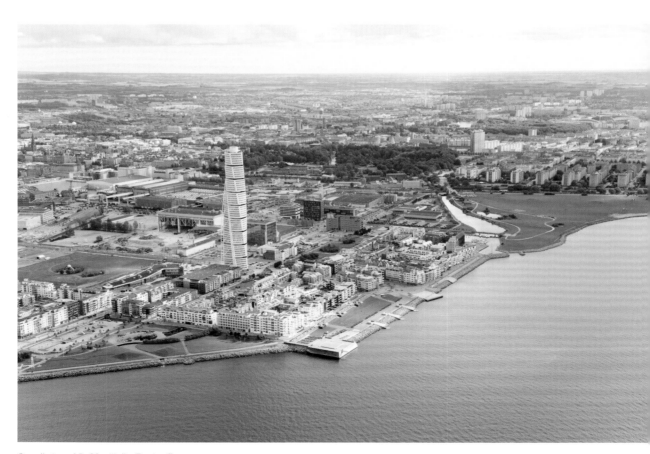

Overall view of Bo01 with the Turning Torso

A quick guide to
Sweden

1 TYPES OF CLIENT

Local authorities (*kommuner*)

Although larger municipalities usually have their own staff handling planning and design projects, private firms are increasingly getting commissions

Developers

....

2 TYPES OF PROJECT/WORK

Most frequently, the production of detailed plans (the legal plans and documents) and smaller design/redesign commissions for public spaces such as parks and streets

Larger schemes, such as masterplans

....

3 APPROACH NEEDED TO WORK IN COUNTRY

No need for authorisation or registration in order to work in urban design or planning

Most international urban design firms team up with a Swedish partner (firm or person) who knows the language and regulations

Some municipalities use a tender procedure to choose firms they will use over the following years

Larger schemes are usually commissioned through competitions, which can be combined with a developer competition:
- Competitions can be open, restricted to invited participants, or two-stage
- 'Parallel task' means that the municipality gives a few invited firms different tasks for the same area in order to have a wide array of perspectives. The municipality may then ask one of the firms to proceed, or develop the task in-house
- Developer competitions may be used when the municipality owns the land. Developers team up with a urban design team to make a proposal in order to win the right to develop the land

....

4 LEGISLATION THAT NEEDS TO BE REFERRED TO

Planning and Building Act

Environment Code

Local structure plans, detailed plans and special area regulations

The municipalities procurement process is regulated by the Public Procurement Act (*Lagen om offentlig upphandling*, LOU)

....

5 SPECIFIC TIPS
FOR SUCCESS

Most architecture and urban design competitions are announced by the Swedish Architects' Association (*Sveriges arkitekter*)

....

6 USEFUL WEBSITES

Government Offices of Sweden: www.sweden.gov.se

Nordic Urban Design Association: www.nuda.no

Swedish Architects' Association: www.arkitekt.se

....

SELECTED FACTS

1	area	449,964 km^2
2	population	9,379,116
3	annual population growth	0.9%
4	urban population	85%
5	population density	21 p/km^2
6	GDP	$458,973,278,964
7	GNI per capita	$50,110

Source: The World Bank (2010)

CZECH REPUBLIC

Veronika Sindlerova, *engineer–architect*

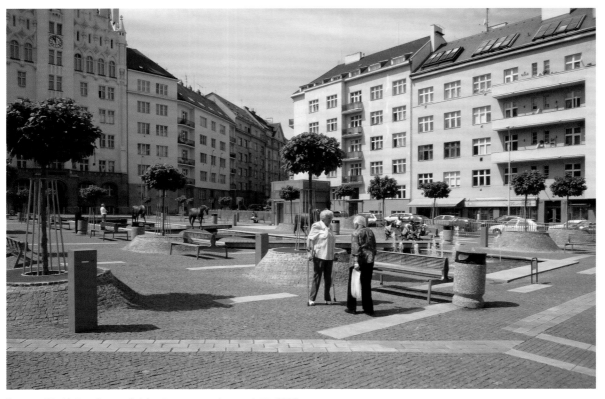

Prague – Wuchterlova Square, Dejvice, former car park converted in 2008
into an urban living space. Parking is now underground

THE CZECH REPUBLIC is a parliamentary republic, divided into
14 regions, one of which is the capital city of Prague. The parliament has two
chambers, the chamber of deputies and the senate. In turn each region has its own
assembly, though Prague has a different status. The country was created in 1993
after Czechoslovakia was divided into two, the Czech Republic and Slovakia.
In its present form it is therefore a very young country, but one with a very
long history.

The importance of Czech towns is not the result of their size (the largest city
is Prague with a population of only 1.2 million) but of their millennial history and the
high level of preservation of their monuments. Unlike many other European centres,
Czech towns were not seriously damaged during the second world war. Their essence,
the repository of historical values, was therefore preserved. However, the communist
regime that followed, and which lasted more than 40 years, left significant scars on the
face of Czech towns; insensitive restoration of historic cores, a difficult relationship
between established urban areas and large new housing estates, and a greater regard

for the political order than for the quality of the home environment led to serious and often irreparable damage to the structure of towns and cities. Today, 20 years after the fall of the regime, Czech towns are still dealing with the negative consequences of communist planning but they also have to address new problems and new issues: key changes in property relations and private land ownership, the unprecedented expansion of urban areas and the new demands of their inhabitants. As a result of changes in the economic, social and political contexts, the work of architects, planners and urban designers is having to evolve as well.

The fundamental basis of the Czech Republic's urban structure is its system of medieval towns, which evolved from ancestral settlements or were established in the period of rapid urbanisation from the 11th to the 14th century. Most Czech towns thus feature intact medieval cores, which still represent their most important and established centres. As a result, urban design – as a theoretical and practical activity – has a long tradition, arising from the care needed to preserve a valuable urban cultural heritage and to ensure its consistent future development.

Definitions

As towns expand and spread into the countryside, spatial organisation, land uses and transport links have become increasingly complex. Research and practice related to urban areas can no longer be the concern of one single discipline. What was originally one scientific field has now split into several disciplines which, however, remain in close relationship with one another. In order of scale, spatial range and subject of interest, the division is as follows:

Architecture (building design)
▲
▼
Urban design (urbanism)[1]
▲
▼
Urban planning (spatial planning)
▲
▼
Regional planning + landscape planning

Urban design, both as an academic discipline and as an applied activity, overlaps with architecture and urban planning. Furthermore, it affects and is affected by regional planning and landscape planning. In the wider sense, urban design deals with issues of urban form and the development of urban units and their components. Therefore a complex multidisciplinary approach is needed: urban design draws on the knowledge of the social, technical, environmental and economic sciences. It is also concerned with the evaluation of spatial layouts, land uses and the aesthetic aspects of developments.

Every development represents a complex system consisting not only of objects organised around streets, squares, riversides, parks, courtyards and other spaces, but also of the required transport and technical infrastructure, and natural and environmental components. The primary aim of urban design is to create favourable conditions for the development and coordination of all these elements. In doing so, it interacts with both the material environment and the needs and interests of its inhabitants, with the objective of shaping a liveable urban environment. Thus urban design makes the link between the more contextual work of urban planning and the design of buildings. The former operates in the long term and at a scale that goes beyond the boundaries of one single development; it provides the framework for the more local urban design which deals with a district, a street, a block or a group of buildings. Nevertheless it is almost impossible to demarcate precise boundaries between architecture, urban design, urban planning and regional planning because they are all interconnected and blend together.

The professional position of urban design

As architecture becomes more diverse and all-encompassing, greater demands are imposed on its practitioners. In the Czech Republic, the architect is still viewed in the old traditional way, as an expert who should be able to respond to a broad spectrum of commissions from building design, restoration and interior design, through urban design and urban and regional planning, and even to investment, development or building management. Furthermore, architects must be well informed in all related disciplines.

When it comes to urban design practice, the architect operates as a coordinator and is usually the head of a team consisting of various professionals. Depending on the range and complexity of a specific commission, the project team must have access to experts from other disciplines. Transport specialists in particular can play an essential role, as they assist in ensuring the accessibility of a particular area, assessing the parking requirements and advising on the necessary transport infrastructure. Other team members may be landscape architects, responsible for the detailed design of green areas, water elements or related environmental components; experts in technical infrastructure, sociologists or demographers.

In practice, an architect is almost always the author of the overall scheme, its composition and morphology, the land-use distribution, the hierarchy of open spaces and the aesthetic considerations which have an impact on the quality of the townscape. The architect is responsible for the design as a whole and his/her main task is to reconcile the demands emerging from the various experts, comply with the laws in force and avoid any conflicting solutions. Therefore, the traditional view of the architectural profession as the agent for urban design is also reflected in the education system and the post-education professional registration process, legally required in order to practice.

Architects belong to the Czech Chamber of Architects, an autonomous professional organisation. Its mission is to supervise the architecture and built environment professions, including urbanism and urban planning; to protect the public interest and to license (or, if necessary, withdraw or suspend) practitioners.

For architect–engineers (graduates of architectural faculties in technical engineering universities) or graduates in related disciplines, three kinds of licence are available: architecture, urban planning (which includes urban design) and landscape architecture. Each type of licence is conditioned by the education followed, length of practice after graduation (three or five years, depending on the discipline) and proven experience in a defined number of projects. One person may obtain a licence to practise in all three disciplines.

Urban design education

Education follows the professional pattern described above: architectural faculties within technical engineering universities offer a comprehensive and general curriculum in architecture and urbanism. This includes theoretical subjects and participation in design studios, with a balance between technical disciplines and the humanities, and covers a wide spectrum that ranges from architecture to planning. Individuals can specialise by choosing from a number of options and projects without altering the qualification that they eventually obtain.

In recent years, changes in scientific knowledge and advances in technology, materials and procedures have led to animated debates on the future of the architecture profession and the related education system. The demands from practice are constantly changing, and require new and wider knowledge which education institutions are supposed to impart. The position of urbanism in relation to the other subjects is one of the most important topics of discussion within the profession. One of the options considered is the separation of architecture, as the design of buildings, from urban design, planning and landscape design, but the professional community is far from unanimous on this possibility and its consequences.

The architecture faculties also offer a doctoral programme in architecture with the possibility of specialising in a field such as urbanism. Research in urban design depends largely on the special interests of a specific department, and tends to produce guidelines or recommendations for practice which occasionally help to modify the legislation on urban planning.

The legal position of urban design

All development, at any scale, is primarily controlled by the 2006 Czech Planning and Building Act and its regulations. The main aim of this legislation is to create the conditions for sustainable development and an efficient use of land, whilst respecting the natural, cultural and social values of a given area and its aesthetic character. To fulfil this aim, the act requires all administrative units of the Czech Republic, ie municipalities and regions, to prepare planning documents with the necessary regulations for the control of development such as environmental protection, conservation of historic buildings, transport infrastructure and national security. There is a hierarchy of plans, with the higher-level ones being binding on the lower-level ones: regional plans are at the top of the hierarchy, followed by masterplans at municipal level and more detailed local plans, which are the basis for granting planning permissions.

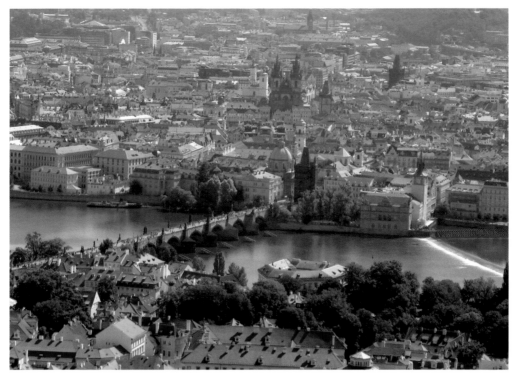

Historic Prague was not damaged during the war

Historical development

Czech towns and cities represent a unique example of urban and architectural design covering virtually all stages from the middle ages to modernism. As they were not heavily damaged during the second world war, urban renewal in the postwar period was relatively quick in comparison with that in other countries, and did not involve major demolitions or interventions.

The totalitarian period (1948–89)

Urban planning and urban design are always closely connected with the political and economic situation of a country. After the second world war, Czechoslovakia became a people's democratic state allied to the USSR. In 1948, the Czech Communist party came to power and its leaders started to implement their ideas about a new, socialist society. Private properties were largely nationalised and individual parcels of land could be amalgamated into larger plots. All design, planning and construction activities were gradually nationalised and centralised under the monopoly of state-owned building enterprises.

   One of the main objectives of the regime was to remedy the considerable housing deficit caused by the lack of maintenance and construction during the war. 'Adequate housing for every family' was the slogan of the 1948 government, and this meant quantity rather than quality. Fast and cheap building was the only way to fulfil the quotas required. The functionalist theories of the time helped by offering standardisation, industrialisation and prefabrication together with open free-standing development. The results were large housing estates, panel-built and located in the outskirts of cities or adjacent to their historic cores. These estates were characterised by their uniformity, dullness and architectural poverty, and a lack of response to their context. The traditional design of streets, clearly defined courtyards and squares, was completely abandoned, resulting in a loss of identity and a degraded environment. Although the estates provided services such as schools and shops, and health, cultural and sports facilities, they did not offer job opportunities and became 'dormitories'. Residents had to commute for work to distant industrial areas or to town centres.

This period of development is known as 'Panel Story', and it has marked virtually all Czech towns and even some villages. Most estates were never successfully integrated into the organically developed town, and therefore their relationship with historic cores is deeply problematic. In addition, new buildings of inadequate scale or form were often inserted in gap sites within the traditional city.

New phenomena after 1989

The fall of communism in 1989 meant not only fundamental political, social and economic changes but also the advent of new processes of planning and urban design. The abolition of central economic planning, the restoration of rights to all forms of ownership and the introduction of private entrepreneurship were the first results, and they deeply influenced planning practice. Soon after, autonomous local governments were elected and price controls were abolished.

All properties nationalised after 1948 were returned to the original owners or their legal heirs. The process of privatisation started in 1991 when retail shops, restaurants, hotels and some services were included in the scheme known as 'small privatisation', in which these outlets were auctioned to private buyers. The 'big privatisation' which followed converted state enterprises into stock corporations.

Urban design therefore operates in an entirely new context, in a market economy with private ownership. Planning is no longer centrally commanded by the state, but delegated to local authorities; similarly, investment does not come exclusively from the state but from diverse private sources as well. Private property owners, often motivated by profit, and the public, previously excluded from the design process, are now active participants in it. Thus, new urban planning instruments are needed in order to guarantee the coordination and regulation of development.

Urban designers face the challenge of having to undertake previously unknown tasks: not only the protection of built heritage and the maintenance and repair of large ageing housing estates, but also dealing with new phenomena such as suburbanisation and out-of-town shopping and service centres. Urban areas are becoming fragmented, and pressures for more land from developers and investors are on the increase.

Humanising panel-built housing estates

The construction of large housing estates – a relatively short episode in the history of western Europe – lasted until the first half of the 1990s in the former Czechoslovakia. Panel-built blocks of flats represent roughly one third of all apartments in the Czech Republic, and they house more than three million people. They are out of date from every point of view and need adapting to current standards; 'humanising' the residential environment cannot be achieved through mere insulation or by colouring the grey facades, however. It is a much more complicated and contextual problem and

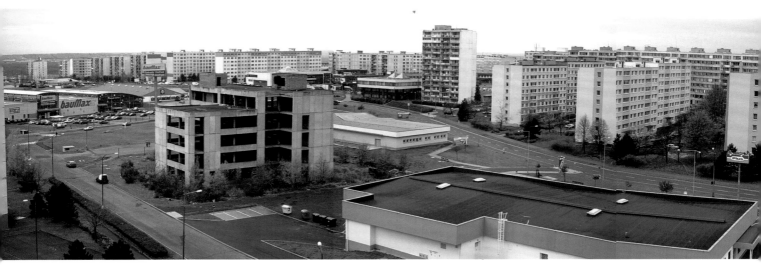

Photomontage of Most (north-west Bohemia): panel-built housing estate 'Vidrholec'

one of the main challenges for urban designers. The current solutions are infilling and making the areas more compact, densification and intensification; redefining spaces by enclosing them into blocks and giving them a clear identity; and creating transitional zones between urban areas and the surrounding open landscape. But this process of humanisation is often slowed down by complicated legal and property-ownership issues, and by the lack of agreement between owners.

Gap sites in urban areas – infilling

Whereas before 1989 development in Czech towns was mostly concentrated on the outskirts, from 1990 onwards activity focused on town centres, historical cores and former 19th-century suburbs which still have free space – either vacant since the war or resulting from neglect and subsequent demolition during the years of

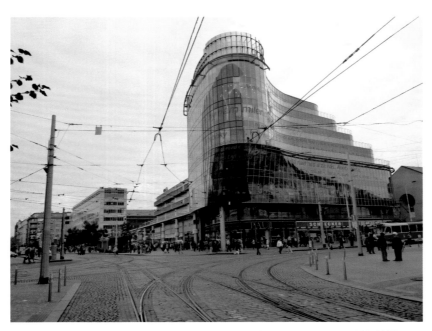

Prague – Golden Angel administrative and commercial centre (Architect Jean Nouvel, 1999–2000) in 19th-century suburb, replacing historical block partially demolished in the 1980s

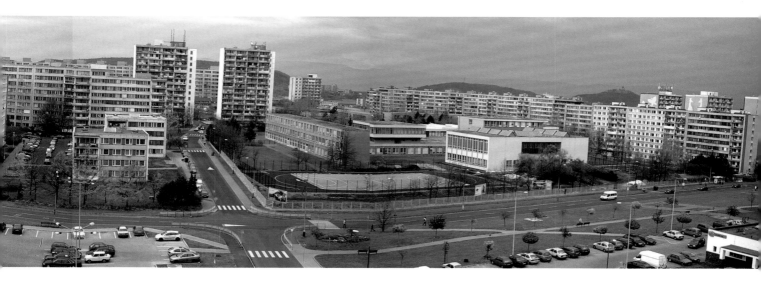

communism. Placing a new building in an established context requires a sensitive approach, particularly in a historic area or in the vicinity of landmarks. Gap sites can vary in scale from single plots to part or even whole blocks, the functions are mostly residential or commercial, and in each case all aspects of the context must be taken into account.

Brownfields – symbols of post-industrial town

Whilst prior to 1989 the economy was based on heavy and manufacturing industries, a fundamental transformation took place after the fall of communism, with a resulting decline in industrial production and the increasing importance of the service sector. Many enterprises closed down, leading to the emergence of extensive areas requiring radical transformation not only on the outskirts but also within urban areas.

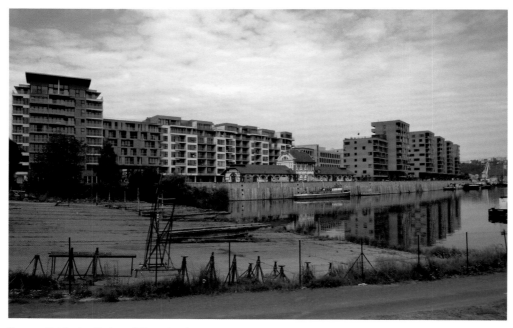

Prague – Holešovice, Marina – 19th-century former docks on the edge of workers' suburb, recently redeveloped into a luxury housing complex

Urban designers thus have a new task: to find new functions for these abandoned industrial estates, docklands and empty warehouses, and to incorporate them spatially and functionally into their surroundings. Although the sites are often polluted and have various constraints, such as protected historic structures, they are well served and accessible and their economic value is constantly increasing.

Public spaces – the image of a new society

In the European tradition of urbanism, public spaces are a reflection of society, its cultural values and economic development. In the past two decades, public spaces in Czech towns have acquired renewed relevance, and they are increasingly appreciated.

During the communist period, the role of public spaces was devalued: most of them became transport corridors, car parks, blighted historic cores or leftover green spaces between housing blocks. The provision and creation of public space stood outside the interests of government, and it was understood purely as residual space between buildings. Consequently, another role for contemporary urban designers is the transformation and adaptation of public space. It is a long-term and demanding process, complicated by the aforementioned issues of property ownership (particularly in cases of restitution) and by the high cost of this kind of investment.

Local authorities' priorities are first of all the regeneration of central areas, where residential and recreational activities are located; new pedestrian areas, commercial streets and promenades are created; and squares, parks and other public spaces are revitalised for everyday relaxation. The uses on the ground floors of the surrounding buildings are of increasing importance as generators of activity with the spaces.

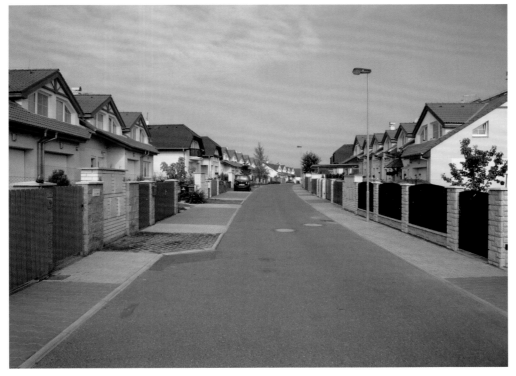

Hostivice, suburbanisation around Prague

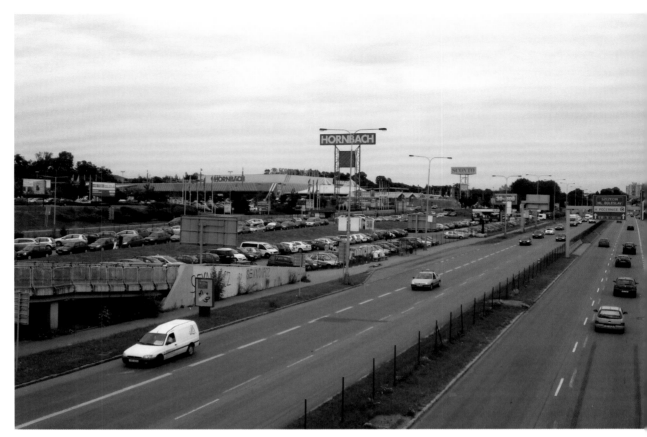

Cerny Most commercial centre alongside a motorway

Urban sprawl – a step into the unknown

Although the population of the Czech Republic is stable, the demands for development and related infrastructure are increasing. Since the fall of communism, rising living standards have increased people's demands for spatial comfort at all levels; mobility is also growing, and with it a level of car ownership previously unattainable. The 'American dream' of a family house with a garden in the suburbs is now what Czech people aspire to, and this leads to rapid suburbanisation around all big cities. Unfortunately, brownfield sites and those within urban areas that are difficult to deal with are not the ones being developed. Instead, new settlements spread into the countryside, particularly if they are near main roads. Such greenfield sites are abundant and have fewer constraints for investors than the brownfield ones.

Natural and rural areas are thus invaded by urban sprawl, scattered, unregulated and leading to a poor-quality environment, whether for family housing, commercial or service precincts. These suburbs present a huge problem and a risk for the future development of Czech towns. They do not lead to a sustainable way of life, are not self-sufficient but parasitic on core towns or rural villages, and are usually entirely dependent on the private car. They are inhabited by people with no relation to the locality, and are becoming places without identity.

Practice and concerns

Since 1989, responsibility for urban development has been delegated to municipalities. The two key participants in the process are the public sector (for infrastructure and public spaces) and private investors – each one with their own interests, which can be in conflict. To perform their tasks, urban designers are caught between the two; their duty is to implement the legislation and other regulations in order to protect the public interest, but private stakeholders also have an influence on their work, particularly if their land is affected.

The work commissioned from urban designers can either be public, where the client is a municipality, a state organisation, a region or another public entity, or private. The cooperation between the two sectors in public–private partnerships is still in its infancy in the Czech Republic.

According to the legislation, every municipality must have an approved masterplan; some may also have detailed 'regulatory plans', similar to the German *Bebaungsplan*, or additional studies. Urban designers usually participate in the preparation of all such documents. In addition to plan preparation, urban designers may work on a broad spectrum of studies to do with public spaces, central-area regeneration and historic areas, or increasingly on the renewal of the public spaces in housing estates.

Private commissions relate mostly to the urban extensions described in the previous section. However, the recent economic crisis has affected the level of activity: many projects and studies were stopped or considerably slowed down. The previous boom of studies and projects has been replaced by stagnation and uncertainty.

Most urban design work is undertaken by private consultants and these are almost always architects, in keeping with the traditions of the profession. Hardly any consultant offers urban design services exclusively, and most of them cover the whole spectrum of work.

Within the mass of housing estates built between the 1950s and 1980, South-West Town stands out as exceptional. The design was chosen in 1968 through a national design competition which was won by architect Ivo Oberstein's team, and it is based on strong urban principles which were implemented throughout construction. Although the revolution of 1989 changed some of the characteristics of the development, the basic concepts embedded in the competition project continue to be respected and nurtured to this day, which is a sign of its resilience.

The urban concept

The urban composition of South-West Town was predetermined by the exceptional landform, the links to nearby Prokopske and Dalejske Valley Nature Park, and by the idea of a linear city developed along a public transport line. Thus the scheme avoids an endless and monotonous series of grey panel blocks. Instead it is divided into individual and independent housing units, each one with its own identity, differentiated through form and spatial configuration, and resembling beads strung along the metro line which connects South-West Town to the centre of Prague. Each metro station is the focus of a neighbourhood with a public square surrounded by shops, schools and other services. It is also where pedestrian routes and bus lines serving other parts of the estate, converge.

The main centre and the gate into South-West Town is Sluneční Náměstí (Sun Square), where administrative, cultural and other public and private activities are concentrated. The housing

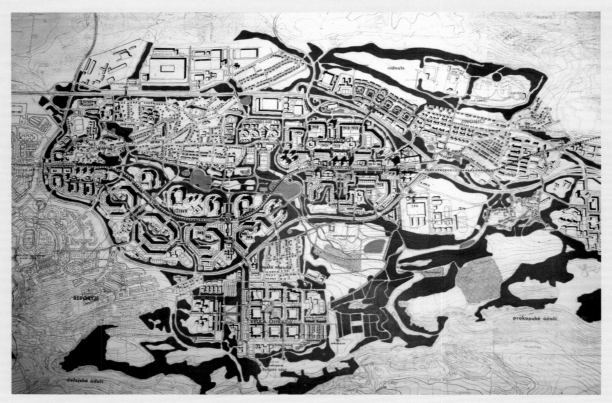

South-West Town (Ivo Oberstein et al, 1990)

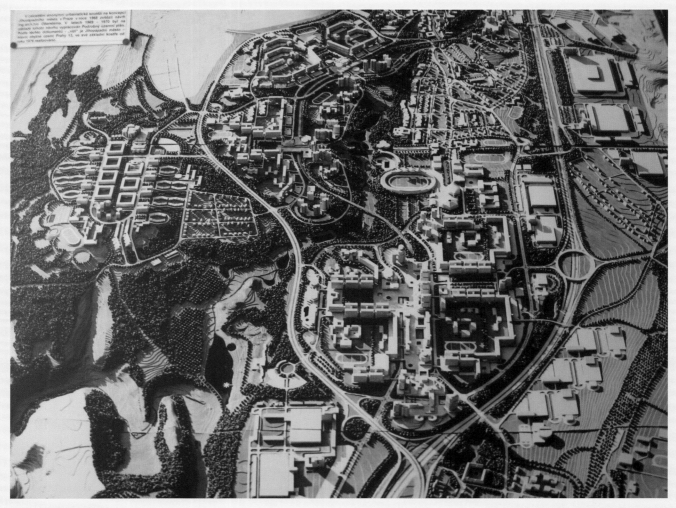

1970 model of South-West Town

density is higher in this neighbourhood than in other parts of the town, and a group of tower blocks contribute to this.

A green spine, the Central Park, meanders through the whole scheme linking the various housing units with the surrounding nature reserves. It follows the river valley and includes water reservoirs used both for recreation and as retention basins protecting the surrounding housing from flooding. The metro line crosses the valley above ground through an elevated tube.

From the start, South-West Town was conceived as a town on a metro line, giving priority to pedestrians and public transport, with the cars placed on the periphery of the settlements. The housing units are sensitively adapted to the terrain with attention given to environmental and ecological issues.

Changes: present and future

Development of South-West Town continued until 1990, by which time the basic structure of the town was established, together with its transport and other infrastructures, and the natural spine. These can now evolve, even if the overall coordination that existed until then has now been lost as the land is broken up into individual private parcels.

Today more than 50,000 people live in South-West Town, and it has become an attractive residential area with great development potential. Since the political changes of 1989, such well-equipped and accessible neighbourhoods have become a magnet for private investors. Gap sites are gradually being filled with housing or mixed-use developments; thus the grain of the area is thickening and missing functions are added. Each new scheme, with its individual characteristics and diverse spatial

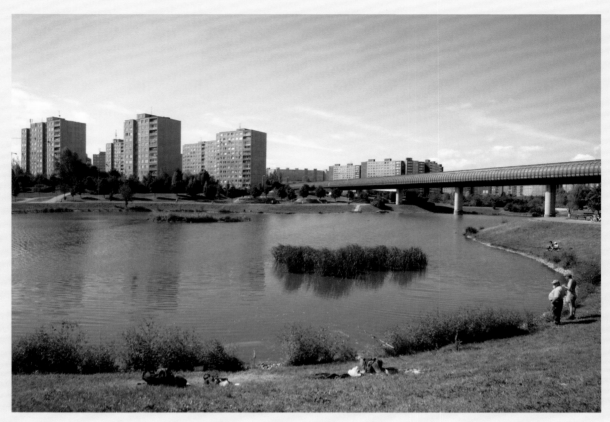

View of Central Park, with retention basin and the metro tube

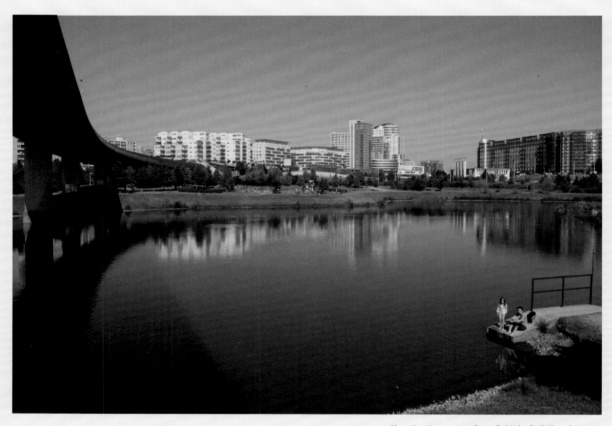

New development at Sluneční Náměstí (Sun Square);
the new town hall between two residential towers

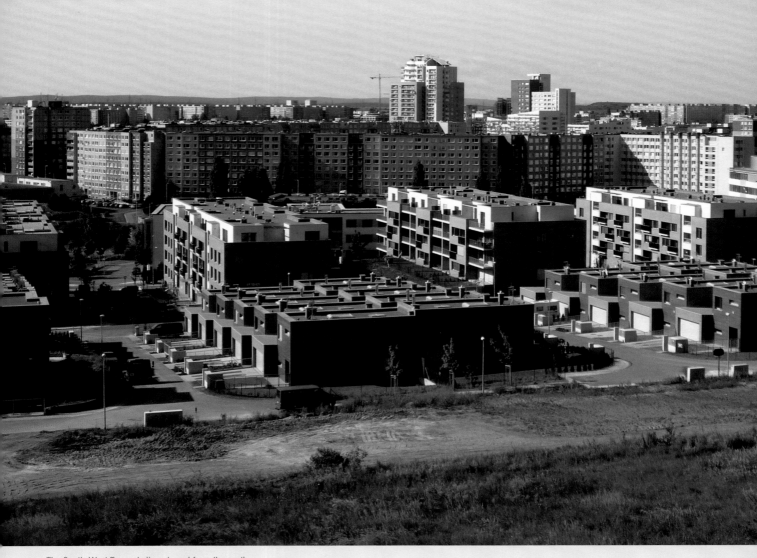

The South-West Town skyline viewed from the north

solutions, contributes to the identity of the town. Architects, urbanists and other designers search for the best ways to integrate the new buildings into the established development.

Since 1990, most large development has been focused on the central area of Sluneční Náměstí, a space that was never completed. The original idea of creating an entrance gate and a centre to South-West Town is gradually being implemented; the town hall, the church and community centre, a private clinic and a number of mixed-use structures have been built in the last two decades. However, space is still available for a future library, a concert hall and sport facilities linked to the Central Park. Sluneční Náměstí therefore represents an important challenge for urban designers.

South-West Town is also expanding along its edge: new developments are being inserted, taking advantage of the well-serviced original estates. These peripheral developments are mostly housing, but there are also higher-end office buildings and shopping centres. The town is going through a new phase of change; spaces between traditional panel-built blocks are being regenerated; new service centres are growing around the metro stations, where in the past unregulated or illegal uses had become established, and the authorities are looking for new functions to replace them. So gradually, South-West Town is adapting to new needs and new demands.

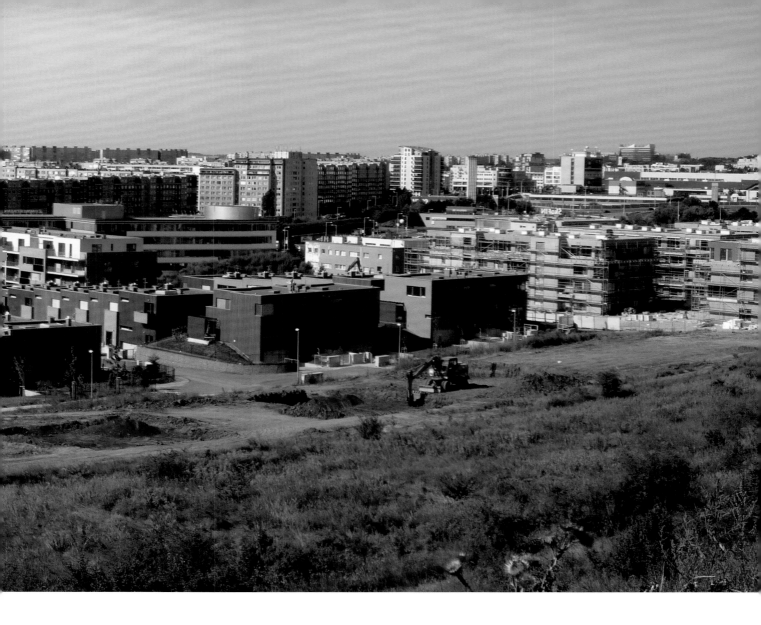

The future of the profession

The population of the Czech Republic is currently stable, and a small decrease is expected. For urban design this will probably result in attention being focused further on inner urban areas, as their renovation will make economic sense; the regeneration of brownfield land will increase, particularly in areas with good infrastructure. Traditional ideas of urbanism will be complemented by economic, ecological and engineering issues, and the increasing social dimension of urban areas will be reflected in the importance of public spaces.

The creation of an environment that reflects local culture, that is ecologically responsible and that functions satisfactorily is increasingly the goal to be achieved. Sustainability has become an integral part of the work of urban planners and designers. Equally, the participation of the public as residents, users or simply as citizens is becoming central in turning the designers' ideas into realities.

A quick guide to
Czech Republic

1   TYPES OF CLIENT

Municipalities

Regional authorities

Various kinds of investors

2   TYPES OF
PROJECT/WORK

Masterplans
- Urban renewal in city centres and housing estates
- Urban extensions

Design guidelines

Local urban studies

3   APPROACH NEEDED
TO WORK IN COUNTRY

Contact with mayor/regional governor

Partnership with local firm

International competitions

Direct negotiation with client

4   LEGISLATION
THAT NEEDS TO BE
REFERRED TO

The 2007 Spatial Planning Act

Spatial development principles (regional)

Local plans

Regulatory plans

Public Contracts and Concession Act, dealing with procurement

5   SPECIFIC TIPS
FOR SUCCESS

Consultation with various stakeholders is important

Concern for and understanding of environmental issues and sustainability

6   USEFUL WEBSITES

Czech Association for Urban and Regional Planning: www.urbanismus.cz

Czech Chamber of Architects: www.cka.cc

Ministry of the environment of the Czech Republic: www.env.cz

All the above legislation information can be accessed through: www.portal-vz.cz
(Public Procurement and Concession Portal)

1	area	78,866 km^2
2	population	10,525,090
3	annual population growth	–0.1%
4	urban population	74%
5	population density	133 p/km^2
6	GDP	$192,151,584,569
7	GNI per capita	$17,890

Source: The World Bank (2010)

SECTION 2

AFRICA AND THE MIDDLE EAST

DUBAI

Tim Catchpole, *development planning consultant*

Manosh De, *urban design and masterplanning professional*

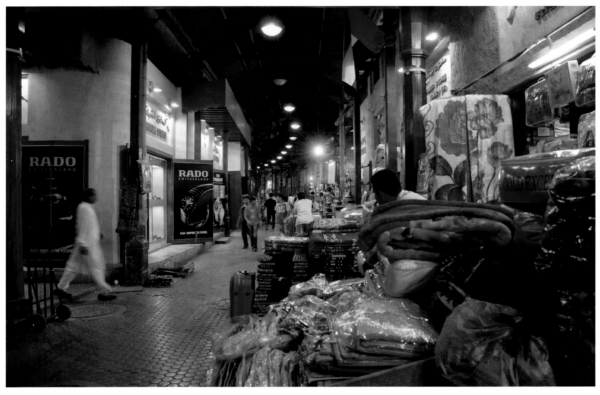

The traditional souqs were designed around a fluid street form
that connected the old trader homes

DUBAI, a constitutional monarchy, is the second largest emirate of the United Arab Emirates (UAE) by population and land area. Its rise from humble trading post to world city in the last 50 years has been meteoric. This has been due in large part to the vision of its ruler Sheikh Rashid bin Saeed Al Makhtoum and his son, the present ruler, Sheikh Mohammed, who have taken full advantage of the strategic location of their city at a crossroads between Europe and Asia and between the Middle East and north Africa.

Dubai is among the most urbanised of the emirates, with an urban population density of around 70 persons per hectare. Dubai City's population has risen from a few thousand in 1960 to over 1.5 million today, and is expected to double by 2020. Despite this growth, only 12% of the population remains local or Emirati, and by 2020 this proportion is expected to fall further. The rest of the population is drawn from all over the world, with a predominance of people from the Indian subcontinent and the neighbouring north African countries.

Unlike in neighbouring Abu Dhabi, where the main contributor to the GDP is oil revenue, the most significant contributors to the Dubai GDP are the port and airport, trade, real estate, financial services and tourism. Oil was a significant contributor to the Dubai GDP in the 1960s but its supply was limited, and the result has been a highly successful diversification of the city's economy.

Dubai City is governed by the Dubai Municipality, which has produced a succession of structure plans for its expansion. Parts of the city are also governed by separate free-zone authorities. The Dubai government oversees the city and the rest of the emirate. The ruler of Dubai, Sheikh Mohammed, is also Vice-President and Prime Minister of the Federal Government of the United Arab Emirates.

Definitions

Although not defined as such in the Structure Plan for the Dubai Urban Area, urban design in Dubai would appear to be the art of laying out a land development framework and public realm that can attract development of the highest quality.

Successive masterplans have defined the expansion of a road grid from Dubai Creek eastwards to the Sharjah border and westwards through Jumeirah and Jebel Ali to the Abu Dhabi border. The overall development strategy was to guide future development of the urban area based on growth-management principles to encourage cost-effective use of Emirati resources. This coastal grid is interrupted by open-space corridors extending between the coast and hinterland. The grid sets out the structure for development along this coastal stretch, and for each grid square there are development guidelines for plots.

As the grid has expanded, so it has taken on new forms. The old parts of Dubai around the creek are organic in layout; the 1960s' grid is rectilinear, edged with development of a uniform height and massing; the 1990s' grid is more fluid, and uniformity has been replaced by a proliferation of iconic towers. The 'backbone' of the 1960s' grid is the Sheikh Zayed Road, which connects Dubai City to Abu Dhabi City and which became an impressive corridor for tall buildings in the 1990s. Prior to this, the gateway development to the Sheikh Zayed Road was the landmark World Trade Centre, at one time the tallest building in the Middle East. It has since been eclipsed in this respect by the Emirates Towers and the Burj Khalifa.

A recent addition to Sheikh Zayed Road and to other streets within the city is the Dubai Metro, the world's longest driverless system at the time of completion, which stitches together the different communities through two metro lines and a network of feeder buses.

The professional place of urban design

Dubai's urban design practitioners are drawn from around the world, having been attracted to the city by the prospect of unbridled creative 'imagineering'. Many of the world's top design firms are either represented here, or have been involved with a project for the city. The practitioners include the range of the design profession, architects, planners, engineers and landscape architects who have been trained and have practised in different physical contexts and climatic regions as well as economic conditions.

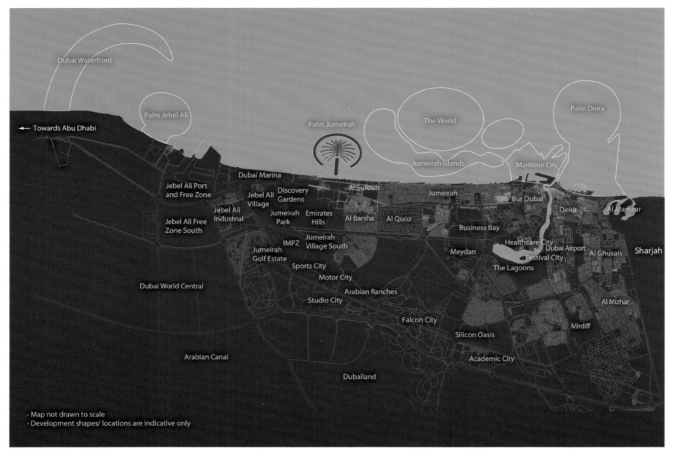

Map showing the location of the various proposed projects

The Dubai Municipality is the key formal body that recognises architects and engineers practising in the city. While there is no separate institutional body that recognises either urban designers or planners, there are loose industry groups that meet regularly to discuss and share ideas from new practice and research, and their impact on developments in Dubai. These societies, groups and councils promote the design fraternity both within the emirate and regionally, using various forums – the World Architecture Forum at Cityscape is an important annual event – or media, through one of the many magazines published from Dubai. Important organisations include the Dubai Municipality Historical Buildings Society, the Institute of Chartered Engineers and the Royal Institute of Chartered Surveyors.

A key group among these is the Green Building Council (GBC) set up in September 2005 to be among the first such bodies in the world. Given the diminishing supply of oil in the emirate, and with a view to long-term economic sustainability, Dubai sought to address its growing carbon footprint by focusing on energy-efficient buildings and context-sensitive site design. The GBC comprises industry professionals who have been collating a body of knowledge specific to the region, in relation to both 'green' building and urban space design, focusing on the interrelationships between manufacturers, consultants and the government. The subsequent establishment in 2009 of Estidama – based on the Arabic word for sustainability – both in Dubai and Abu Dhabi has also had an impact on the local designers with respect to sharing best-practice methods in sustainable planning and urban design in relation to the local climate and cultural context of the region.

The discipline

Given the relative age of the nation, there are very few established universities within Dubai itself. The initial economic growth of the emirate focused academia first on various elements of engineering and infrastructure, with the 'soft' sciences and liberal-arts programmes developing later. In fact, the prominence of using Dubai's buildings as global branding icons changed the way that architecture and design came to be perceived within the emirate. Soon, as the city grew there was a rapid demand for locally trained designers.

Many schools, each with their own focus, have been established within the UAE in order to deliver a high standard of architectural and urban design education. The American University of Sharjah (AUS) is one such prominent school set up by the ruler of Sharjah in 1997: it offers both architecture and urban planning at the undergraduate and master's level. It is accredited by the Commission on Higher Education of the Middle States Association of Colleges and Schools, USA. Although there is no known specialist urban design programme within the nation, there are architecture programmes at the University of Ajman, the University of Ras Al Khaimah and the Islamic Azad University in Dubai, and urban design is a component of their educational curriculums.

In recent years, the Masdar Institute in Abu Dhabi, established with the support of the Massachusetts Institute of Technology (MIT), has also had an impact on the conceptual development of urban design and planning within the UAE. It has been focusing on the science and engineering of advanced alternative energy, environmental technologies and sustainability, each of which have an impact on current paradigms of spatial and built-structures delivery.

While academic institutes account for much of the research that is taking place in the city, the level of information sharing through events in Dubai's Meetings, Incentives, Conferences, Exhibition (MICE) calendar cannot be overstated. Dubai is home to Cityscapes, one of the more prominent real estate events in the region, which is also associated with the World Architecture Congress (WAC), a forum for designers working within the region to share current thoughts and trends in design. As many of the key participants of the WAC have worked in Dubai, the result has been a contextual sharing of ideas, particularly around the treatment of climate and culture. A number of architectural, urban design, landscape and construction magazines – such as Architect, Urbanism and architecture, and Landscape and Construction Weekly – are also published from the city, documenting the evolution of the local and regional craft.

Legal status

The overall urban development of Dubai has been guided by various underlying spatial structure plans dating back to the 1950s. The most recent plan, issued in 1998, has been given further definition by the development plans of the individual free-zone development companies, such as Emaar, Nakheel and Limitless, which have been established since the ruler decreed changes to the land ownership rules in 2002.

As a result, the urban areas of Dubai have come to be broadly managed by two types of authorities, the Dubai Municipality and the free-zone developers. Both bodies follow a similar basis in their approach to planning and urban design, although it

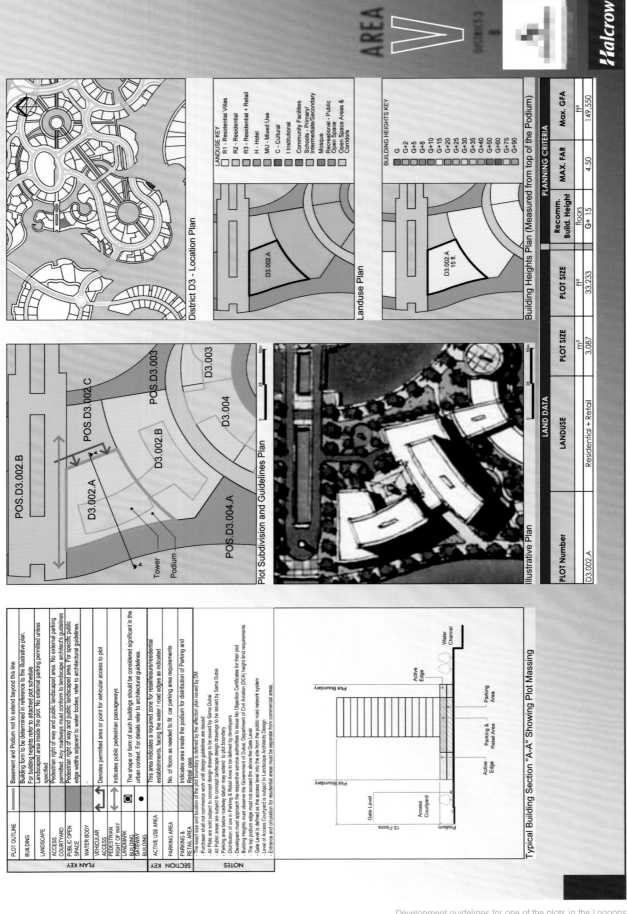

THE LAGOONS - PLOT DEVELOPMENT GUIDELINES

AREA V

DISTRICT 3

Halcrow

PLAN KEY

PLOT OUTLINE	Basement and Podium not to extend beyond this line
BUILDING	Building form to be determined in reference to the illustrative plan. For building heights refer to attached plot schedule
LANDSCAPE	Landscaped area inside the plot. No external parking permitted unless specified
ACCESS COURTYARD	Pedestrian right of way and public landscaped area. No external parking permitted. Any roadways must conform to landscape architect's guidelines
PUBLIC OPEN SPACE	Pedestrian right of way and public landscaped area. For specific public edge widths adjacent to water bodies, refer to architectural guidelines.
WATER BODY	-
VEHICULAR ACCESS	Denotes permitted area or point for vehicular access to plot
PEDESTRIAN RIGHT OF WAY	Indicates public pedestrian passageways
LANDMARK BUILDING	The shape or form of such buildings should be considered significant in the urban context. For details refer to architectural guidelines.
GATEWAY BUILDING	

SECTION KEY

ACTIVE USE AREA	This area indicates a required zone for retail/leisure/residential establishments, facing the water / road edges as indicated
PARKING AREA	No. of floors as needed to fit car parking area requirements
PARKING & RETAIL AREA	Indicates area inside the podium for distribution of Parking and Retail uses

NOTES

- The exact size and location of the plot boundary is defined by the affection plan issued by DM
- Purchaser shall not commence work until design guidelines are issued
- All Plots are sold subject to concept design drawings to be issued by Sama Dubai
- All Public areas are subject to concept landscape design drawings to be issued by Sama Dubai
- Parking area below roadway datum may extend to plot boundary
- Distribution of use in Parking & Retail Area to be defined by developers
- Developers must approach the respective service authorities to issue No Objection Certificates for their plot
- Building Heights must observe the Government of Dubai, Department of Civil Aviation (DCA) height limit requirements.
- The top podium edge must not exceed 8m above the Gate Level
- Gate Level is defined as the access level into the site from the public road network system
- Level of Access Courtyard is subject to Landscape Architects Design
- Entrance and circulation for residential areas must be separate from commercial areas.

District D3 - Location Plan

LANDUSE KEY
- R1 - Residential Villas
- R2 - Residential
- R3 - Residential + Retail
- H - Hotel
- MU - Mixed Use
- C - Cultural
- I Institutional
- Community Facilities
- Schools - Primary/ Intermediate/Secondary
- Mosque
- Recreational - Public Open Space
- Open Space Areas & Corridors

Landuse Plan

BUILDING HEIGHTS KEY
G, G+2, G+5, G+8, G+10, G+15, G+20, G+25, G+30, G+35, G+40, G+50, G+60, G+75, G+90

Building Heights Plan (Measured from top of the Podium)

Plot Subdivision and Guidelines Plan

POS.D3.002.B
POS.D3.002.C
D3.002.A
D3.002.B
POS.D3.003
D3.003
D3.004
POS.D3.004.A

Tower
Podium

Illustrative Plan

LAND DATA

PLOT Number	LANDUSE	PLOT SIZE m²	PLOT SIZE ft²
D3.002.A	Residential + Retail	3,087	33,233

PLANNING CRITERIA

PLOT SIZE	Recomm. Build. Height floors	MAX. FAR	Max. GFA ft²
33,233	G+15	4.50	149,550

Typical Building Section "A-A" Showing Plot Massing

Plot Boundary
Active Edge
Water Channel
Parking Area
Parking & Retail Area
Active Edge
Plot Boundary
Gate Level
Access Courtyard
15 Floors
Podium

Development guidelines for one of the plots in the Lagoons

might be argued that the free-zone developers are likely to be more lenient in the event that a new planning precedent is being sought. For example, in areas like Palm Island or Dubailand, special-purpose planning departments were set up to monitor and regulate development, based on criteria established by consultants during the masterplanning process.

These planning regulations were based on a compendium of urban design principles, namely plot development guidelines that included the maximum allowable built-up area, and acceptable building heights and setbacks. In some areas, described as Planned Unitary Developments (PUDs), strict aesthetic guidelines were also established to suggest a particular architectural style that would give an area its character. To avoid the continued proliferation of smaller planning agencies in the region, some of the individual planning departments within the free-zone development areas were brought together under Technology, Electronics, Commerce and Media (TECOM), a companion to the Dubai Municipality, particularly where these developments were owned by the same holding company.

The Dubai Municipality has a similar planning role for the non-free-zone areas of the city. However, a key distinction between the municipality and the free-zone authorities is that the former has a much wider planning remit, which includes architecture/building permits, environmental impact assessments, landscape and park designs, green building regulation, and maritime and infrastructure requirements. At the time of writing, the government was in the process of considering a complete change to the system of planning and urban design delivery to the city, focusing on a potentially well-knit multidisciplinary body that would have executive powers over both the free and non-free zones of Dubai.

Historical development

The definition of urban design has not changed in Dubai over the past 50 years, but the results on the ground today are different from those of earlier eras. This has occurred through a combination of changes in the urban structure, in building technology (including the advent of green buildings) and in urban management.

When Dubai started to expand in the 1960s, its grid was essentially rectilinear. Plot development guidelines in each grid square ensured a uniformity in height and massing, and this has led to a pleasant, if somewhat monotonous, built environment. Any variation in height was seen as unfair; nevertheless, in certain strategic locations a few developments have been allowed to exceed the uniform height and become landmarks, giving the place identity.

Changes occurred in the 1990s when a new central business district was established along Sheikh Zayed Road in Jumeirah. Within the rectilinear grid, buildings were allowed to rise to 30 storeys in order to emphasise the importance of the new centre. In fact many have exceeded this height, and the overall effect of this cluster of towers is dynamic, with varied heights as well as diverse iconic designs, rooftops, silhouettes and facing materials. The new Burj Khalifa tower is part of this cluster, though not on Sheikh Zayed Road itself, and it rises to over six times the 30-storey height limit.

Changes have also occurred in the new areas of expansion. As the grid has extended from the coastal area into the inland desert, so its structure and public realm have had to take on new forms in order to attract potential occupiers. The grid has

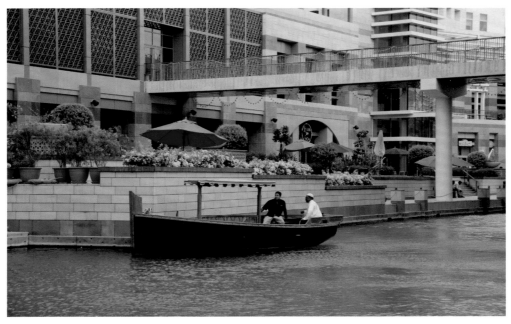

An artificial internal lake in Festival City with boat rides

become curvilinear rather than rectilinear, and the public (actually semi-private) realm now includes green golf courses, which provide a setting that can compete with the waterfronts in the coastal areas.

Waterfronts are much sought after and command high land values, so much so that new developments are emerging offshore in spite of their huge infrastructure cost. The grid structure and public realm in these offshore developments are unique. Most of them are managed by the new free-zone development companies rather than the Dubai Municipality.

Practice and concerns

Dubai's initial development was commissioned directly by the ruler of the city. However, these commissions were small and predominantly located around key pieces of infrastructure such as a port or the airport, where the scope for masterplanning and urban design, though present, was limited.

Over the course of the last decade, the primary driver for large-scale masterplanning and urban design has been a mixture of quasi-government and private developers such as Sama Dubai, Dubai Properties, Nakheel, Limitless, Emaar, Union Properties and Damac. These companies were entrusted with helping to spur development within various parts of Dubai under a spatial framework plan, each project with a particular emphasis related to its geography. For example, given Nakheel's expertise in coastal development – it is a sub-company of Dubai World, which manages and builds ports worldwide – it was entrusted with developments that had a strong waterfront component, such as the Palm or The World.

Emaar and the others were entrusted with inland development, to help create value on desert tracts. These projects sought to raise land value by introducing key planning and infrastructure interventions, such as the creation of lakes to offer water frontage, golf for landscaped frontage, or even key iconic towers and buildings – such as the Burj Khalifa, the tallest building in the world, which became a nucleus around which the subsequent development could be arranged.

In addition, a fundamental aspect of planning was the creation of a theme for each development in order to target potential customers. These themes or lifestyle options resulted in the creation of a polycentric or clustered structure for Dubai's conurbation, with a number of mini-cities such as Motor City, Business Bay, Uptown, Downtown and Internet City.

Given that all these changes were happening rapidly, urbanists and planners were mindful of the nature of the social engineering that was taking place. While whole cities were being constructed overnight, the same could not be said of the societies and communities within the developments, as their opportunities were limited by the rates of industrial growth and job creation, and by local residency laws.

In an effort to provide more 'sustenance' to these developments and protect them from becoming just a speculator's market, the government introduced regulations giving residency rights to people who purchased property above a certain value. Given the political instability within the region, this provided a powerful reason for people to invest in Dubai and resulted in strong cash flows that in turn helped fuel further development.

A key government commitment during this period was that of delivering infrastructure to support these developments. Spending on the airport, the port, roads, public transport, power and water utilities, and community facilities was increased in order to create a framework for the development around them. The infrastructure was future-proofed, designed to handle high capacities and giving developers and residents the confidence that, economically, the government was also investing in Dubai's success.

Unfortunately, the sudden arrival of the recession crippled many of these private developments and exposed the weak relationships between commerce and society. So while the quality of the infrastructure is high, the social fabric is still lacking. Cities, particularly in their formative years, cannot just be a collection of architectural objects or a continuous urban fabric. Density and urbanisation, leading to sustainability, are at least as important.

The new polycentric development of Dubai with discrete packages affecting the cost, the dimensions and maintenance of its infrastructure, became a barrier to the formation of society. The city form, with developments at different stages of completion and occupancy, directly affected its performance, and has led to a review of the structure plan and development framework.

Green building initiatives are now being promoted in order to conserve power and water; cost-share agreements on infrastructure are being drawn up to force developers to consider whether their projected development is a reflection of cash flow or true demand; and communities are being entrusted with the development of homeowner associations that are protected under local laws, to help them actively manage and promote their own urban spaces.

Global cities are characterised by their demographic diversity, and this is no different in the case of Dubai. However, given that the population profile of the city is skewed towards males and to the under-40 years of age range, and that the native population is in a minority, achieving a balance on all counts is a key challenge. Other countries have also been developed on the foundations of immigration, and communities' contribution to society can be measured by the sense of belonging that people have towards a place. The leadership of Dubai is currently trying to tackle this sensitive issue in order to maintain the social glue that binds the place together.

CASE STUDY

LA VILLE CONTEMPORAINE

Background

This case study examines a major project undertaken in 2004–6, namely the masterplanning of a 36 km² area south and south-west of Dubai International Airport, approximately 12 km from the old central business district. The government set out an ambitious plan to tie together existing developments, densify the existing creek area and to create a new extension that would add a further 16 km of waterfront development, by dredging the new creek all the way back to the Gulf, and crossing the Sheikh Zayed Road.

The project, called *La Ville Contemporaine* (LVC), focused on the creation of additional industries in order to diversify and modernise Dubai's current offering; it comprised three distinct development areas:

- Business Bay: a new central business district designed around the extension of the creek
- Lagoons: a mostly residential development designed across seven islands, with typologies ranging from villas to multistorey apartment blocks
- Dubai Healthcare City II (DHCC II): the second phase of the successful medical economic zone that included among other key institutions the Harvard Medical School (Dubai Centre); it borders the Ras Al Khor Wildlife Sanctuary

The first of these projects is being developed by Dubai Properties, the other two by Sama Dubai. Together these schemes seek to challenge the existing planning paradigms in Dubai by taking over large brownfield land and waterfront areas for new private development. For example, the combined projected resident population expected in these developments was estimated to be around 220,000, more than a tenth of the existing population of the Emirate of Dubai.

Process

The original masterplan vision for LVC was prepared by a consultant appointed by Sama Dubai (then Dubai International Properties), which was then validated and re-engineered in order to facilitate its implementation. Initially the project was expected to be delivered by one company, but given its complexity and size it was later split between two sister companies in order to achieve a more robust solution.

Although the area had always been considered for development, none of the previous plans envisaged the building of a grand canal that could link the historic creek to the Gulf, creating a continuous water body. Once this vision was established, the plan evolved from the necessity to ensure that high-quality water could be maintained within both the main creek and its offshoots. Extensive water modelling and flushing studies were conducted in order to test various configurations for their efficiency.

The evolution of the waterfront and its shape led to the setting of landside boundaries and edge conditions, which helped to define the morphology of the spaces. For example, the softer edges along the wildlife sanctuary, essential to preserve the area's biodiversity, confirmed the need for the replanning of buffer and core zones in the sanctuary, and for the creation of a floating pontoon to dampen the waves resulting from water taxi movements along the new creek. Along Business Bay, these edges were harder, with straight quay walls that permitted boats to dock and maximised the space of the waterfront promenade.

Transport

Once an agreed creek form was established, the transport infrastructure was devised to support the masterplan's ambitions. A variety of transport modes was envisaged in order to maximise modal

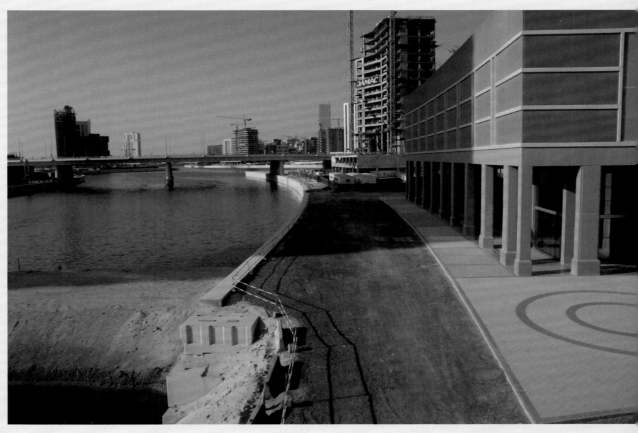

Business Bay: new waterfront edge and promenade

change opportunities between land and waterside connections, including a link to the airport via a metro system. In particular, the network of waterways offered the opportunity to revive the connection that the city had originally had with the creek. A variety of bridge designs was intended to connect the banks, and in some cases allow direct access to podium structures at the base of the multistorey towers.

Urban design

Given the complexity of the engineering solutions required, once the design and physical fixes had been agreed the urban designers and planners reassessed the design of spaces, keeping in mind the principles that were required of a modern city. Such elements as focus, variety, scale and drama were used to offer a range of solutions that would lead to a distinctive settlement. The key objectives drew upon streetscape design and the use of urban forms that created a sense of scale at three distinct levels: the street or pedestrian scale, the scale of the district and the scale of the city in the context of greater Dubai.

The street scale was designed to provide a comfortable year-round environment by encouraging the use of landscape and environmental design, urban art and lighting to complement the architectural initiatives and to develop an experience of the public and private spaces within the development.

Although the use of modern designs was not discouraged, designers were asked to incorporate vernacular elements so as to ensure a strong connection to the context. These included colonnades, screens, shaded structures, controlled use of glazing, thermal convection techniques such as wind towers, and the extensive use of water features such as fountains and watercourses.

At the district scale, the guidelines identified potential sites for the creation of new urban landmarks, either towers or plazas. A high standard of design for individual buildings was to be achieved, but again, reflective of the local context and climatic conditions, without resorting to pastiche. Another key consideration was the connectivity between

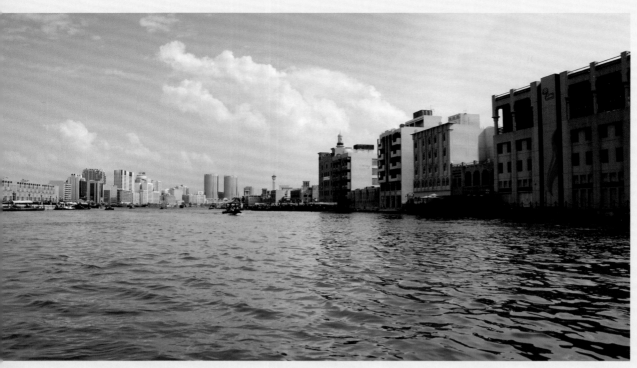

A view of Dubai City from the water

developments, which over the years had been lost owing to the influence of cars on the landscape. Thus mixed-use and linked podiums, sky bridges and other similar devices were explored at the planning stage to develop ideas and draw guidelines that could be taken on board by the architects. Amongst these, many internationally known names can be found such as Koolhaas, Hadid, Reiser + Unomoto and Thompson, Ventulett and Stainback (TVS).

Finally, at the urban scale the development was seen as a city-within-a-city and in the broader context of Dubai. By guiding the massing and skyline in the three development zones – DHCC II, Lagoons and Business Bay – a network of view corridors and 'breezeways' was created that connected back to the creek. The overall silhouette of the skyline and the sculpted urban forms, emphasised by locating these blocks alongside the major public transport interchanges, were aimed at drawing people into the area.

Evaluation

The delivery of the whole plan was achieved through a series of detailed masterplanning documents that included planning, transportation, environmental, infrastructure and architectural guidelines, some of which were specific to the chosen theme for each development. Given the multidisciplinary character and large scale of the project, implementation has been slow. At the moment, the creek extension has been dredged in order to give shape to the islands in the Lagoons, so that the underlying structure has been established.

At Business Bay, the new central business district is taking shape and, together with the nucleus of the adjoining downtown development by Emaar, the area is becoming the hub that people are expecting it to be. Highway and metro infrastructure have also seen rapid progress, with the Green Line being extended to Al Jadaf, a site neighbouring the DHCC II development. This prepares the area for more transit-oriented opportunities in the future, linking the area back to the core of Bur Dubai and Deira.

Environmentally, the Ras Al Khor Wildlife Sanctuary has been declared a *Ramsar* (convention) site, ensuring a more careful treatment of the creek extension in line with the convention laws that guide new development close to and around the core wetlands area. The current financial recession has, however, affected the pace of the development, and many of the plots although sold have not been built upon.

Conclusion

In recent years, Dubai's prominence as an international city has been unprecedented. Its long-term goal is to position itself as the central economic hub between the world's leading global cities. It has attracted a considerable amount of public attention over its fantastical scale of urbanism and development that challenges cost, climate and cultural mores, which is made all the more impressive given its context within a strife-torn Middle East.

While Dubai presents an extreme example of a rapidly emerging global city, its roots are still founded on some very simple principles comparable to other developing cities. Thus, although some people see Dubai as a luxury playground in which clients have magnanimous budgets, it is in fact a very difficult place in which to implement visionary schemes since designers have to develop trust with their clients before they are given the budgets for their work.

Dubai's urban development focus over the past few years has overemphasised the creation of infrastructure and of gated communities, which have been presented as exemplary models. Ironically, it is the lack of connection between these two elements that has led to the 'underachievement' of the city's public realm and urban design.

The older parts of the city, developed organically from the roots of a small fishing village – self-sufficient, integrated and reflective of the local society – succeed as its more engaging areas. In contrast, the eclectic new Dubai, a statement of modern consumerism where human connections have been weighed down by the requirement to provide obvious tourist attractions, state-of-the-art and 'in-your-face' infrastructure, offers an extreme but fractured experience.

The global slowdown has exposed the polycentric nature of development in the city, as large tracts of vacant land between densely built pockets still await infilling. The aim of Dubai's urban designers should be to creatively connect these areas so that the feeling of a splintering city is mitigated. The challenge is how to achieve this given the reliance on private cars, which prevents the drivers whizzing past from noticing these spaces.

However, the key to a successful city is its ability to promote walking, not by compulsion but by choice. The solution may lie in history. Cities grow and mature very much in the way people and relationships do. Perhaps the least appreciated aspect of Dubai's emergence as a Middle Eastern city is its fundamentally liberal underpinnings: much of what has taken place would have been impossible if it were not for the foresight of allowing foreigners to participate in its economy, and to stay in the city through a set of renewable residence visas.

Dubai's unusual brand and scale of urbanism needs time to mature; after all, it is just a few years old compared with more established cities like New York, London or Delhi. These cities benefit from age, and despite being paradigms of urbanism they were once like Dubai, a constellation of isolated events waiting to be linked. Dubai needs time to burnish its shiny new feel, time to let people get to know it and to develop the conventional devices of compactness, connectivity and integration that arise as populations grow and naturally need to link together.

A quick guide to
Dubai

1 TYPES OF CLIENT

Executive Office/Council

Dubai Municipality and associated departments

Infrastructure authorities (Roads and Transport Authority, electricity and water companies)

Local and international developers, both quasi-government and private

....

2 TYPES OF PROJECT/WORK

Masterplans
- Urban renewal and regeneration
- New communities, gated/not gated
- Urban extensions

Design and development guidelines

Concept architecture

Landscape and public arts/public realm strategy

....

3 APPROACH NEEDED TO WORK IN COUNTRY

Good track record and experience of having delivered quality/prominent projects either internationally or locally

Contact with local authorities

Local office (preferred)

Partnership with locally registered firm (licence to trade/practice architecture or engineering)

International competitions

Tendering process (limited or open)

Direct negotiations with client

....

4 LEGISLATION THAT NEEDS TO BE REFERRED TO

Structure plan for the city

Local development plans/urban design and development guidelines

....

5 SPECIFIC TIPS
FOR SUCCESS

Sustainable approach to development in order to reduce heat loads, water use, traffic, energy consumption

Focus on high-quality public realm, local amenities, pedestrian and cycle movement

Adherence to local cultural standards

6 USEFUL WEBSITES

Dubai Government official website: www.dubai.ae

Dubai Development Board: www.dubaicity.com/government-departments/Dubai-development-board.htm

Dubai Municipality portal: www.dm.gov.ae

SELECTED FACTS

1	area	4,114 km^2
2	population	2,260,000
3	annual population growth	7.32%
4	urban population	86%
5	population density	50 p/km^2
6	GDP (2009)	S$82,110,000,000
7	GNI per capita	Not available

Source: Dubai Statistics centre (2011)

EGYPT

Dr Noha Nasser, *architect and urban designer*

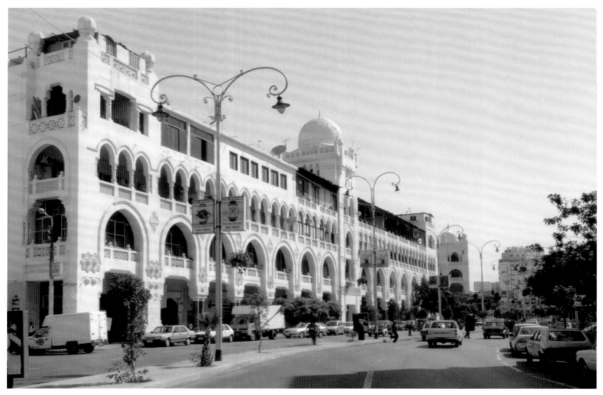

One of the Beaux-Arts-inspired buildings in Heliopolis
with Moorish detailing

EGYPT is a republic; following the 2011 revolution, a new constitution is to be drafted. The country is divided into 26 governorates, 188 city administrations and 808 rural councils. Seven regions with planning responsibilities were created in 1977. There are a number of additional institutions with responsibility for planning. A National Five Year Plan (2008–13) sets up the government planning strategy for the country.

Like many developing nations, Egypt has experienced the practical and physical consequences of the current conflict between conventional forms of modern development and the contrastingly structured urban fabrics of historic and cultural traditions. A somewhat artificial polarisation between tradition and modernity characterises the analysis of Egypt's approach to urban design. Diverging philosophies, ideologies and cultural attitudes, imported during colonisation in the form of European models of urban design and planning, created a break with traditional urbanisation processes. Urban design in Egypt evolved from the first spurt of urbanisation under Islamic dynasties in the middle ages, to the urban sprawl characteristic of megacities such as today's Cairo, with a population of 11.6 million (nearly 20 million for the metropolitan area). Throughout these periods of development, it was primarily private sector led initiatives that shaped significant parts of the capital, where urban design models are best exemplified.

Definitions

In Egypt, the expression 'urban design' is used in education and professional circles and its definition is derived from European and North American models. Conceptually, urban design is grounded in the physical improvement of public space, as well as overall concerns with the layout, arrangement, appearance and functionality of parts of cities.

In the absence of a formal definition in planning legislation, it is apparent that urban design plays a less important role than that outlined above as a discipline in its own right. Nevertheless, the masterplan as a tool for guiding the development of an area is widely used by government bodies such as the General Organisation for Physical Planning (part of the ministry of housing, utilities and urban development), and by the private sector.

Within university courses, urban design is not taught as a separate discipline, but understood as being interdisciplinary. Good urban design is closely connected with a positive human experience of housing layout patterns, the upgrading and conservation of historic areas, neighbourhood design, and the form and meaning of urban spaces.

The academic discipline

As in many countries, urban design in Egypt borrows from and integrates the two disciplines of urban planning and architecture. Within both these traditions, it has developed either as a more detailed approach to planning (an approach rooted in faculties of urban planning) or as a three-dimensional expression of buildings, urban spaces and the human experience (led by departments of architecture).

On the other hand and in contrast with the situation in many European and North American countries, urban design is taught at undergraduate level as a series of courses. Following the political shift in the late 1970s from a socialist to a more western regime, urban design teaching was introduced as faculties realigned themselves with North American schools. Newly trained staff first began teaching the subject in the department of architecture at Cairo University. Unsurprisingly, the theoretical content

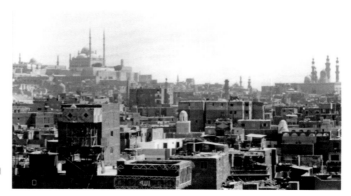

Historic Cairo has been designated a UNESCO world heritage site

of the syllabus developed at that time was strongly based on western theories and models of development. However, with the designation of the historic part of Cairo as a world heritage site in 1979 and the related explosion of interest in the conservation of Islamic heritage, more contextual approaches ensued.

In spite of this emerging interest in traditional environments, the application of western methods and techniques continued: urban-tissue studies, visual perception, townscape, urban form analysis, mental maps and community development were all used in projects in the historic neighbourhoods. More recently, courses have increasingly focused on the Egyptian context and the problems of Cairo as a sprawling megalopolis, particularly in the field of housing. Indeed, informal housing, the urban poor and their infrastructural needs are major issues of concern. More recently, the field of landscape design has emerged, with courses in site landscape and plantation being taught at Cairo university.

The professional place of urban design

Academia holds an important position in the education and practice of urban design in Egypt. Urban designers associate themselves more with university centres than they do with formal societies or associations. The majority of graduates of architecture or urban planning belong to the Syndicate of Engineers, equivalent to the Royal Institute of British Architects (RIBA) or Royal Town Planning Institute (RTPI) in the UK.

The majority of practising urban designers are faculty members who have gained PhD qualifications from schools abroad, and who use their skills to teach as well as consult on government-led projects. The competition is relatively small, and success depends mostly on involvement with international agencies such as the World Bank, United Nations Habitat or Development Programme or the Aga Khan Foundation. Therefore, urban design professionals employed by these organisatons tend to be academics or graduates, mainly with architectural backgrounds, or planners who have worked in architectural practices. There are very few independent Egyptian urban design consultancies not connected with university staff. This explains why a large number of international agencies and consulting firms are working in Egypt, on both public- and private-sector schemes.

The planning system

Since 1986, the General Organization for Physical Planning (GOPP), established within the ministry of housing, utilities and urban development with the support of the United Nations Development Program (UNDP), has made concerted efforts to decentralise spatial planning in Egypt to four tiers:

- National Spatial Development Vision
- Regional Strategic Plans at governorate level, or for several governorates making up an economic region
- Strategic Urban Plans for cities and villages
- Local Authority Detailed Plans (supervised by GOPP)

GOPP, as a national body, is involved in preparing planning guidelines, managing and monitoring urban development programmes, conducting and supervising urban studies (concerning transportation systems, infrastructure, waste handling, treatment plants and environmental issues), proposing and developing planning related legislation, monitoring urban extensions to stop urban sprawl taking over agricultural and environmentally sensitive areas, and preparing village planning strategies. It has published physical-planning manuals related to the legislation, but these are mainly concerned with land use and rarely use the term urban design. The Urban and Detailed Plans are undertaken by consulting firms.

Historical development

Within Egyptian legislation, urban design has always been considered a subset of urban planning. From as early as Mohammed Ali's reign in the late 19th century, an endogenous urban reform process called the *Tanzimat* introduced institutional and legal structures to regulate planning and building, and by implication to influence urban design. At first, these structures were fairly autonomous, though as early as 1834 an agency called the *Commissione di Ornato* was created in Alexandria, followed by a similar one in Cairo in 1843, entrusted with city beautification and the improvement and straightening of streets. After independence from British rule in 1952, a central planning body, the Tanzim Higher Advisory Council, was created to coordinate the activities of the various departments in charge of municipal affairs (*Tanzim*, city police, public health, drainage and public buildings), as well as advise on all projects involving city improvement and embellishment.

During Mohammed Ali's rule, European-modelled schools and factories, importing foreign teachers and advisers, chose western – and, more specifically, French – methods as their model. Therefore, regulations dealing with land subdivisions and street layouts were introduced as part of a more centralised and standardised control over property and public space.

Egypt's last ruling Islamic dynasty, the Ottomans, allowed modern institutions to develop in parallel with traditional ones. The social, religious and cultural structures established since the 8th century continued under a powerful religious–legal framework that secured a high degree of law and order in all civil and criminal affairs, including the urban environment. This framework laid down the principal legal precepts in order to find optimal solutions to an accretion of individual decisions. In its simplest form, the law permitted building as long as no harm was inflicted on neighbours or passersby. The expression 'no harm' was interpreted as the following:

- no obstruction of passage
- no intrusion on neighbouring privacy
- no deprivation of light and air
- no disturbance with noise or smells
- no neglect of condition of property to increase likelihood of collapse or destroy life or neighbouring property

These simple precepts meant that building took place in a highly self-regulated manner. The resultant urban fabric was a dense assemblage of buildings, an efficient use of land and compact inward-looking residential buildings with protected internal private courtyards.

Similarly, religious and public buildings were located side-by-side in mixed-use compact areas, with minimal public open space. Indeed, public space under this religious–legal framework lacked the structured layout imposed by highly formalised institutions, as was the case in Europe. Rather, public space allowed for a high degree of interaction between various social activities, including religious functions. Since Islam conceded a large amount of autonomy and responsibility to various social groups, they 'were always allowed to take charge of the respective sections of public open space running through their territory, in both residential districts and market areas' (Bianca 2000, p. 39). The mosque, the focus of public life, along with other public buildings such as *madrasa* (colleges), *wikala* (caravanserai for trade), *maristan* (hospitals) and *sabil kuttab* (schools for orphans) were all integrated seamlessly with the marketplaces. The public street network was reduced to the sheer minimum required to provide connections between the main city gates and the central markets.

Ever since the middle ages, Egypt's feudal system relied on an urban, economic base in order to maximise returns from the major trade routes. The wealthy ruling class contributed significantly to the permanence and resilience of the urban fabric with religious and political patronage. They invested in real estate, urban development and regeneration projects. They established prominent public buildings to convey symbolic meaning and foster identity, and commercial buildings to house the burgeoning international trade. State-owned land was given or sold to the ruling class to develop as residential and commercial neighbourhoods, along with the public facilities required for social welfare. This pattern of private investment in large-scale development continues to be a hallmark of Egyptian masterplanning today. Although the state does fund the establishment of new towns (for example, 6 October City and Nasr City), public housing and urban improvements, the private sector has created the most visible urban design examples, largely because of upfront investment and shorter construction timescales.

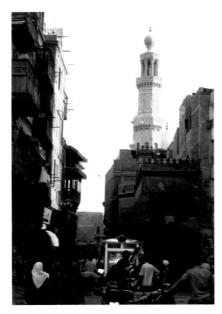

A street in a traditional neighbourhood of Cairo

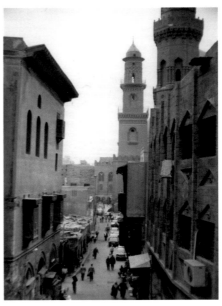

Public buildings are the focus of the traditional neighbourhoods

Imported urban design models

> In the current transformation processes imposed by an unilateral concept
> of 'progress', the issue at stake is the continuity of local cultural identities,
> as materialized in the built environment. The correlation between man's
> identity and his environment implies that the question to be addressed is
> how to foster significant architectural forms which both solicit and express
> identification with deep-rooted human values.
>
> (Bianca 2000, pp. 325–6)

This statement reflects a point in Egypt's urban history when the continuity of local
cultural identities, as materialised in the built environment, was broken by the French
(1798–1801) and British (1882–1952) occupations. A statement by the Ottoman ruler
Khedive Ismail also captures the transformation: '[the] country was no longer part of
Africa, but belonged to Europe'.

Such new attitudes meant that the 900-year religious–legal framework that had
shaped traditional urban patterns was dismantled in favour of the more European-
styled and centralised Tanzim Higher Advisory Council. During this period, privately
developed suburbs such as Ezbekiya, Maadi, Garden City and Heliopolis were inspired
by Beaux-Arts and Picturesque models. Heliopolis for example, a 240 ha garden
suburb, combined an arrangement of picturesque architectural detailing styled in
Moorish or Indo-Saracenic traditions with a more rectilinear urban layout of higher-
density arcaded apartment blocks and wide tree-lined boulevards .

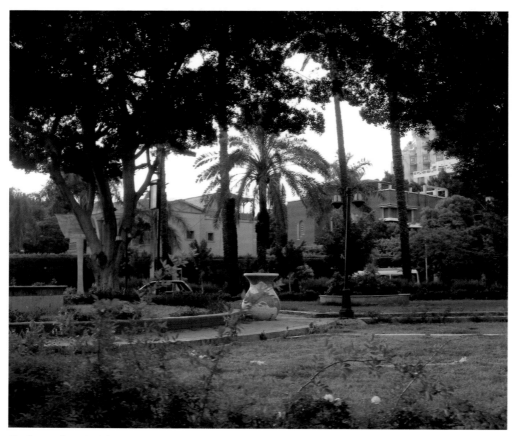

Maadi, a garden suburb from the early 20th century

Ezbekiya, one of the first urban extensions, imported European urban and architectural typologies: parks (designed by a French gardener), commercial street arcades, large single-use public buildings such as ministries, an opera, a circus, a French theatre and a grand hotel. A new morphology was also introduced, with an orthogonal street grid attached to a star-shaped pattern centred on a circular public space. Long esplanades and wide diagonal tree-lined streets were laid out, and building plots were planned for low-density single-family 'palaces'. New zoning laws meant increasing specialised land-uses, leading to a segregation of economic activity and social organisation.

Almost all suburban developments under British rule resulted from the initiatives of private companies, without the control of the state: Heliopolis and Koubbeh Gardens by Belgian financier Edouard Ampain; the garden suburb of Maadi by Egyptian Delta Land and Investment Company; the island of Rawda and the left bank of the Nile by Alexandrian entrepreneurs, the Zervudachi brothers; and Garden City suburb by Charles Bacos, a wealthy merchant and landowner from Alexandria, through his Nile Land and Agricultural Company.

A new type of imported urban model appeared following Egyptian independence in 1952. The energy of the new socialist state was focused on housing the masses: a public company built large numbers of housing projects inspired by Soviet-styled monolithic blocks. One of these is captured by F. Steinberg (1991, p. 75), when she writes:

> with its monotonous order of rows of apartment blocks it is a complete break-off from the prevailing architectural and urbanistic tradition. Known as an almost 'negative case' of public housing in the 1950s, it is presently in a pitiful state of degradation and dilapidation in terms of both its physical structure and its services. The area is marked by intensive overcrowding and rather abandoned 'public space', which as a 'no man's land' is far from attracting Cairene outdoor life.

Another ideological shift started in 1973, as Egypt followed an economic transition policy to a free-market system. This coincided with the development of an extensive new towns programme to relieve Cairo of its burgeoning population, stop the sprawl on to rural land and channel it towards the desert. Ten new settlements were planned in the 1980s. Six new cities and satellite towns are now established, and ten more new urban extensions have been added around the Cairo middle and outer ring roads. However, the new towns have not achieved the objective of shifting population away from Cairo. Those closest to the capital have largely accommodated the wealthy seeking a better quality of life, less pollution and lower densities in contrast to the city centre. Private developers and land speculators have seen this as an opportunity to construct luxury housing within gated communities, inspired less by European than by North American suburban models. They have been accompanied by a proliferation of new shopping malls, modern high-rise blocks, large expanses of artificially created lakes and golf courses, and private educational institutions and services. New Giza, one such urban extension, is the focus of the following case study.

ocated 7 km north-west of the Giza pyramids, and 16 km west of the centre of Cairo, New Giza is a 610 ha site situated along the Cairo–Alexandria motorway. Billed as a 'new traditional community' with an abundance of public open space and amenities, its advertising emphasises the contrast with the overcrowding of other Cairo suburbs (www.newgiza.com):

> A welcoming environment that leaves the stress of the city far behind and a sanctuary away from the hustle and bustle, NEWGIZA will pioneer the next generation of integrated community living.

The New Giza Real Estate Development Company was set up primarily by Mahmoud Al-Gammal and Partners, a group that has a track record in

similar luxury projects. In New Giza, the vision according to Dover, Kohl and Partners (DKP) is to create an:

> up-market, mixed-use community that will include eight residential neighbourhoods with townhouses and single-family homes, parks, a sports complex, schools, a university, luxury hotels, mixed-use centres, and a hospital. The new community will also feature a tram that will link the neighbourhoods to one another, and will connect to a regional transit system leading to the Pyramids, The Grand Egyptian Museum, and one day, Downtown Cairo.

Like many private developers in Egypt, Al-Gammal has chosen to engage international consultants to undertake some of the key roles, including overall

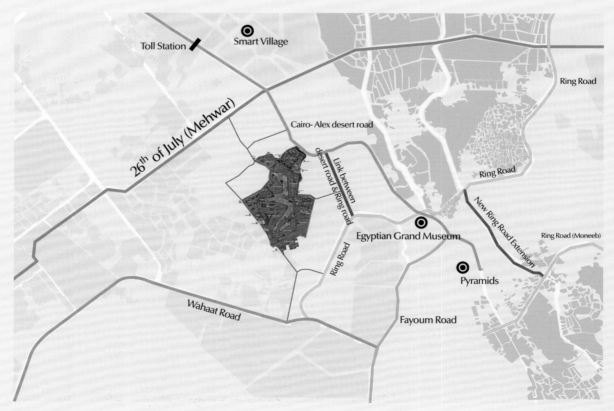

New Giza is located along the Cairo–Alexandria motorway

conceptual masterplanning (DKP), masterplanning for the downtown area (Gensler), retail consultancy (Colliers International), landscaping (HJA Design Studio) and golf course design (Thomson, Perret and Lobb). Nevertheless, Al-Gammal has also created Egyptian teams in order to liaise with the international agents, including Earth Architecture and Planning (EAP), commissioned to develop the

detailed masterplan for the area (excluding the downtown); Degla, to provide project management and engineering services; and New Giza Design Studio, for architectural design.

Contrary to the European models that inspired Egyptian designers in the past, such new developments are strongly Americanised. The

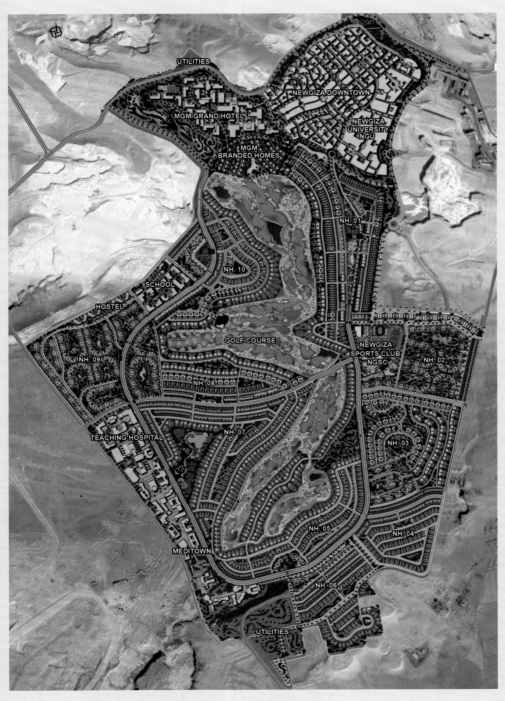

Masterplan of the New Giza community by Earth Architecture and Planning for New Giza Real Estate Development Company

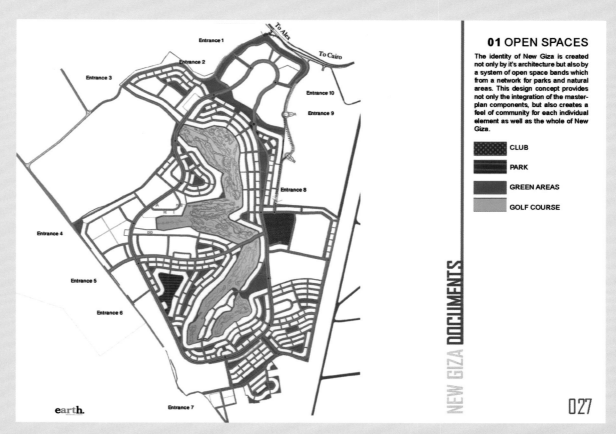

01 OPEN SPACES

The identity of New Giza is created not only by it's architecture but also by a system of open space bands which from a network for parks and natural areas. This design concept provides not only the integration of the masterplan components, but also creates a feel of community for each individual element as well as the whole of New Giza.

CLUB
PARK
GREEN AREAS
GOLF COURSE

NEW GIZA DOCUMENTS

027

Open spaces network at the core of the New Giza masterplan

majority of consultants are either based in the US or are multinationals. Unsurprisingly, they bring to Egypt the ideas and models they learned in the US. DKP, designers of the New Giza masterplan, have close connections with EAP, whose president, the Egyptian architect Ibrahim Mohasseb, trained in urban design at the University of Miami and worked with DKP for four years before setting up his own practice in Egypt. Inspired by the prevalence of the New Urbanism (NU) school of thought in Miami, New Giza reflects NU principles.

DKP's conceptual masterplan proposes eight neighbourhoods of distinct character based upon their location within the site, their topographic features and natural views. Most neighbourhoods will be residential, featuring single-family residences and town houses, laid out in a system of blocks and streets that respond to the natural topography of the site. Their design carefully balances the desire for long views with that of privacy and the need for a street grid to ensure walkability. An important feature of the project is the system

of interconnected parks created to enhance the public enjoyment of each neighbourhood. Many of these are strategically located in order to provide an uninterrupted view from the private terraces of homes, and will be accessible to families and visitors. The park system also connects the neighbourhoods to adjacent shopping centres, schools, recreation facilities and mixed-use centres.

EAP's design intends to accommodate 30,000 people at low densities with generous setbacks, 30% built-up area and large open spaces and streets. New Giza has been conceived as a middle-class suburb with very little social mix, as the masterplanners argue that the neighbouring new town, 6 October City, provides for all social groups. At least the mixed-use downtown, located adjacent to the Cairo–Alexandria motorway, is accessible to a wider public. It includes New Giza University, a sports club, a medical centre, two hotels and a mall. The commercial buildings, however, though not gated are controlled through front-door access from a podium.

Case study: New Giza urban extension ~ **EGYPT**

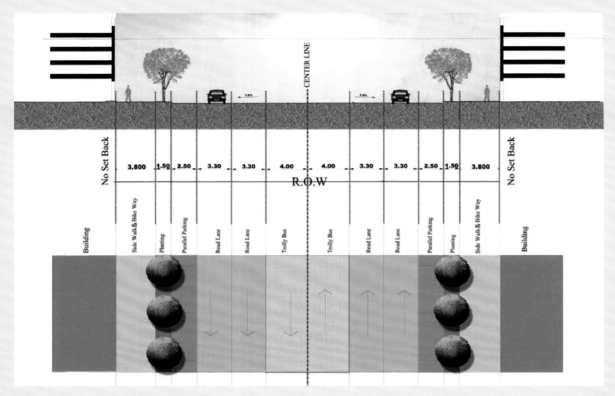

Example of the design code for the Boulevard,
one of the streets of New Giza

The remainder of the site, in particular the public open spaces and neighbourhood centres, are also accessible to a wider public via the street and tram network. Compared with other similar new suburbs currently being developed, New Giza is almost the only development to include publicly accessible mixed-use areas. This is an important development, modelled on the historic suburbs of Maadi and Heliopolis that were used as successful precedents of community building. However, the residential streets themselves are gated.

Design decisions on urban layout have been influenced by two sources: North American NU schemes and the colonial suburbs of Maadi and Heliopolis. No reference has been made to the more traditional urban principles of the Islamic middle ages. This is probably understandable in view of the high density and overcrowding that these parts of Cairo suffer from, though in terms of walkability and climatic adaptation they are far superior. During the masterplanning process, Gensler and EAP debated the cultural precedents for mixed-use centre typologies: EAP wanted to adopt the arcaded

typology from Heliopolis for climatic reasons, and as a means of softening the edge of public–private space. Gensler did not follow this advice because arcades might have obscured the shop signs, but their analysis of the traditional marketplace typology (souk and mosque ensemble) did influence their designs.

Design codes regulate street sections and plot arrangements for the various housing areas. The streets follow North American dimensional standards, paying little attention to climatic requirements. The central Boulevard is 40 m in width with a dual carriageway, other minor streets are 26 m and 17 m wide. The majority of streets are tree-lined with high landscaping specifications and parallel parking. Architectural styles, according to principal architect Amr Ghaly, are supposed to follow neo-classical, Moorish-inspired or modern styles, similar to those adopted in the colonial neighbourhoods of Garden City and Heliopolis.

The site was formerly a rock quarry and it is characterised by flat, sandy areas and rocky outcrops, with a number of sheer cliff faces. The topography includes slopes of 20% or more. This pattern of parallel ridges and valleys allows for developments with dramatic vistas, including a potential for views of the Great Pyramids. To take advantage of this feature, the residential suburbs have been placed on higher ground. However, because of the plot layouts the need for cut and fill has been extensive, indicating that topographical ridges and valleys have not always been carefully followed. On the other hand, the level change of approximately 30 m between the mixed-use zone and the residential areas has been used as a form of natural separation.

The central Boulevard connects neighbourhood centres and key services, and the new tram runs along it. A proposed extension of the existing metro line from Cairo to New Giza will connect to it as well.

The basic principles of DKP's earlier conceptual plans have been retained, ensuring that each residential suburb is served by a transit stop and a small local centre, as have 13 acres of public open space. However, in developing detailed designs some changes, largely related to land-use requirements, have been introduced by EAP.

When asked whether the number of people living in the settlement would be able to support the services and amenities provided, EAP argued that employees of the hotel, university, school, and Meditown (a hospital complex), as well as visitors from Cairo and neighbouring 6 October City, would generate the critical mass required. When queried about the impact of climate on New Giza's layouts, the masterplanner acknowledged that wind and shade had taken a secondary role in relation to views, as these were considered to add greater economic value.

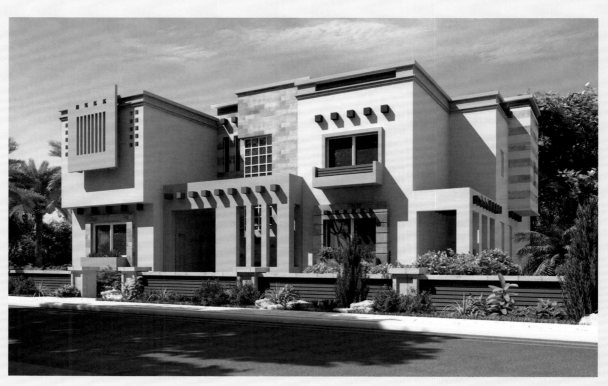

A typical modern grand villa in New Giza

Conclusions

The most significant recent urban design initiatives in Egypt have been characterised by the move from traditional models of urban development to those inspired by western ideas. Traditional urban design was largely decentralised and unregulated: accretive interventions on public space over time guided by simple religious–legal codes, and many small-scale decisions by individuals, shaped organic growth and created dense and continuous urban forms of narrow winding streets with mixed uses. The strong connection between culture and the built environment was reinforced through the social, economic and political patronage of the ruling class. These interdependent relationships were gradually eroded as greater control and a new political context were modelled on urban planning examples from Europe.

The result of this shift was urban patterns that placed greater priority on public open space, wide streets and building typologies adopted from Europe – in particular, from Paris. Stylistically, the climatic imperatives that guided traditional architecture were dropped in favour of neo-classical styles and detached villas set in private gardens. The Beaux-Art grand manner, the Picturesque and the orthogonal grid were combined in various ways to create distinctive new suburbs.

Another feature of urban design in Egypt is the long-standing leadership of the private sector in developing new parts of the city. Even under the Islamic dynasties, the ruling class and those closely connected with the state-initiated major urban projects. Most noticeable was the strong underpinning of social welfare functions such as mosques, colleges and hospitals, which to some degree continued during the colonial period, though with a more zoned layout. Later, during the neo-liberal economic period, the mix of uses decreased as profiteering in residential real estate became the norm. The involvement of international or foreign-trained urban designers in many of these privately led developments has been largely responsible for the appropriation of new foreign lifestyles and their resultant urban patterns. This had begun during the colonial period with the creation of parks and esplanades, and has resulted in the more recent creation of middle-class neighbourhoods centred on golf courses and entertainment hubs.

Arguably, an increasing economic and social segregation can therefore be attributed to urban design practice. Although the public sector played an active role in urban development, particularly during the socialist period, planning never catered equally for all sectors of society. The 'gated street' is not an entirely new concept and was utilised traditionally by communities to provide security, privacy and control over public space. In the guise of the 'gated community', it has reappeared as a North American import in contemporary developments like New Giza for precisely the same reasons, although marked by greater economic variances than historically.

Finally, Egyptian urban design practice still remains unresponsive to the needs for sustainable development, particularly with regard to climate change. New Giza has implemented a transit system to support more car-free environments, but in middle-class suburbs situated at some distance from the centres of employment in Cairo it is unlikely that residents will abandon their cars for a tram system. Moreover, adaptation to climate has not been attempted in street layout or by the clustering of urban form to maximise shade. On the contrary, landscaping and open views have been prioritised as they add higher commercial value to a project.

The current Arab Spring taking place in Egypt may challenge the acceptability of this existing contrast in lifestyles and built forms. Whether international or western models, which have inspired new cultural identities, can continue to influence urban design practice is also a question that remains to be answered.

A quick guide to
Egypt

1 TYPES OF CLIENT

General Organization for Physical Planning (GOPP)/ministry of housing, utilities and urban development

Egyptian developers and investment groups

United Nations, Aga Khan Foundation and other international development agencies

....

2 TYPES OF PROJECT/WORK

Masterplans
- Public housing
- Urban extensions
- New towns

Village planning strategies

Urban and detailed plans (including design codes)

....

3 APPROACH NEEDED TO WORK IN COUNTRY

International competitions

Partnership with Egyptian practices

Subcontractor to another international consultancy firm working in Egypt

Invited tenders or joint ventures with private/public sector

International practices who wish to set up a branch in Egypt to carry out a specific contract need to register with the General Authority of Investment and Free Zones (GAFI)

....

4 LEGISLATION THAT NEEDS TO BE REFERRED TO

National Spatial Development Vision

Regional Strategic Plans at governorate level or for several governorates making up an economic region

Strategic Urban Plans for cities and villages

Local Authority Detailed Plans

....

5 SPECIFIC TIPS FOR SUCCESS

Understanding of traditional urban form and its adaptation to contemporary living

Consideration of all aspects of sustainability

....

6 USEFUL WEBSITES

Society of Egyptian Architects: www.sea1917.org

....

1	area	1,001,450 km^2
2	population	81,121,077
3	annual population growth	1.7%
4	urban population	43%
5	population density	81 p/km^2
6	GDP	$218,894,280,920
7	GNI per capita	$2,420

Source: The World Bank (2010)

MOROCCO

Gwenaëlle Zunino, *architect–urbanist*

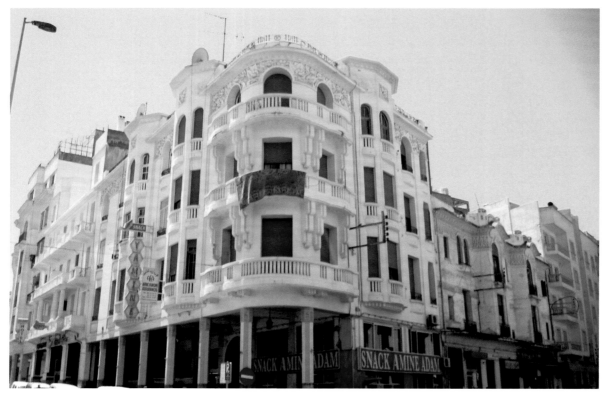

View of the art deco district of Casablanca

Morocco is a constitutional monarchy with an elected parliament of two chambers, the Assembly of Representatives and the Assembly of Councillors. The country is divided into 16 regions, 62 departments and 1,547 municipalities (*communes*).

A country undergoing major changes

Morocco is currently undergoing profound demographic, social, urban, economic and political change. The country has chosen to make significant efforts to open up internationally, by establishing strategies for modernisation and human development. Its demographic evolution has been significantly fast: life expectancy extended from 60 in 1980 to 71.8 in 2008; spectacular fall in birth rates; increase in school attendance, particularly for girls; participation of women in the workforce; etc. This has been closely related to the growth of urban areas, particularly along the coast. Today, over half of the population is urban and it is expected that by 2050 this proportion will have reached two-thirds. The number of cities in Morocco grew from 112 in 1960 to 350 in 2004, 54 of which had more than 50,000 inhabitants. Casablanca, the country's economic capital, is the largest metropolis with some 3.4 million inhabitants (4 million for Greater Casablanca). Most of the other large cities, including the national capital Rabat, are on the coast. Only Marrakech and Fès are inland.

One of the consequences of the country's rapid urbanisation is the massive transformation of the cities' outskirts. Their development creates problems, particularly because most of it is spontaneous, with significant numbers of substandard housing projects in spite of the fact, that in order to deal with this situation, a number of planned social housing developments and new towns have recently been built. Urban sprawl is further complicated by the fact that many schemes that are in conflict with a comprehensive planned vision for the future of an area are nevertheless approved as 'exceptions', thus leading to problems related to land use, social and functional mix, and a lack of services.

The Moroccan Planning High Commission – a government organisation in charge of planning – predicts that, whilst the rural population of the country will have stabilised by 2030, the urban population will have grown by more than 7 million, thus requiring a long-term planning strategy specifically for urban areas. This strategy must strengthen and multiply urban centres in rural areas, and establish a structure for metropolitan areas in order to avoid an increase in land speculation and in social division. It would appear that the regional structures – the *wilayas* – are the most appropriate for planning the country's urban development as they have the capacity to make the link between national policies and those of other stakeholders, and to implement these policies through local initiatives.

The large urban project, another way of developing a city

Morocco wishes to place itself as a 21st-century country, particularly by strengthening its economic appeal and its urban character. As a result, a number of large cities – Rabat, Tangiers and Casablanca – are changing their image and positioning themselves in a global market through the realisation of major urban developments. These cities want to embody modernity and present a new face to the world through a changed skyline and the rediscovery of their seafronts. Large schemes such as Bouregreg in Rabat; Tangiers' Med; and Marina, Anfa and others in Casablanca indicate that urban design is central to the conception of current Moroccan metropolises. These projects are commissioned from well-known international architectural offices as their 'brand' is easily recognised and is the reason for choosing them.

It is, however, clear that a city is not just a series of iconic urban projects that embody its international presence. Cities also have to be regenerated and the daily lives of their inhabitants has to be improved. With this in mind, specific policies established by the government for social housing, new towns and the removal of shanty towns are being implemented through numerous schemes conceived in a very different manner from the ones marketed internationally. Unfortunately, in the case of these projects quantity is a greater priority than quality: standards are applied without reflecting on the coherence between different projects, or their integration in the wider urban context. Additionally, public space is rarely taken into account in the conception of these schemes.

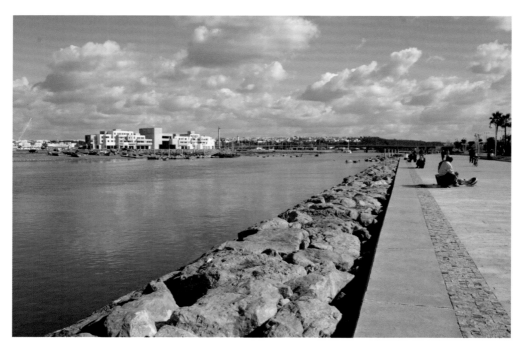

Morocco wishes to compete internationally through large urban schemes such as the Bouregreg in Rabat: seen here, the marina and the Hassan tower

Morocco has therefore to confront two different approaches to city development: one based on international models, the other trying to let the cities evolve within the local traditions. In summary, the concept of urban design translates for current Moroccan practice as the large urban project. Architecture and the image given by it retain their priority, even though urban composition and grand vistas, symbols of power, are also very important. Concerns about sustainability are gradually impacting on the above, and the needs of the population are also increasingly taken into account, but participation remains limited to the major stakeholders and lacks any significant involvement of the general public. Hence, some questions remain to be answered before urban design can become a reality in Morocco: how can urban projects be integrated within their urban context? How can cities be for all?

Professional networks

The architecture and engineering professions – the latter remaining very technically oriented – monopolise most of the conceptual urban work, whether related to large projects or to more routine urbanism. They follow the French model of professional bodies: the national Order of Architects, the College of Architects and Urbanists of Morocco, the recently established Association of Moroccan Landscape Designers (founded, February 2011) and Majal, the Association of Planning Agencies for the major cities (source: Fédération des agences urbaines du Maroc). Architects are very well organised and represented, their role is recognised and their opinions are listened to in all relevant debates. Landscape designers on the other hand are not really established; they are involved mostly in the design of gardens and parks, even though their wider vision should be fundamental in order to place urban schemes within their wider geographic and environmental contexts. Their participation in the conception of the city should be essential.

An additional significant fact is that Morocco gives priority to its native professionals. Therefore, international architects or consultants need to have Moroccan partners in order to participate in local tenders. This can be very beneficial for the exchange of ideas and expertise. In addition, the country's large urban projects are frequently private developments with international financial backing, or are funded by subsidiaries of the *Caisse des Dépôts*, a public financial institution acting in the collective interest. For the time being, these projects are almost exclusively located in Casablanca, Rabat and Tangiers, even though all the other large cities are also rethinking their planning.

Urban design education

At present, hardly any courses related to urban design are offered in Morocco. In fact there is only one school of architecture, the National School of Architecture located in Rabat, and one planning school, the National Institute of Planning and Urbanism (INAU), also in Rabat. A second school of architecture is to open in Casablanca in the autumn of 2011. However, many Moroccans go to study abroad, mostly in France but increasingly in the US or other Anglo-Saxon countries. It is therefore conceivable that a number of Moroccan professionals will obtain their formal education or their practical training in urban design abroad, and thus acquire a wider and more holistic approach to the urban project.

A legislation evolving towards greater pragmatism

Because of its history, the Moroccan legislative context closely follows the French one, and it is now evolving to respond to the challenges of urban expansion. Current planning documents are the National Land Management Plan (Snat), the regional Structure Plans (SDAU), the Local Plans at the municipal scale and, more recently, the Urban Transport Plans (PDU).

Historically, the range of legislative instruments in Morocco constituted a forerunner for the former colonial power: the French tested their first planning laws in Morocco before applying them to France. So, a decree of April 1914 instituted planning documents to manage urban extensions and created instruments for the control of urbanisation. With regard to urban design, this fundamental act made possible the drafting of regulations concerning the public realm, building alignment and the conservation and enhancement of the country's built heritage. A decree of June 1933 allowed and regulated land subdivisions, at first only for the provision of housing; in 1953, this was widened to include commercial and industrial activities. Another decree, of July 1952, widened the scope of planning documents to include outskirts, suburbs and rural areas.

The main current legal instruments are Law No. 12-90 on planning and No. 25-90 on land subdivision and housing, both dating from 1992. Their importance lies in the fact that they introduced regulatory planning documents, urban management, development control and enforcement against non-compliance. They are complemented by a decree of 1993 establishing the Planning Agencies, the equivalent to a city's planning department but only charged with research and masterplanning. Building permits and other authorisations are granted by the president of the local council.

The daily practice of Moroccan urbanism suffers from some malfunctions. The first is the length of time taken to prepare and update planning documents, and as a result the frequent and systematic use of 'derogations' (exemptions from the regulations) which end up harming urban, architectural and social coherence. In fact, because at the moment the whole regulatory system is in a state of flux, the vast majority of large urban projects are approved using these exemptions, thus escaping any constraint. As a result, the Moroccan system operates at two different speeds: small schemes are often delayed awaiting a plan's revision, whilst the large schemes that comply with no regulations are approved using derogations.

Other problems relate to the paucity of investment in public infrastructure, the cumbersome procedures needed to obtain a permit, the lack of overall building regulations and the multiplicity of people involved, resulting in no overall responsibility being taken. Additionally, complex systems of ownership make it difficult to assemble land and nearly impossible to build up land reserves.

In order to try to solve these problems and to allow cities to evolve, the planning system is currently being overhauled. However, care has to be taken not to simply transfer legal systems from elsewhere – from France, in particular. Moroccan legislation may be – or may become – progressive in certain fields such as social matters, sustainable development or administration, but new legal instruments may have trouble adapting to local situations. In that case, conflicts may become more frequent in the future. The solution is to have a more pragmatic approach made up of well-focused laws that encourage innovation in the way projects are financed and urbanisation is managed, in planning regulations, and in the collaboration between authorities or the setting up of local development companies. Planning documents better adapted to the current urban context, and approved without delays, would also avoid the systematic use of derogations.

Finally, sustainability must be a fundamental issue in the review of the planning system. This should result in a consideration of the environment in all planning documents, the establishment of environmental impact studies and the general application of the principle of urban compactness. Additionally, a national energy strategy, a national charter for the environment and sustainable development, and climate strategies are being prepared. Consideration of the energy efficiency of buildings is yet to be incorporated into the regulations. At the same time, sustainable development must not be made an excuse for forgetting economic or social issues. The whole point of sustainable development is that it cuts across sectors and across spatial and time scales.

A Moroccan urban design tradition

As a result of its history, the Moroccan city is made up of a series of layers that correspond to different periods and images. The *medinas*, symbols of traditional Arab cities, sit adjacent to the European cities, symbols of the French presence in early 20th century, and to the much more recent neighbourhoods built to respond to the urban explosion.

The *medina* is the historic centre of the Arab city. Its coherent form is enclosed by the surrounding walls; the mosque is in the centre, from which radiate strategic routes. A very tight network of spaces is structured through a form of zoning wherein all urban functions can be found: intellectual (Koranic schools or *medersa*), economic (markets or *souks*) and public. From the centre outwards, successive enclaves correspond on the one hand to economic activities in decreasing order of importance and increasing degree of nuisance, and on the other hand to residential neighbourhoods, more or less enclosed. Family life takes place in private houses with internal patios and high walls with few windows, and which are accessible through a chicane that protects the family's intimacy. Several such houses are grouped around a *derb*, a cul-de-sac approximately 3 m in width, which opens into the wider streets of the *medina*. Children play and residents meet in, and identify with, the *derb*, a semi-public and intimate space. Several *derb*s form a *hawma*, a neighbourhood with a few additional functions

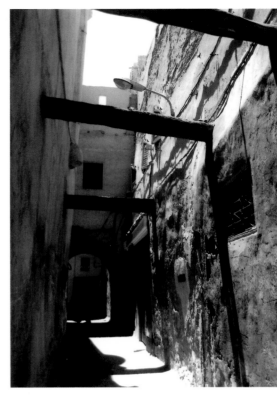

A residential street in the *medina* of Marrakech

and still identifiable by its residents. The simple external aspect of the Arab-Muslim buildings, their scale and the materials used, give the city an amazing architectural unity. Only public buildings offer diversity, through their shapes and colours.

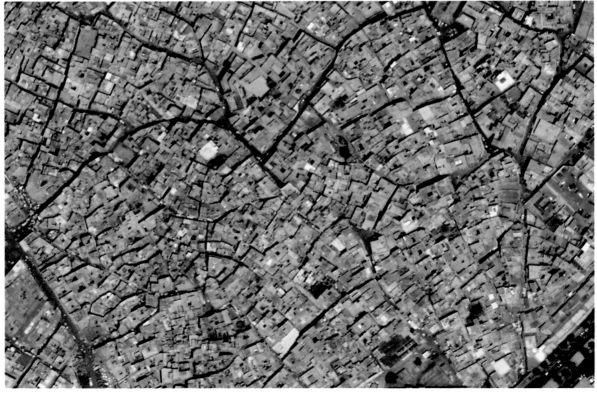

Aerial view of Casablanca's *medina*

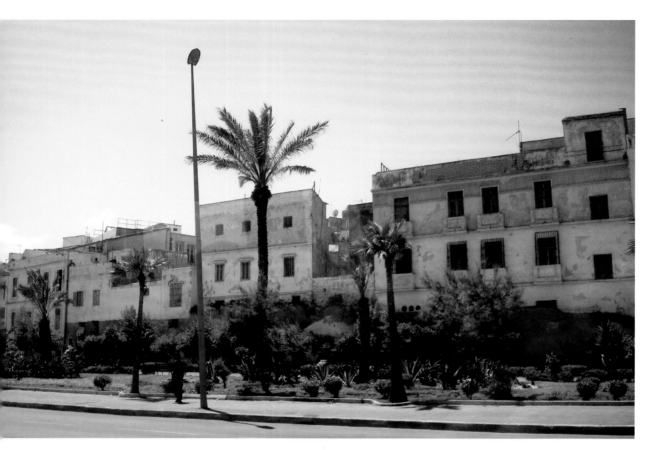

In the European city, regular openings
and aligned cornices characterise the volumes

Commenting on the Arab city, Le Corbusier said: 'The *medina* is compact, functional, efficient and fast: you exit its doors and there is nature's splendour.'

When the French Protectorate was established in 1912, the Resident General Louis-Hubert Lyautey decided to stimulate urban development and asked Henri Prost to prepare the first planning documents. These have left their mark on history because of their numerous innovations: instead of adopting a grid as in so many new towns, Prost's was a radial plan adapted to the topography and taking account of existing structures. His idea was that on exiting the *medina*, new sensations and new behavioural patterns would correspond to a different light, a different scale and different vistas: a new, more European, kind of landscape, with building lines, pathways and carriageways, and functional separation. The resulting new hierarchical system of boulevards linking the major city nodes continues to be effective to this day. The urban functions – central, industrial, leisure and health – are distributed in zones with distinct morphologies. Within this scheme, urban design had an important role, in particular because of the inclusion of principles of city embellishment and the requirements for quality and unity between architecture and public space. Prost gave priority to quality, coherence, function and harmony both for buildings and for the spaces in-between. A large number of public spaces were created: esplanades, promenades, urban parks, exhibition grounds, avenues and corniches. Equally some large projects were developed, such as the art deco district in Casablanca, representative of the urban vision of the day, or its new *medina*, the Habous, which successfully reinterpreted the traditional urban layout.

During the 1950s, the head of planning, Michel Ecochard, broke with the local planning tradition, in Casablanca in particular. As a result of industrialisation, large population movements from rural to urban areas had created many shanty towns. Ecochard prioritised quantity, encouraging the development of suburbs and introducing a typology of social housing based upon an evolving cellular unit. The objective was to find an alternative to the traditional Arab patio house adapted to the local context, and the answer was to build western-type apartment blocks opening on to superimposed patios. Therefore, concerns for functionality and efficiency replaced those for quality and morphology. Ecochard also favoured linear development along major routes. Nevertheless, in parallel and at the same time, many architectural schemes of high quality were built – in particular, private villas and public buildings.

During the 1980s, planning became more concerned with the ownership and the provision of neighbourhood services, though some large urban projects and major public spaces were also planned. Today, most large new town developments or the ones aimed at relocating shanty towns return to geometric grid patterns and zoning, resulting in urban areas of low intensity and poorly connected to existing neighbourhoods or to the history of the existing city.

An important point to remember is that in the Arab tradition people do not necessarily use public spaces except for those in their immediate neighbourhood (the *derb*). Other public spaces are neither shared nor respected. Therefore, the challenge is to consider how people use spaces currently (for parking or informal trading) and to offer them new possibilities, in particular their use for leisure (Casablanca's corniche, Rabat's Bouregreg promenade, etc). This requires finding a way to give the project a new meaning that can best respond to the local context.

In summary, a concern for innovation and for architectural and urban quality can be found throughout Morocco's history. This is particularly true of Casablanca, which was during the 1930s and 50s a kind of architectural and urban laboratory whose experiments were mostly successful and have made this city a model of innovation. Nevertheless, the question 'is there an urban tradition in today's Morocco?' needs to be asked. The traditional city model has been abandoned, and its replacement is yet to be found; can Morocco invent new urban models that are adapted to the local context and that reinvest in the cultural wealth of the country?

Who does what?

The wish to establish a seamless planning system at all scales does not always correspond to the Moroccan reality, with projects split between those that are the result of government policies, such as shanty-town eradication or school-building plans, and the large urban schemes designed by international architects. This division can also be found in professional practice between mostly foreign consultants, in charge of masterplanning and large projects, and local ones that deal with more routine daily matters. Frequently, the large projects are commissioned by international investment groups while the other schemes are the result of either public initiative (the state or a local authority) or a private individual. All schemes need to be approved by the president of the municipal council or, in the case of large cities, the *Wali* (regional government), following the advice of the local planning agency.

In addition, Moroccans have realised that masterplanning – in particular, that involving large projects – positions them in the global market. The danger is that the contrast between large cities and small rural settlements will be widened, as well as the gap between rich and poor. This problem is obvious in the area around the Bouregreg project in the Casablanca region. Politicians are well aware that urban quality is essential in achieving sustainable development and improving the life of people, but they have difficulties in ensuring this quality.

Sustainability as a concept is now starting to be considered in some projects, but it remains to be seen whether concrete actions will follow, and especially whether a more sustainable lifestyle will be achieved in the new neighbourhoods. The traditional building methods in Morocco are based on a very efficient energy-saving know-how which needs to be applied once again. In addition, the level of awareness regarding natural risks (tsunamis, earthquakes, erosion, droughts) is lacking in current projects, and needs to be raised. Equally, social or economic issues are rarely taken into account in new projects. Without too much exaggeration, it can be said that these large projects seem to be based on a kind of dream city meant for the rich who work in service industries and spend their leisure in luxury shops or international shopping malls. There is therefore a substantial amount of work still to be done in order to reach the ideal of sustainable development as an integral part of a city for everybody.

CASABLANCA, A LABORATORY OF URBAN DESIGN

In contrast with other Moroccan cities, and because of its history, Casablanca is a model of architectural and urban innovation. Ever since the first Prost plan of the early 20th century plans have followed plans, enabling the city to evolve. Today, as the largest city and the economic capital of Morocco, Casablanca wishes to be a player on the global market scene. In order to become a 21st-century metropolis, it needs to respond to several challenges: how to envision its large urban projects? How to become a city for everybody? How to satisfy the needs of the population whilst enhancing the city's competitiveness? How to develop this new vision of the city, respecting its tradition and being 'modern' at the same time? To answer these questions, Casablanca has decided to prepare new planning documents (such as the Structure Plan, SDAU) in order to enhance the life of its population, and to implement a number of large schemes that will revitalise the skyline of the metropolis.

The new SDAU, presented to the king for signature in 2008, asserts the global positioning of Casablanca through the development of tertiary nodes, and attempts to make it a sustainable city. It establishes a regional polycentric armature and aims at achieving a balance between the city and its seafront, through a number of urban regeneration policies. To this end, it puts forward large mixed-use developments offering a new skyline and high-quality public space. Casablanca aims to project to the world an image of daring, innovation, sustainability and international urbanism.

Many new large schemes are emerging, particularly on the coast. In order to reinforce its appeal, the city has chosen to develop primarily the service, leisure and luxury retail sectors according to international standards. So new districts are being created, for example the Marina, Anfa 03-21 and the sustainable neighbourhoods at Sindibad; new strategic amenities, such as the CasArts theatre or the Morocco Mall shopping centre; or seaside resorts, such as Anfa Place. The proliferation of these new urban centralities with similar profiles seems risky, as they will have an impact on existing urban life and on neighbourhood shops.

Casablanca today is a collection of neighbourhoods with varying morphologies. The *medina*, the traditional Muslim city with a very characteristic form, is next to the European city, built between 1915 and 1940 with a radial plan and well-ordered and harmonious buildings. On the hill west of the city centre, the villas of the better off line up along large picturesque avenues and display examples of innovative 1950's architecture. Further out, residential areas for the middle classes and large social housing estates are located on the urban periphery.

Although some of the new schemes reinterpret the traditional Arab city (as is the case for CasArts or the Sindibad neighbourhoods) or follow the established morphology but not its architectural typologies (as in the case of the Marina), others, such as Morocco Mall, are breaking completely with their context, asserting their modernity and looking to the future. In addition, increasing numbers of high-rise towers are establishing new landmarks on the skyline. The SDAU has identified potential locations for these towers and suggested criteria for their contextualisation in terms of design, density, environmental quality and liveability.

A fundamental principle of urban design is that any new project needs to fit in the existing urban armature and respect the local identity. The Anfa 03-21 scheme positions itself within the existing structure in its own particular way: located on the site of an old airfield adjacent to existing neighbourhoods, it continues the urban structure, connects with its networks and respects the old airstrips. The scheme also gives top priority to the

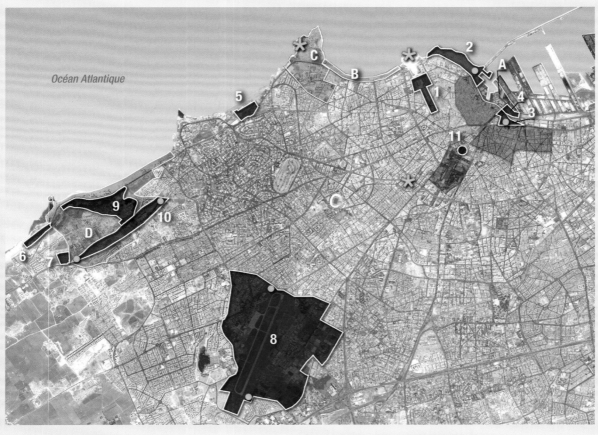

The large projects in the centre of Casablanca

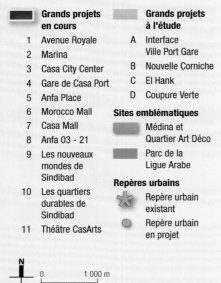

Grands projets en cours

1 Avenue Royale
2 Marina
3 Casa City Center
4 Gare de Casa Port
5 Anfa Place
6 Morocco Mall
7 Casa Mall
8 Anfa 03 - 21
9 Les nouveaux mondes de Sindibad
10 Les quartiers durables de Sindibad
11 Théâtre CasArts

Grands projets à l'étude

A Interface Ville Port Gare
B Nouvelle Corniche
C El Hank
D Coupure Verte

Sites emblématiques

Médina et Quartier Art Déco

Parc de la Ligue Arabe

Repères urbains

Repère urbain existant

Repère urbain en projet

0   1 000 m

quality of the public realm. As a new centre for the Casablanca metropolis, Anfa aims to be a symbol of the city's transformation. The new district will be an intense and attractive service centre including housing, major urban amenities, universities, retail units, parks and gardens, and a multimodal transport node with the arrival of a new TGV-style rail line. Its specific geographical character and the existing natural spaces have informed the design; the largest public space is based on the landing strips of the old airfield and is bookended by two towers that will be urban landmarks. The major institutions and the high-intensity activities will be located along this main symbolic axis, around which five neighbourhoods will be created or renewed, each one with its identity and form. A range of

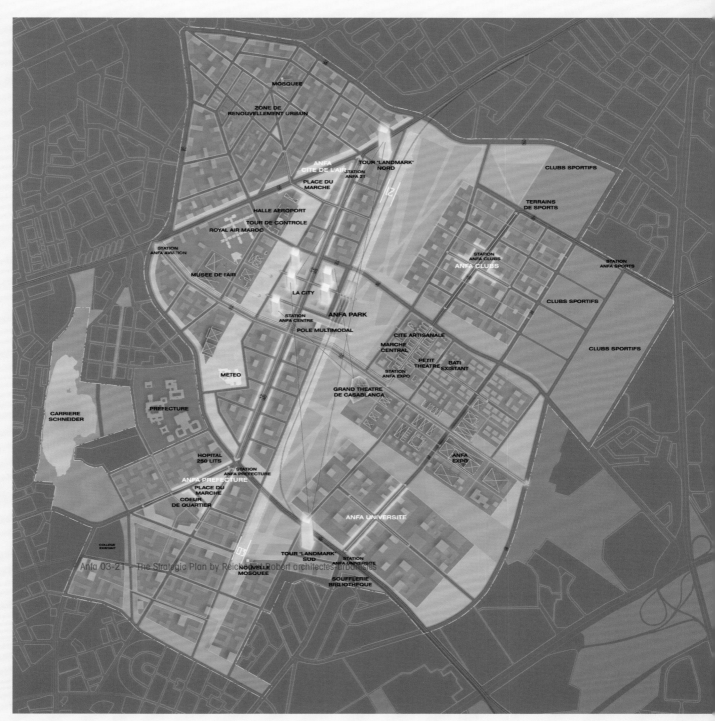

Anfa 03-21 – The Strategic Plan
by Reichen et Robert architectes-urbanistes

typologies adapted to the character of each of the parts and emphasising the role of open spaces has also been defined. Equally, the building heights are prescribed according to the area: the lower town adjacent to public spaces, 10.5 m; the middle town, introducing the concept of green roofs, 20 to 25 m; and the taller town with heights of 50 m for apartments and 150 m for offices.

In summary, the Anfa 03-21 project wants to be part of the new image of Casablanca, using international architectural models but adapting them to the local context. It aims to attract a wealthy clientele, predominantly from abroad, and is marketed accordingly. It hopes to help position Casablanca nationally and internationally within the 'circle' of global metropolises.

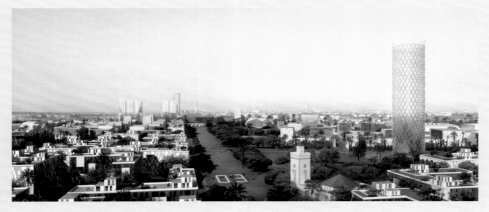

Anfa 03-21 – panoramic view,
Reichen et Robert architectes-urbanistes

Facts and figures for Anfa 03-21

CLIENT: *Agence d'urbanisation et de développement d'Anfa* (Auda), a branch of the *Caisse de Dépôt et de gestion du Maroc* (CDG)

MASTERPLANNER: Reichen et Robert & Associates, architectes-urbanistes

AREA (FORMER AIRPORT): 365 ha

PROGRAMME INCLUDES:

4,300,000 m² of commercial area

2,300,000 m² of housing (100,000 inhabitants)

1,300,000 m² of office space (100,000 jobs)

500,000 m² of metropolitan services

200,000 m² of local services

55 ha of parkland

78 ha of public spaces

In order to be attractive, Casablanca must also become a sustainable city where social and local issues are taken into account. Environmental concerns and the landscape cannot be ignored when designing a city, particularly along the coast. The large projects currently being proposed or developed assert the position of Casablanca as a service centre and give a contemporary and international image, but they also need to respect the existing population and the environment in which it is positioned. The challenge is whether these projects can really make it a city for everybody.

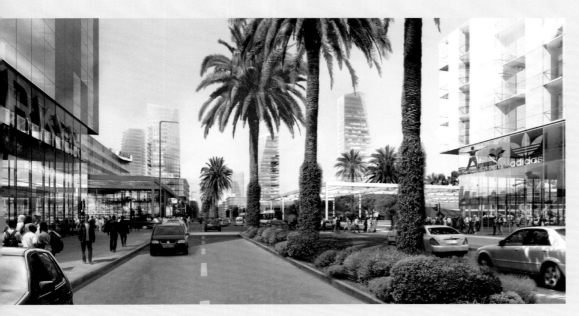

Anfa 03-21 – view of the future main street,
Reichen et Robert architectes-urbanistes

Morocco: a two-speed but evolving urbanism

To this day, the Moroccan city is divided. Its conception and design are implemented at three levels:

- The large urban projects, responding to an international elite
- The renewed neighbourhoods and the new towns, destined for the middle classes
- The shanty towns, for which there is no economic model that could assist their transformation and which are therefore difficult to change

These three different approaches to city creation can be complementary, but can also respond to conflicting objectives.

The large projects with global ambitions are conceived by international consultants, aimed at well-off international clients, and they need to show a 'brand' that can be recognised. Most of these schemes are located along the coast or in the centres of the main cities, and are approved without concern for the regulations, but they offer possibilities for high-quality urban design.

A more routine urbanism is the norm in the case of urban renewal, which aims at improving the life of the inhabitants. This is mostly the result of public initiatives, and includes the building of new towns and social housing schemes as well as the relocation of shanty towns and edge-of-town business parks, but also private individual developments. All these activities are subject to controls through the existing planning system, and involve a heavy bureaucratic management process that needs to be simplified. Fortunately, legislation is being revised in order to respond to practice, avoid derogations and take a more holistic approach than hitherto. It is to be hoped that this will lead to a real change in practice.

Mentalities and methods of work also need to be changed at every level – professional, administrative and political – as a city with two different faces can no longer be acceptable. Creativity must be applied equally to the ordinary city, to urban renewal and to resolving social problems. The fact that the city's global image and appeal are given by all of its constituent parts, and that the population is an essential contributor to them, needs to be understood. Therefore the methods applied to the large urban projects must also be applied to the routine management of the city, whilst at the same time maintaining a strategic, global and coherent view for the long term. Ad hoc management of a succession of large projects that are subject to investment market fluctuations and in competition against each other is not the way to build a city. Innovation in urban design could help create a city that is not just global but also continues the Moroccan urban tradition.

A quick guide to
Morocco

1 TYPES OF CLIENT

For large-scale plans, the city authorities (*communes*) and the *Agences Urbaines*

In some cases, the *Caisse des Dépôts et de Gestion du Maroc* (public financial institution)

For major development schemes (*grands projets*), the *Agences Urbaines* and private developers (international development groups).

....

2 TYPES OF PROJECT/WORK

Large-scale plans
- Structure plans and urban development plans
- Masterplans for *grands projets* and urban regeneration
- Transport plans
- New towns

Design guidelines
- Urban and architectural codes
- Conservation plans for the *medinas*

....

3 APPROACH NEEDED TO WORK IN COUNTRY

Partnership with a local firm is compulsory

An international competition is, in most cases, the way to obtain a commission

International tenders are frequent, and a partnership between local and international firms is the best way to respond to them

Contact with the mayor and/or the head of the regional administration is advisable

Some small jobs can be negotiated directly, either with the local authority or in cases where a developer chooses a designer

....

4 LEGISLATION THAT NEEDS TO BE REFERRED TO

National Land Management Plan (Snat)

Regional Structure Plans: *Schéma Directeur et d'Aménagement Urbain* (SDAU)

Local Plans

Urban Transport Plans (PDU)

....

SPECIFIC TIPS
FOR SUCCESS

Checking the launch of international tenders is important, as the *Agences Urbaines* are outsourcing much of their design work

The following is a warning, rather than a tip:
Not long ago a French consultant in association with a Moroccan one won the tender for the *Schéma directeur* of Marrakech; as their work was deemed unsatisfactory, the contract was cancelled and a new tender launched; this was won by a Korean group in partnership with a Moroccan consultant

6 USEFUL WEBSITES

Ministry of housing, urbanism and the city/Ministre de l'Habitat, de l'Urbanisme et de la Politique de la Ville: www.marocurba.gov.ma

Moroccan Order of Architects: www.ordrearchitectes.ma

SELECTED FACTS

1	area	446,550 km²
2	population	31,951,412
3	annual population growth	1.0%
4	urban population	57%
5	population density	72 p/km²
6	GDP	$90,804,562,196
7	GNI per capita	$2,850

Source: The World Bank (2010)

SOUTH AFRICA

Liezel Kruger, *architect and urban designer*

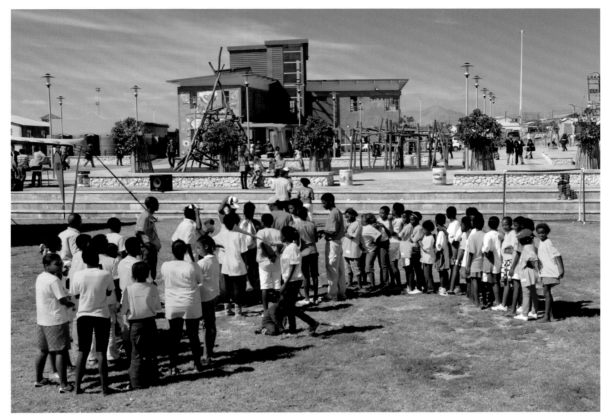

Harare Urban Park I with the Active Box in the background

South Africa is a parliamentary republic with a written constitution; the positions of head of state and head of government are merged in a parliament-dependent president. The country is known for its diversity of cultures and languages: 11 official languages are recognised in the constitution. It is one of the founding members of the African Union, and has the largest economy of all the AU members.

South Africa is divided into nine provinces, 47 districts and 245 municipalities. It has three capitals: Cape Town, the oldest, is the legislative capital and the seat of parliament; Pretoria is the administrative capital and the seat of the president and the cabinet; and Bloemfontein is the judicial capital and seat of the supreme court of appeal.

South Africa can be described as a developing country still experiencing growing pains, having had a much shorter time than European nations to adapt to changes in technology, immigration and politics. In order to understand the position and role of urban design in South Africa, the social and political context as well as the urban morphology within which it has to function must first be explained.

Founded in 1652 by the Dutch, who established Cape Town as a refreshment station, South Africa can be described as a nation of immigrants – both white and black. Great Britain took over the management of the Cape in 1795, colonising it in 1806. The Union of South Africa was established in 1910, granted independence from Britain in 1931 and became an independent republic in 1961, when it also left the Commonwealth. In 1994, the country took a whole new direction when Nelson Mandela became president and sealed the end of apartheid.

Urban development is localised mainly around four geographical areas: Cape Town, Port Elizabeth, Durban and Pretoria/Johannesburg. Beyond these four economic centres, development is less significant and poverty is, despite government efforts, still widespread. The availability of land and a long history of segregation and migrant labour have led to an urban environment characterised by dispersed low-density settlements. Current patterns include on the one hand ex-colonial elements in city cores, and on the other suburban developments, towns and large informal settlements known as townships. The last-named are laid out in distinct and fragmented cells, isolated from each other by roads or ill-defined spaces, usually along some type of grid structure.

Formal townships, which result from providing informal settlements with services and gradually transforming them, are one of the most significant factors in urban growth in South Africa. They mostly house migrant labour, and grew initially in the 1950s and 60s on urban fringes. In the 1970s and 80s, as a result of apartheid, segregated urban areas known as 'homelands' followed, together with the unparalleled growth of informal settlements (squatter camps) around large urban centres. This meant that the poorest people were located furthest from economic opportunities, whilst the wealthiest enjoyed preferential access to transport networks and urban amenities.

The context for urban design

The main function of urban design in South Africa today is to assist the urban transformation of the country's historical and political legacy. This distinguishes South Africa from most other countries, as the challenge is to generate integrated communities from those that were once segregated. Segregation resulted in towns where communities were established on the basis of culture, race and income. The objective now is to make cities equitable and sustainable for all.

In 1994, the newly elected South African government of Nelson Mandela and the African National Congress (ANC) recognised the need to introduce enlightened policies concerning land, housing, employment, education and equality. However, the settlement patterns originally shaped by historical forces remain largely unchanged, and as a result extreme disparities in degrees of access to land, adequate services and housing still exist. It is unfortunate that the majority of settlements continue to grow and develop following historical patterns, and resist the introduction or influence of new policies. The result is ever-increasing unsustainable low-density sprawl on the urban edges.

The shortage of affordable housing in appropriate locations has meant that the building of new housing for low-income communities has become a priority for the country. New settlements are for the most part built even further from city

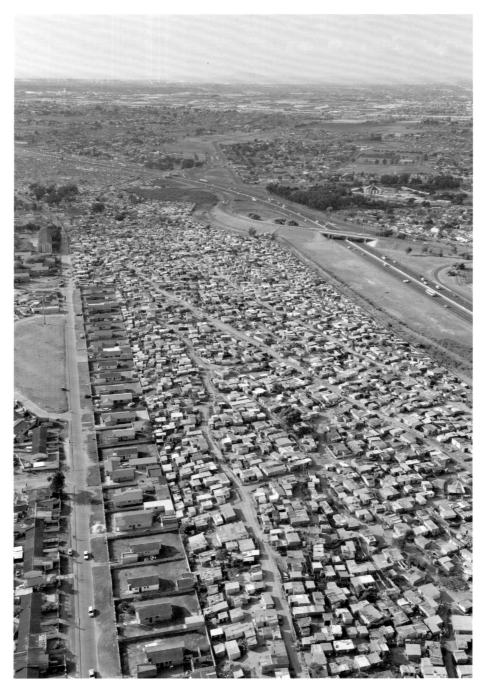

Informal settlements with shacks built from corrugated iron and wood.
Next to them are new houses: the aspiration

centres than before, and on open land on the periphery rather than on underutilised brownfield sites. The urgent need and demand for formal housing, seen as a basic human right, is a main reason for this, fuelled by the incredibly high levels of migration from the rural areas to cities. Whilst the objective of the production of new housing is the removal of informal settlements, this is rarely achieved because movement from the latter to new housing stock is followed by the occupation of the vacated informal housing by new urban migrants. Overall the poor are the ones most affected by these changes, and the settlement patterns generate unsustainable movement patterns.

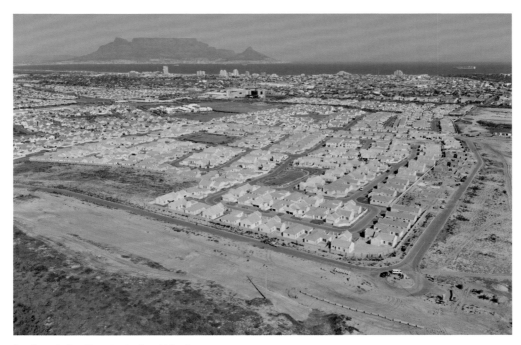

Developers' offer of housing for the middle classes

Another form of housing self-provision widespread in South Africa's low-income settlements is the building of temporary structures in backyards, in order to provide additional accommodation and rental income for the main owner. These structures are mostly illegal and difficult to regulate or to service. Government-provided low-cost housing aims to prevent this activity by positioning houses on plots in a way that makes it impossible to build additional accommodation. This type of urban building appears nevertheless to be a significant part of the hidden economy, and is probably no different from what happened in the past in first-world countries. The main problem in South Africa is that unregulated building, using poor-quality materials, creates health and safety hazards – especially that of fires, which regularly displace thousands of people and render them homeless.

At another end of the social spectrum, sprawling suburban housing developments alongside large shopping malls are spread throughout the country. Unfortunately, this is also the dream model for those in lower income groups who demand the same unsustainable typology, the single-storey dwelling located in the middle of the plot and defended by walls. This is what people expect, and what the market demands and delivers. Higher-density affordable housing, built as two-storey maisonettes or three-storey walk-ups, is frowned upon by the lower income groups for it still sparks memories of apartheid-era flats with limited space, overcrowding and inadequate services. Such negative emotional links with a sustainable urban form hampers the establishment of higher-density nodes for lower income groups closer to resources and access to public transport.

Market forces dictate the design process in other instances as well. As crime in South Africa is a major issue, those that can afford it choose to live in secure complexes surrounded by high walls and electric fences, which they perceive to be safer. Houses in sought-after 'security villages' often appreciate in value more than free-standing dwellings nearby. Developers know this, and as a result this is likely to remain the

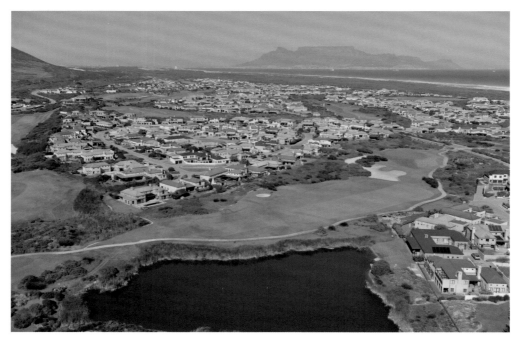

One of the many security villages, in this case with a golf course as an additional amenity

residential model of choice for the foreseeable future. Instead of trying to resist the security-village concept, planners and designers may be better advised to minimise its impact on the environment, by, for instance, encouraging 'green' permeable fencing rather than continuous solid walls.

With limited budgets and a challenging political context, public-sector investment focuses on the essentials: improving quality of life through better housing provision, and to some extent upgrading the public realm in order to first make it safer rather than necessarily beautiful. Water, for instance, is a basic necessity, and cannot be used as a 'mere' art feature in a public space.

Having these issues in mind, and in order to be effective, South African urban designers have to create frameworks or structures within which to apply good practice. Achieving this within a system that is geared towards service delivery is a lengthy process, but success stories are increasing and mindsets are gradually changing. The greatest impact of urban designers is seen in the upgrading of the public realm and through their campaign for awareness of context and design, which aims to halt the mere subdivision of any available land.

Unfortunately, a democratic country within a developing context has to deal with political challenges and propaganda, which can result in the delay of many well-designed initiatives. Service strikes and vandalism of property are still frequently used as legitimate tools to demand action. This can make the consultation or participation process very difficult to handle. To put this in context, South Africa has 11 official languages, various political alliances and one of the highest levels of illegal immigration in the world. Here, the mediation or facilitation role of the urban designer can and is skilfully being used to improve what is perceived to be public: the revitalisation or, in many cases, the creation of the public realm. Success lies in its principle-based approach, which echoes the needs and desires of the local population.

Definitions and the status of urban design

> Urban Design is at the same time a specialised and an overarching, integrating profession aimed at joining the various natural and built form professions in achieving good quality places for people to live, work and play in.
> (UDISA, Urban Design Institute of South Africa's website)

Within a South African context, the unique focus of urban design lies in facilitation; it has a developmental role in a rapidly changing, post-apartheid society and aims to create a better-quality living environment for all. Urban design is perceived as an emerging, specialist profession whose members mediate between the various scales of the urban environment and influence the planning system through the creativity acquired by an architectural education. Because urban design is as much a process as a product, it requires knowledge and skills in decision making, and an understanding and shaping of the interaction between people and places, and between the natural and the built environments. Urban designers can offer awareness and understanding of contexts: the landscapes, the needs and dynamics of society, the fundamentals of economy and the three-dimensional form of place and space.

The practice of urban design is based on principles. The first of these is the promotion of the public good. The second, sometimes overlapping principle, is the enhancement of property values through investment in the public environment. In practice this translates into the improvement of public space as an element of dignified social enrichment, offering a sense of belonging, safety and community; and into the preparation of large-scale spatial frameworks as key structuring guidelines for future growth. As a result, both the public and private sectors can use this principle-based approach and need not be in competition with each other. There is, however, a tug of war between the needs and wishes of developers and those of the authorities trying to achieve an outcome acceptable to all.

The planning process is mostly led by town planners, engineers and land surveyors; each one of these disciplines comes laden with its own value system and operates within a political context. Increasingly, the urban designer plays a facilitating role in bringing the various professions together by applying good principles in order to help structure both large-scale frameworks and smaller precinct plans, and to promote a human scale for building projects and site development plans.

Currently no South African legislation relates explicitly to urban design. Zoning and subdivision dominate the planning process; the built form and the context are secondary to regulations and property rights. The perceptions of developers and authorities are often in conflict, and there is neither a vision for urban areas nor for urban design guidance. Nevertheless, although not made explicit urban design principles underlie a good part of the legislation. Publications such as Design for Safer Environments, by the Council for Scientific and Industrial Research (CSIR), or Breaking New Ground, a housing policy document, are essentially urban design documents aimed at improving quality. Environmental and transport legislation is also starting to incorporate urban design principles, coordinating the various elements of the public realm.

The request for development frameworks supported by urban design guidance and a package of plans (hierarchy of scales) is becoming more frequent. In this way planning and design issues are being addressed, such as integration with the context, physical development constraints and opportunities, density standards, heritage, environmental resources, and standards for the provision of services infrastructure. In addition, the demand for a more transparent way of dealing with planning applications reinforces the need for local authorities to have clear urban design guidelines. To this extent, the City of Cape Town, the local authority for the Cape Town metropolitan area, is in the process of developing its own guidelines that aim to integrate urban design principles into decisions taken by land-use management officials. This should serve as an important example for other local authorities and provide much-needed alignment between urban design aims and land-use management decision making.

Sustainability

Although the South African planning system is not yet fully equipped to deal with the major urban challenges of a developing nation, a very positive national policy framework has been established for moving towards sustainable design practice. As part of the discourse on sustainability, South Africa has successfully organised and prepared for the Conference of the Parties (COP17) Climate Change talks that took place in Durban in late 2011.

What is missing, aside from specific emissions targets, is the education of the local authority personnel responsible for approving planning applications. Although national policy supports sustainable design, local guidelines and standards often contradict this and need to be updated. Innovative planning and design practices, more responsive to the requirements of sustainable urbanisation, are also needed. One of the tasks of urban designers is to motivate authorities to adopt sustainable designs.

As sustainability covers a broad spectrum of issues – transport, energy, water, etc – a variety of approaches is also needed. One initiative currently being proposed by the CSIR and the Council for the Built Industry (CBE) is mandatory energy efficiency education for government officials, aimed at replacing the culture of urban sprawl by the adoption of integrated and energy-efficient urban development. This means not only investing in alternative energies, innovative materials and smart technologies when designing or retrofitting buildings, but also carefully considering land allocation. Recent examples of innovative initiatives include the Kuyasa Project in Cape Town, Africa's first Clean Development Mechanism project, which will be scaled up to a National Sustainable Development Facility (NSDF); and the Integrated Energy Environment Empowerment – Cost Optimised (iEEECO) project taking place in Atlantis, a town 50 km north of Cape Town.

Although no specific legislation is yet in place in respect of 'green' building requirements, the Green Building Handbook provides practical advice on design, technologies and materials, and on the environmental impact of buildings, offering solutions relevant to the South African context. The focus of this manual is primarily on energy and resource efficiency and on environmental responsibility, and it includes the ways in which buildings are used after completion. The implementation of the green buildings concept is still evolving, and it is being promoted by a monthly e-journal which provides news and information regarding green building both locally and internationally (www.alive2green.com) and shows the links with other elements such as transport, energy, water and waste.

In this connection, the annual Green Building Conference and Exhibition, established in 2007 and showcasing green building products and services, offers to South African participants presentations from the world's leading experts, and innovative design charrettes centred on the notion of collaborative design and giving an opportunity to apply theory to a practical example.

South African urban areas are growing at an alarming rate and the need for viable and sustainable mobility and energy solutions has never been greater. A radical rethink of how to transport people and goods is a top priority, and regulations concerning emissions, safety and efficiency have already been introduced. Now the aim is to increase mobility capacity while reducing pollution, time spent travelling and the transporting of energy. Transit Oriented Development (TOD), not a new concept but one that has not been applied with any conviction in South Africa, is being debated in the context of city planning and densification, particularly around activity nodes and corridors.

An example of this is the densification strategy for the metropolitan area of Cape Town (not including the rural areas), which supplements the Spatial Development Strategy for Cape Town. It identifies nodes that have the potential to serve a multitude of objectives, not least to optimise transport operations and steer private property investment in directions that support community development objectives, and ultimately contribute to the overall objectives of sustainability. In the absence of incentives, there is a long way to go to make transport and mobility truly sustainable. For the time being, the decision-making processes of the various organisations dealing with transport lack coordination and guidelines. Some success stories can be found in the newly introduced Bus Rapid Transport system in Cape Town and the Gautrain in Johannesburg.

Another major sustainability issue in South Africa is sensible water management. Clean water, or the lack of it, is a crucial contributor to the quality of life of the population. Yet in many regions water has been consistently wasted and overused, and there is a real danger that in the next few years some areas could run out of water and become deserts. Sustainability experts Alive2green cc have produced a manual, the Sustainable Water Resource Handbook, that focuses on issues, policies and solutions related to the water sector. Everything from water uses to waste-water treatments, water in agriculture and mining, as well as the urban and rural environments are being looked at in order to understand the true status of what is available and how it is used. Alive2green 'embraces the notion of "sustainability by design" and as such seeks to give inspiration by creating platforms that enable leading designers to share their insights and achievements. Design technologies are imperative for the growth of every sector' (www.waterresource.co.za).

In addition, the Water Research Commission of South Africa is a national body that aims to find solutions to issues such as provision of water for all, and a sustainable environment – all essential parts of the country's priorities. Finally, the National Water Act of 1998 and the related national water strategy emphasise the importance of good water management and call for research support.

Academic discipline and the discourse
of urban design in South Africa

South African universities are currently restructuring their academic programmes, and the role of urban design is a very contentious topic. The University of Cape Town (UCT) and the Witwatersrand University (WITS) have two very different approaches to the subject.

UCT's urban design school developed through the thinking of Professors Uytenbogaardt and Dewar, who promoted the principle of integration (a socialist approach) within an apartheid-driven planning environment. The UCT school had generally only admitted architectural students. In their South African Cities: A Manifesto for Change (Dewar and Uytenbogaardt 1991), the main lecturers developed an approach to urban design based on the knowledge they had acquired at the Pennsylvania School of Design, and it became the backbone of most of South Africa's urban design philosophy. This approach is now dated, and although many of the principles are still valid, a new direction is essential in order to remain relevant. The UCT school is therefore restructuring its courses, taking into account the current academic debate on how integrated or unique urban design as a profession should be.

The other main institution offering a postgraduate course in urban design, the WITS in Johannesburg, has a broader approach, attracting members of other professions such as planners to their courses. The outcome is a more process- and policy-orientated urban designer, more suitable for the demands of public service and monitoring the development process.

Research in urban design is limited in South Africa, where basic needs still drive development and the budgets of educational institutions are already under strain. There is no specific body of research dealing with urban design, but the establishment in 2007 of the African Centre for Cities (ACC), with sponsorship from UCT amongst others, is a new and positive development. The ACC 'seeks to facilitate critical urban research and policy discourses for the promotion of vibrant, democratic and sustainable urban development in the global South perspective'.

ACC's predecessor, the policy-driven Urban Problems Research Unit (UPRU), was established in the mid-1970s in connection with UCT: the unit's approach to design was influenced by some of its members' education in Europe and the USA, which they applied to South Africa. Its publications, in turn, influenced future generations of the country's urban designers.

Another research organisation, the Council for Scientific and Industrial Research's Urban and Regional Planning research group, aims to make a contribution towards the sustainable development of cities, towns and regions and towards the enhancement of the quality of life.

Changes in the profession

South African urban designers are starting to differentiate themselves as a stand-alone profession of city makers who have studied design for a minimum of six years. The current debate is about whether urban design should be narrowly or widely defined, bearing in mind that a common understanding of the principles of city making by all professionals is still needed.

In the last few decades, and similarly to other countries, South African planning has moved from large-scale 'city beautiful' masterplans to a more principle-driven approach which results in a process driven by a 'package of plans' and frameworks. Lately, smaller towns and municipalities throughout the country are following the example of larger cities in specifically drafting urban design frameworks for growth. Thus, a better understanding of urban design is spreading to many more communities than hitherto.

A new wave of urban design practice is also generated by professionals who have been studying or working abroad, and are now returning and applying their experience to the specific South African context. They have joined with local colleagues to establish the Urban Design Institute of South Africa (UDISA), a voluntary, non-profit association of urban designers and associate members. Its aim is 'to promote greater public awareness of the value of and need for urban design as well as developing the educational, institutional and professional capacity and potential' of urban designers throughout South Africa.

UDISA is currently engaged in discussions with the South African Council for the Architectural Profession (SACAP) concerning its formal recognition as a voluntary organisation. This is the first step towards becoming a professional organisation, and could lead to the recognition of urban design under the Architectural Profession Act. These discussions highlight the issue of where the correct 'home' for urban designers is, and contribute to a government initiative of formalising professional bodies through their identification of key areas of specialisation and responsibility.

Urban designers work in both the private and the public sectors. Most are employed by planning consultants offering urban design expertise, but architectural/urban design practices are also growing. The public sector does have some limited in-house urban design expertise, but consultants are usually appointed to assist with projects.

In summary, South Africa is striving to create sustainable, high-quality settlements and at the same time to meet the challenges of urbanisation and addressing the legacy of segregation and economic exclusion. The skills of urban designers are therefore an essential resource. But while South African urban designers are ready to meet the challenges of city making, they cannot fully resolve the issue of sustainable growth while unrestricted immigration results in the spread of illegal settlements. Not only do these settlements create the impression that South Africa does not care about its citizens, but they also put great pressure on local resources. This constant expansion – resulting out of necessity, but also a type of profiteering through land claims – limits the possibility of creating urban places that will be valued by their users in a way that the inhabitants of European or American cities understand it. Because of these challenges, the impact of good urban design can be greater in South Africa than in other countries. Fortunately, its value is now being recognised not only by built environment professionals but also by politicians, business leaders and the wider community.

CASE STUDY

VIOLENCE PROTECTION THROUGH URBAN UPGRADE IN KHAYELITSHA

Violence Protection through Urban Upgrade (VPUU, www.vpuu.org) is a systemic approach to neighbourhood improvement currently run in Khayelitsha, Cape Town. It is a public–private collaboration between the local authority of Cape Town and the German Development Bank, which aims to deal with key concerns such as safety and the legacy of restructuring cities in a very challenging environment. Other partners from governmental organisations, civil society and the private sector are involved, and community participation is actively sought. It is implemented by a Consortium of AHT Group AG, its South African Partner SUN Development and a host of other partners in cooperation with the VPUU unit of the City of Cape Town.

Khayelitsha, or 'new home' in native Xhosa, is a large, predominantly black African area of Cape Town, about 30 km from the city centre. It has an estimated population of 600,000 inhabitants living in an area of approximately 2,300 ha. Problems of violence, safety, inadequate service provision, illegal immigration, squatting and low incomes have led to a dysfunctional urban environment which deprives its residents of dignity.

The aim of this programme is to combine crime prevention with the restructuring of the built fabric. It incorporates and promotes the support of local organisations to take ownership of public spaces and create so-called Safe Node Areas where communities can interact and engage in a safe environment. In doing so, they help support the local authority's integrated planning, budgeting and implementation of projects. The strategy in turn informs individual interventions, and utilises local people and their skills as resources.

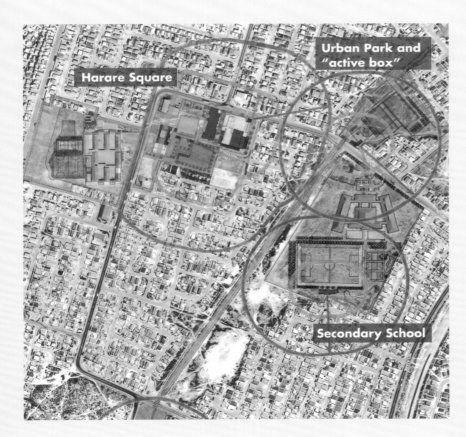

The Violence Protection through Urban Upgrade area

A package of plans (from precinct plan to site plan, to building plan) is utilised in order to ensure a clear understanding of the various scales of design, and to address community issues such as crime at each of these scales. The work starts with an analysis of the current situation and is carried out by urban designers, social development and local economic experts, public participation experts, and professionals who understand the multidimensional character of space in a specific neighbourhood context. The baseline information helps developing an area-based community action plan – a strategy to transform a 'dormitory' into a thriving neighbourhood. From a wider urban management perspective, the programme aims at the establishment of financial viable neighbourhoods that can stand on their own.

Crime prevention through good design assumes that positive changes in the physical environment ultimately lead to safer communities. Safety principles and design guidelines for development in low-income neighbourhoods include: 'eyes on the street'; 'owned' space, enabling community participation; clear edges and good lighting for public spaces; well-defined access routes, especially for pedestrians; and good management. In the South African context, this addresses not only the physical aspects of the neighbourhood but also the social aspects of community life, and it aims at giving people dignity.

Specific tools are used to increase safety, such as clear and legible signage, a series of landmark buildings or so-called 'activity boxes' along defined walking routes, and direct-movement routes for walking and cycling safely. They also include the clustering of public activities around public spaces, and active edges and landscaping that reinforce a legible urban structure and encourage the enjoyment of the public realm.

The urban design framework includes several precinct plans: a recreational precinct with playing fields and informal play spaces, a commercial precinct set around Harare Square and a predominantly infill-housing precinct. These are all connected by a pedestrian route that runs diagonally through the grid structure, linking the

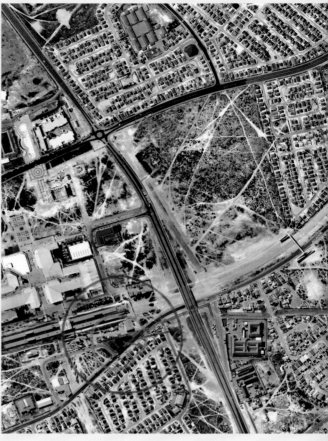

Map showing the location of Harare Square

various areas of activity. Within the wider area, two specific urban design projects are emerging: Harare Square, currently being implemented, and a multipurpose urban park.

Harare Square is a multi-use, multipurpose public space offering services, shops and businesses to local residents in partnership with public, private and non-governmental organisation (NGO) partners, making it the centre of the neighbourhood. Good lighting and 24-hour activity makes this square a safe space that the community can utilise day and night. As the square isn't located on an access route, it had to develop as a destination by attracting uses identified in the Community Action Plan's vision – namely, a space for youth and business. This vision has been implemented through the following:

- A house of learning, which includes a library, an early childhood resource centre, adult-based learning facilities, a caretaker's flat, offices and a community hall. This building incorporates local and provincial departments as well as the Carnegie Corporation.

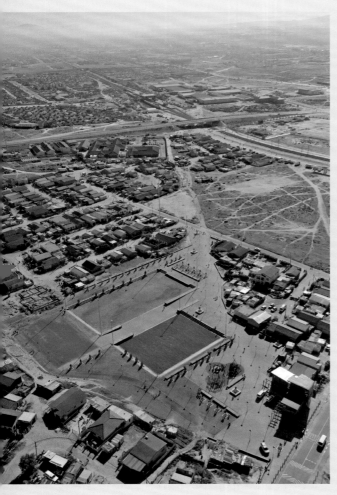
Harare Park seen from the air

an opportunity to generate income whilst living above the ground floor commercial premises, a liberating opportunity in these lower-income areas. The buildings also help to define the public space and offer surveillance on to the square at night.

- A business hub that includes a bulk-buying cooperative for the local convenient stores (*spaza* shops), a business support and advice office, 15 shops for local businesses, a bakery/cafe and an indoor sport facility.
- A three-storey building (known as an Active Box) that provides offices for a local organisation, a caretaker's flat, and a room for surveillance patrols.
- A supermarket.

The mix of uses enables sufficient income streams to allow an effective urban management that employs local residents. The result is a communalisation rather than a privatisation of public space.

The Harare Urban Park is an example of the transformation of a badly managed area (in this case, a storm-water retention pond) from a crime hotspot into a well-managed urban park. Through highly participative processes, the design meets the needs of local residents – recreational areas for various ages, sport facilities, community spaces and opportunities for infill housing are provided.

The process attracted the attention of the international football federation, FIFA, and led to the opening of a Football for Hope Centre. The urban design branch of the city council was able to

- The renovation of a dilapidated building to become a youth centre, including computer rooms and a career-advice centre, in partnership with the largest youth NGO in South Africa – loveLife.
- Live–work units that offer local entrepreneurs

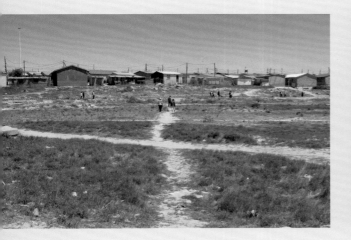

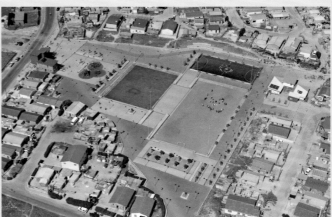

LEFT: Harare Urban Park before improvements
RIGHT: Harare Urban park after improvements

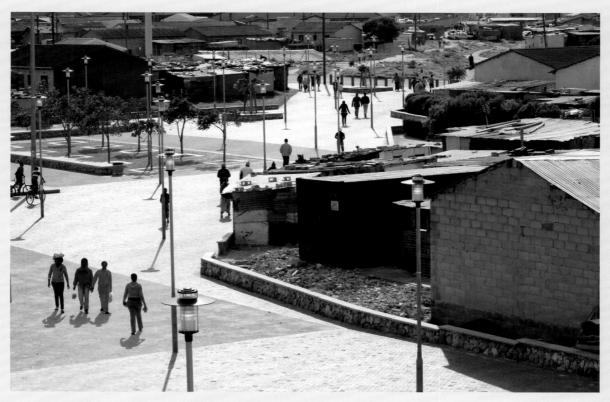

Harare Urban Park is now the core of a safe neighbourhood

convince FIFA to participate in the community-led process and adhere to the locally developed safety guidelines, and by doing so improve the passive surveillance and activities in the park.

Two years after completion, and in spite of the deliberate lack of fencing for any of the buildings, no vandalism has occurred and the trees are well rooted. This proves that the local community has taken ownership of the space, and illustrates the benefits of good landscaping, of creating local jobs and of volunteers guarding the project.

The VPUU programme offers a large-scale example of the way in which urban designers operate in South Africa, and its approach has been replicated in many smaller projects. Having identified the problems, these projects apply urban design principles of safety, involve the community and promote a dignified living for lower income groups. The initial programme was due to last for five years, ending in 2010; four years into the programme, its successes drew the attention of the United Nations. As a result, it has now been extended for another five years and rolled out to additional areas with

the support of Cape Town, the national treasury, the German Development Bank and the federal German ministry for economic development and cooperation, and the residents of the sprawling township themselves. A resource book that explains the process, the experiences and the lessons learned that can be applied to other projects is currently being drafted.

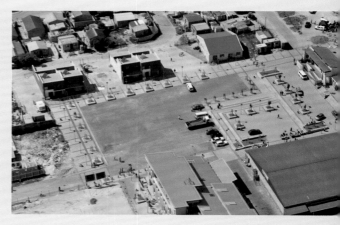

Harare Square: well used as a result of the mix of hard and soft landscape

Case study: Violence Protection through Urban Upgrade in Khayelitsha ~ **SOUTH AFRICA**

A quick guide to
South Africa

1 TYPES OF CLIENT

Local authority or other public bodies

Private developers, local or international

....

2 TYPES OF
PROJECT/WORK

Urban renewal

New communities

Urban extension

Informal settlements

Public space upgrade

Design guidelines

Input towards a variety of schemes, from rural settlement designs to the formulation of design briefs for development (see UDISA website, opposite)

....

3 APPROACH NEEDED
TO WORK IN COUNTRY

There is a determined effort to undo the economic legacy of apartheid through laws governing employment and procurement processes that give preference to historically marginalised population groups

Professionals must be registered in the country

....

4 LEGISLATION
THAT NEEDS TO BE
REFERRED TO

Development planning in general – and spatial planning in particular – is undergoing a process of re-evaluation in post-apartheid South Africa. The principal legislative elements guiding and informing planning are:

The Constitution of the Republic of South Africa (Act 108 of 1996)

National planning policy and legislation
- The Draft Spatial Planning and Land Use Management Bill, 2011
- Others:
  - The National Spatial Development Perspective (NSDP)
  - Comprehensive Plan for the Development of Sustainable Human Settlements (2004)
  - The National Environmental Management Act
  - National Heritage Resources Act
  - The White Paper on South Africa Land Policy (1997)
  - The Green Paper on Development and Planning
  - Municipal Systems Act 32 of 2000, which establishes a framework for planning, performance management systems, effective use of resources and organisational change in local municipalities

Provincial government policy and legislation, each of the nine provinces has its own legislation
- The Provincial Growth and Development Strategy
- Land Use Planning Ordinance (LUPO), 1985
- Provincial Spatial Development Frameworks

Local government policy and legislation – in direct relation to the provincial policy and legislation
- Land Use Management System (LUMS)
- Integrated Development Plan
- Spatial Development Framework
- Black Communities Development Act (Act 4 of 1984)
- The Planning Professions Act (Act 36 of 2002)
- Existing zoning schemes
- Environmental Management Frameworks
- Area management schemes

5 SPECIFIC TIPS FOR SUCCESS

Accept an informal approach to transactions

Ensure local employment opportunities and empowerment

Understand local context and traditions

Ensure participation with local communities and political parties

Plan for low-cost building methods and materials

6 USEFUL WEBSITES

African Centre for Cities: www.africancentreforcities.net

Alive2green: www.alive2green.com

Council for Scientific and Industrial Research (CSIR): www.csir.co.za

South African Association of Consulting Professional Planners: www.saacpp.org.za

South African Institute of Architects: www.saia.org.za

South African Planners: www.saplanners.org.za

South African Planning Institute: www.sapi.org.za

Urban Design Institute of South Africa (UDISA): www.urbandesigninstitute.co.za

SELECTED FACTS

#		
1	area	1,219,912 km²
2	population	49,991,300
3	annual population growth	-0.4%
4	urban population	62%
5	population density	41 p/km²
6	GDP	$363,703,902,727
7	GNI per capita	$6,090

Source: The World Bank (2010)

SECTION 3

ASIA

CHINA

Matthias Bauer, *urban designer*

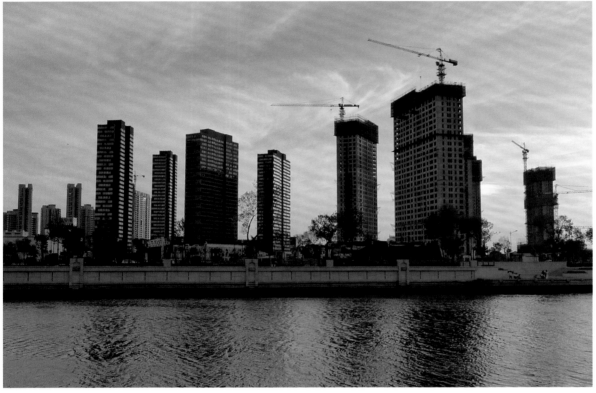

Typical apartment towers under construction in Tianjin, northern China.
High-rise developments like this may be just as likely to appear in the city
centre (as in this case), in the suburbs or in new towns and satellite cities

THE PEOPLE'S REPUBLIC OF CHINA is the world's most
populous country and its second-largest by land area. It comprises 22 provinces,
five autonomous regions, four municipalities and two special administrative regions
(Hong Kong and Macau). The political system is dominated by the 80-million-
member-strong Communist Party of China (CPC).

State power is exercised through the National People's Congress (NPC), the
president, and the state council. Local government is divided into provincial, prefecture
or municipality, or county or township level – with elections only taking place at the
lowest level. The government leadership is represented in two parallel ways: on one
hand the leader of the local People's Government (the mayor), and on the other hand
the local party chief or party secretary of the Communist party.

Urban planning and design projects are usually handled by planning authorities
at the local level, ie by the district or municipal government in urban areas, or by the
county or township government in rural areas. Certain projects such as important

tourism resorts may be handled at the provincial level, while the central government, for example in the shape of the National Development and Reform Commission, only engages in planning for exceptional cases such as pilot and model projects.

Definitions

Urban design tasks in China can encompass the design of a new town for half a million people in a couple of weeks, or a central business district (CBD) in two months. Urban design projects can cover entire counties or districts, and range from Spanish-style villas to cutting-edge high-tech business parks. Projects often measure several square kilometres in size. Urban design in China is certainly different from elsewhere, but defining it is not easy.

In the Chinese language urban design is called *chéngshì shèjì*, which literally means city design as opposed to *chéngshì guīhuà* meaning city planning. The planning process in China starts with strategic plans for very large areas – entire cities, urban districts or rural counties. The results of these planning efforts are large-scale regulatory land-use plans, which are far too large and too abstract to be easily translated into development schemes – let alone architectural designs. This is where urban design steps in: in China, urban design is the essential tool for bridging the huge gap between large-scale urban planning on one hand and the architectural design of individual buildings on the other.

The professional place of urban design

Most urban design practitioners have an architectural qualification or, to a lesser extent, a background in urban planning or landscape architecture. Engineers (including transport, environmental and sustainability experts) are rarely found among them. Urban design is still a very young profession in China, but an increasing number of university graduates with urban design degrees – often from foreign universities – are creating a distinctive professional group. There is, however, no official organisation or institution for urban designers, and most practitioners seek formal recognition as registered architects or registered urban planners.

The discipline

Urban design is also a young academic discipline. The most renowned courses are offered by those Chinese elite universities already well known for either their architecture or their planning degrees, such as Tongji University in Shanghai, Tsinghua University in Beijing and South-East University in Nanjing. Professor Wang Jianguo, dean of the school of architecture at South-East University, has emerged as China's most renowned urban design scholar.

In addition to the universities, the China Academy of Urban Planning and Design (CAUPD) has been established under the jurisdiction of the ministry of construction, and acts as a national institution for scientific research. The most famous classic texts, such as the works of Kevin Lynch and Jane Jacobs, are reasonably well known among professionals and are available in Chinese translation. Current trends and buzzwords in the profession – from 'Transit-oriented developments' to 'Landscape urbanism' – quickly find their way to China and are readily absorbed, though not necessarily well understood.

Legal status

While urban planning and architectural design are strictly controlled by Chinese planning laws and regulations, urban design occupies something of a grey area. The typical end products of urban planning efforts are legally binding plans which regulate road alignments, building plots, green and public spaces as well as land use-classes, building-height restrictions and density requirements for each land parcel. They do not show any massing or the footprints of individual buildings.

The starting point for most urban design projects will be existing regulatory plans, but eventually the masterplan will once again be translated into a new – hopefully more refined and more specific – regulatory plan. This new plan will still lack specific guidance on urban form and urban space, and a substantial part of any design ideas will therefore be lost. In fact, urban design schemes cannot even be adopted as supplementary planning guidance as would be common in the UK. As a reaction to these obvious shortcomings, the concept of urban design guidelines has recently emerged, but so far these are not widely used and have no legal status either.

Compared with many other countries, in China one aspect of urban design is missing: public participation. Its absence does, however, not necessarily mean that the process is more straightforward or that it moves faster than elsewhere. Instead of public hearings or charettes, the urban designer in China has to work his/her way through multiple levels of government, each of which has different goals and agendas. The final word often lies with the vice-mayor in charge of urban development, or the local secretary of the Communist party.

China's notorious breakneck speed of construction is not necessarily preceded by high-speed planning. For example in Shenzhen's New Central District, site selection started in 1986 and a general regulatory plan was set up in 1992. Then, after a series of urban design competitions and endless modifications, the final plan emerged in 2001 and implementation started in earnest in 2002. Since then, most of the buildings have indeed been constructed at lightning speed – after 16 years of planning and design.

Historical development

In the decades of Mao Zedong's government, most development followed highly standardised codes and procedures, leading to endless rows of five-storey residential slabs adjacent to smoke-belching factories. In the 1980s, as a result of the economic reforms and the opening-up of policies under Deng Xiaoping, apartments, offices and shop units became a tradable commodity in a free property market. The emergence of urban design as a recognisable profession is therefore closely linked to the development of a professional real-estate industry.

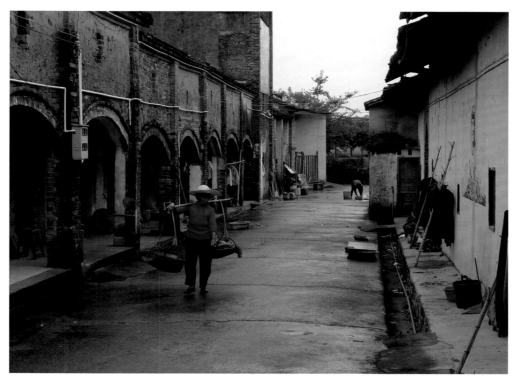

Traditional Chinese courtyard houses created a human-scale living
environment for their inhabitants and fostered a strong sense of
community. This example in southern China's Guangdong province was
built during the 1950s and 1960s; revolutionary slogans and portraits of
Chairman Mao are still visible

During the early days of the Chinese construction boom in the 1980s and
1990s, urban planning was – and to some extent still is – influenced by ill-conceived
functionalism and modernism, defined by a strict separation of land uses, rigid
and oversized road systems, and highly formal green and public spaces. At the
same time, China started to absorb development models and building typologies
from other regions: the high-rise housing estates of Hong Kong and Singapore; the
business districts of Japan; or the suburban homes, business parks and CBDs of
North America.

The 1990s saw the emergence of an increasingly professional real-estate sector,
together with the first signs of frantic growth in places like Shenzhen and Shanghai's
Pudong area. In the southern cities of Shenzhen and Guangzhou (Canton), the local
planning institutes made the first attempts at guiding rampant urban development, not
only through land use but also through building form, thereby giving birth to urban
design with Chinese characteristics.

The profession really got off the ground after the start of the new millennium.
As the purchase of an apartment became a paramount objective for millions of
Chinese, large-scale residential projects started to shoot up – initially only in the
major conurbations, but later also in second- and third-tier cities. In addition the
steady modernisation of the Chinese economy led to the emergence of a vast array of
commercial and mixed-use projects, ranging from purpose-built CBDs to high-tech
zones, retail districts and business parks.

More recently, development 'products' have become increasingly complex,
local authorities and their planning departments are more demanding, and real-

estate buyers or tenants expect world-class facilities for their money. The markets are increasingly driven by fashion trends: one year, every developer wanted to build 'lifestyle' shopping centres and creative-industry 'clusters'; the next year, outlet malls, headquarter office parks or 'cartoon production bases' were all the rage.

Since the opening-up of China's economy, economic development had long focused on southern and eastern China. In the last decade, however, three significant policies have been adopted in order to channel massive investments into China's underdeveloped regions: they are known as Rise of Central China, Revitalise Northeast China and China Western Development (also known as the Go West campaign).

Observers wonder whether this is all a giant economic bubble. The answer is in the fact that between 1990 and 2011, China's urban population increased at a staggering pace: from 254 million to 680 million. Every single year, more than 20 million people continue to move from rural to urban areas. These new urban dwellers create a genuine and massive demand for new housing, shops and public services.

Practice

In order to appreciate the role of urban design in China, one needs to understand that, with few exceptions, all land is permanently owned by the government. A developer who wants to develop a parcel of land has to apply to the local government to purchase the right to do so. The local authority will require an urban design concept for the land parcel in question, and sometimes a development strategy for the wider area. These sales of temporary developments rights (usually for 70 years) are a major source of revenue for local governments.

Three main types of urban design projects in China result from this system:

- Strategic projects for local government
- Conceptual projects for real-estate developers before the actual land sale (so-called 'land-grabbing' projects)
- Realistic projects for real-estate developers after the land sale

Strategic projects for local government

Local authorities in China are under immense pressure to generate revenue from land sales, but also to spur urbanisation and to reach ambitious GDP growth targets. To achieve this desired growth, new citizens and businesses need to be attracted, new communities and industrial parks built. Urban planning and urban design have a distinct role in creating the strategic framework for future development and land sales. Typical government projects will encompass strategic masterplans for entire districts or counties, or for new towns, high-tech zones, economic development areas or tourist resorts. Urban regeneration projects are also increasingly important as older, underperforming areas are subjected to wholesale renewal, and often to demolition.

Conceptual projects for real-estate developers

Developers who want to build on a specific piece of land need to convince the local authority that their project will create the greatest benefit for the public, the government or for the image of the city. The developer will commission an urban design firm to suggest an initial concept, which will be used as marketing material for presentations to the authority. Consequently, urban design work at this stage often revolves around image and branding, and emphasises iconic landmarks, public facilities and impressive cultural or tourism projects. Its typical output will encompass 3D renderings, multimedia presentations, animated movies and huge physical models – all designed to impress the authorities and to convince them to hand over the land.

Realistic projects for real-estate developers after the land sale

If the efforts of the previous stage have led to success, the developer, having secured the land, can pursue his major goal – to create a real-estate product that sells well and generates the maximum profit. As a result, the landmarks and public facilities of the previous stage often disappear one by one, and are replaced by more realistic and more profitable uses: residential high-rises, luxury villas or office towers. Frequently the design follows a more pragmatic path than in the previous stage, using standardised and formulaic approaches that appeal to the local market. At all three stages, exercises in positioning or branding may inform the urban design process; they are provided either by external consultants or by in-house economists within the urban design firms.

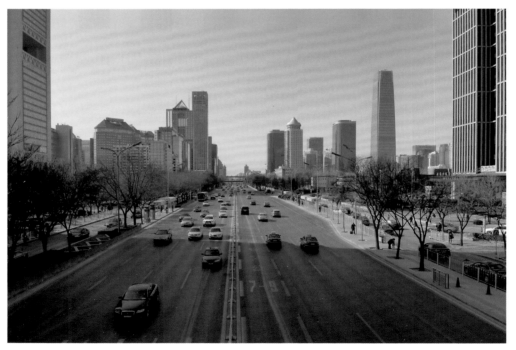

View along Beijing's major east–west artery towards the core of the CBD.
Despite the generous road width, the flow of vehicular traffic will inevitably
come to a standstill at peak hours

By far the biggest players in the market to offer urban design services are the Local Design Institutes (LDI). These are public enterprises, which often employ more than 1,000 people and have – thanks to their excellent connections to local authorities – virtually cornered the local markets for consultancy services. LDIs also hold the necessary licenses – which few private firms possess – to translate urban design schemes into legally binding regulatory plans. Private practices, be they local Chinese concerns, branches of foreign companies or joint venture firms, have only recently started to appear on a sizeable scale, and are becoming significant players.

Main issues of concern

Urban designers in China face many challenges. The sheer speed of urbanisation, combined with the scale and volume of development, leads almost inevitably to myriads of problems. Breakneck urbanisation has created an increasing imbalance between urban and rural citizens. Many of China's large cities face severe problems of overpopulation. In 2010, for example, Beijing had already exceeded the population level predicted for 2020. Consequently municipal infrastructure is often overstretched, as is evidenced by gridlocked roads and overcrowded subways.

Private car ownership has surged tremendously in recent years. The number of cars has recently topped 100 million – about 73 cars per 1,000 citizens. This figure is still relatively low by western standards, but is nevertheless causing severe traffic jams. China is already the world's largest automobile producer and consumer, and in 2010 it overtook the US as the world's largest auto market. Traffic conditions are set to deteriorate even further as more and more aspiring middle-class Chinese fulfil their dream of owning a car.

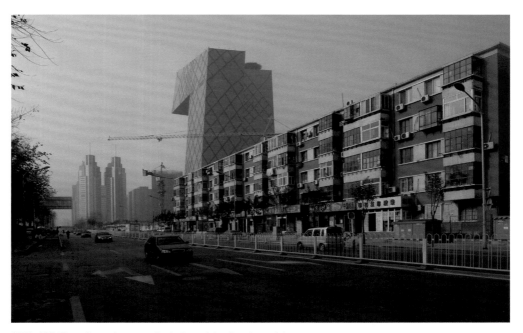

OMA's CCTV Tower looms large over the last remaining five-storey slabs from pre-boom times in Beijing's CBD; the road has been widened and a metal fence prevents pedestrians from crossing

Bicycles, once the predominant mode of transport, have virtually disappeared from Chinese roads; it is no longer convenient or safe to use them, and in China's car-obsessed culture they are not going to raise a person's social status either. Walking is not a convenient option as the new eight or ten-lane roads are difficult to cross, zebra crossings are ignored as merely ornamental features and Chinese drivers treat pedestrians as soft targets.

At the same time as car ownership surged, the government invested heavily into public transport. In 2008, Beijing had only four subway and light rail lines; now it has 14, and seven more are under construction. Shanghai's 11 metro lines now form the world's longest network, and it will be expanded to 22 lines. A number of second-tier cities are joining the construction boom too. Yet despite this massive enlargement of the metro systems, demand frequently outstrips supply and the lines are severely overcrowded. Most second- and third-tier cities (with populations of more than one million) still rely on buses, though new Bus Rapid Transit (BRT) lines have eased the situation in some of them.

Both roads and public transport are used beyond capacity because the need for mobility has increased vastly. In the past, people would live within walking or cycling distance of their work. Nowadays, jobs are often concentrated in certain areas (financial districts, high-tech zones), while affordable housing may be far from them. Unsustainable land-use patterns have forced Chinese workers into long and inconvenient commutes – be they by car, bus or subway.

High-speed railway lines have emerged as a new driver of urban growth. China already has the world's longest high-speed rail network, with 8,300 km of track (as of 2011). New stations, often located outside the urban core, are rapidly surrounded by business parks and large residential communities, or form the nucleus of entire new towns.

New residential compounds almost always feature perimeter fences and guarded gates. Gated communities are indeed the norm, not only for exclusive villa compounds but for any type of residential development. Densities are much higher in China than in the west. Residential neighbourhoods may consist entirely of 33-storey, 100 m tall towers with plot ratios of 3.0 and more. In addition, ancient *feng shui* principles and modern planning codes have conspired to make virtually all Chinese residential buildings face south. East-, west- or north-facing residences are out of the question. The result is highly uniform patterns, where all buildings, regardless of local climate or topography, face in exactly the same direction, towards the sun!

Street spaces are almost always too wide and are further enlarged by additional setback lines on either side. A typical urban road would have at least four, but more commonly six to eight lanes of traffic. The resulting space from building to building may measure 40 to 60 m in width. Major roads and arteries will be even wider. In new development areas these vast thoroughfares are often laid out in mind-numbingly boring rectangular grids, which are superimposed upon huge tracts of land with little or no regard for minor obstacles such as mountains, steep slopes or existing settlements.

Block sizes are far too large, sometimes measuring 300 m or more in length. Development parcels are mostly sold as entire urban blocks, thereby favouring mega-projects by large real-estate companies over small ones by private investors. Individual projects on small parcels of land by independent small landowners, as would be the norm in Japan or Korea, are almost unknown in China – a clear reflection of the land-ownership patterns and the top-down planning process. To build an individual's small house to his/her own specification is nearly impossible in China, and even luxury mansions for millionaires are sold cookie-cutter style 'off the shelf'.

The expectation is that existing legislation is strictly enforced under China's centralised system of governance. In reality enforcement is weak, as can be shown by the example of golf courses. All golf-course developments had effectively been made illegal by the government in 2004. Nonetheless, between 2004 and 2011, the number of golf courses has risen from 170 to 600!

Challenges and restrictions result in a frustrating lack of character and identity that often baffles visitors to China's cities. From the freezing-cold north-east to the subtropical south, modern Chinese cities look strikingly similar. Apart from a disregard for local climate, local materials or local customs among contemporary designers (be they foreign or Chinese), it is the lack of historic fabric that is responsible for this uniformity. While the wholesale demolition of Beijing's old *hutongs* (alleyways) and Shanghai's *shikumen* (terraced housing) has been widely reported in the media, the almost complete destruction of old neighbourhoods in second-tier cities and small towns has gone widely unnoticed. Indeed, Beijing and Shanghai still possess comparatively large swathes of old buildings, while hundreds of other cities and towns have lost their entire heritage to the wrecking ball.

When local building styles are taken as inspiration for new developments, the result is often pastiche design, exemplified in the phenomenon of constructing fake 'ancient culture streets' with little or no genuine historical fabric. And the few old buildings that are successfully restored, often fall victim to their own success: as they are such a rarity, they inevitably attract hordes of tourists. From Shanghai's Xintiandi to Beijing's Nanluoguxiang Alleyway and Chengdu's Kuai Zhai Alleys the result is usually the same: attractive yet crowded tourist traps with a rather predictable array of bars, cafes and overpriced crafts shops.

Finally, sustainability and climate change are also a subject for analysis in China. EcoCities and EcoTowns have started to appear around the country, but so far have failed to live up to expectations. Most of the time, sustainable or 'green' design translates into nothing more than 'lots of trees and flowers'. Genuine sustainable solutions, from Transit-Oriented Development (TOD) to Sustainable Urban Drainage Strategies (SUDS), from live–work units to Combined Heat and Power (CHP), are slowly gaining ground, but are far from being standard solutions. The root causes of unsustainable development – reliance on private cars, insufficient public transport, separation of residential and employment areas, and weak environmental legislation, to name a few – still need to be tackled urgently.

The city of Chengdu is the capital of Sichuan, one of the largest provinces of China, and its administrative and cultural centre. Chengdu has great ambitions: it aims to become the hub not only for Sichuan, but for the entire south-west. In recent years, Chengdu has greatly benefited from huge investments initiated by the China Western Development policy. A large urban extension area – dubbed Chengdu Hi-tech Industrial Development Zone – has sprung up to the south of the existing city centre, and has attracted major high-tech and software companies. The main road link from Chengdu's downtown to the new area is lined with architectural icons, culminating in French architect Paul Andreu's Technology and Science Enterprising Centre. To top it all, Zaha Hadid will add her trademark style with the giant Chengdu Contemporary Art Centre at the southern end of the axis.

The area to the east of the Hi-Tech Zone and north-east of Hadid's futuristic building has been earmarked by the government as Chengdu's future financial district. To achieve this goal, the local authority set up the Company of Investment & Development for the Finance City of Chengdu Ltd, which held an international competition among five top design consultancies. Out of the resulting five proposals, two winning schemes were chosen – one by Atkins (shown here) and one by a Japanese firm in cooperation with a local design company.

The work involved the development of 5.5 km² of land as a mixed-use area including office space for financial services, headquarter buildings for international and local companies, high-quality sustainable housing, and leisure and entertainments amenities.

After careful site analysis and planning-background analysis, four main challenges that the design had to respond to, were identified:

- Creation of a strong image to be recognised internationally and locally
- Creation of a genuine low-carbon financial district
- Integration between the existing commercial areas and the CFD, and interaction between the western and the eastern parts of the site
- New modes of public transportation

In response to these challenges, a clear and realistic urban design framework was established based on the following principles:

- Project branding – International Ecological Mixed-Use Financial District
- Sustainable urban planning combined with sustainable infrastructure
- Robust and flexible urban framework to promote incremental and phased development
- Application of TOD principles in order to create high-density nodes with direct and convenient access to public transport
- Integrated transport nodes and circulation networks to form seamless pedestrian links

The site is divided into two parts (western and eastern), separated by the Fuhe river. An existing island in the middle of the river forms an attractive feature for the development.

The masterplan establishes the key concept of 'One belt, two axes, two districts, three hearts, one street', which is a typical Chinese way to express and summarise a planning concept:

- One Belt: ecological landscape belt along Fuhe River
- Two Axes: urban axis in north–south direction; green axis weaving through the site
- Two Districts: two functional districts, one on each of the eastern and western sides of the river

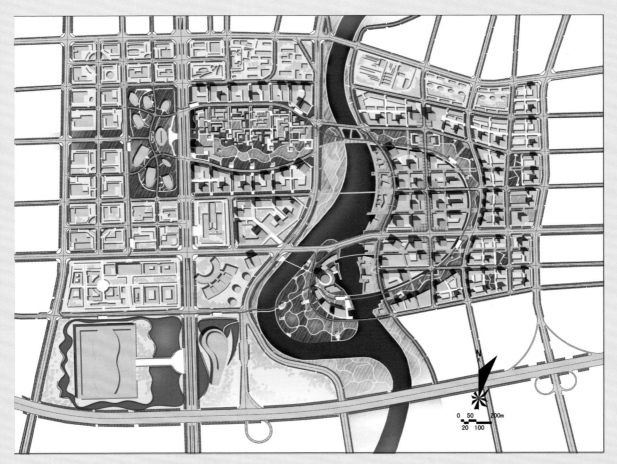

The overall masterplan for Chengdu Financial District. Zaha Hadid's planned art centre is the tear-shaped structure at the bottom-left (next to an enormous rectangular leisure and shopping complex), while Paul Andreu's Technology and Science Centre sits near the top-left of the plan (the group of elliptical shapes)

- Three Hearts: three landscaped spaces at the Financial Service Node (East Area), the Financial Business Node (West Area) and the International Financial Forum Island
- One street: the signature urban space for the CFD featuring a diverse mix of commercial uses, restaurants, cafes and public spaces

The urban blocks have been designed to provide a comfortable walking experience. Each is about 120 m to 250 m in length, smaller than the average urban block in China. In addition, pedestrian links through internal courtyards improve permeability of the blocks.

One significant challenge has been the adequate provision of public transport connections. Chengdu's first metro line has recently opened, yet it runs along the western edge of the site leaving large portions of the project without access to it. Indeed, in the higher-level planning strategy the core area of the financial district would have direct access neither to the existing nor to proposed new metro lines. In order to rectify this fundamental flaw, the urban design plan proposes to realign a planned new east–west metro line to serve the centre of the site, and to add new metro stations and an elevated tram line to run in a loop through the financial district. This tram proposal – unlikely to be implemented – would provide vital connections between several existing and planned metro stations and the different zones of the CFD.

Another challenge frequently faced by urban designers in China is that the alignment and width of major roads are planned prior to the masterplanning and urban design stage. Consequently, the resulting road systems are based on transport engineering

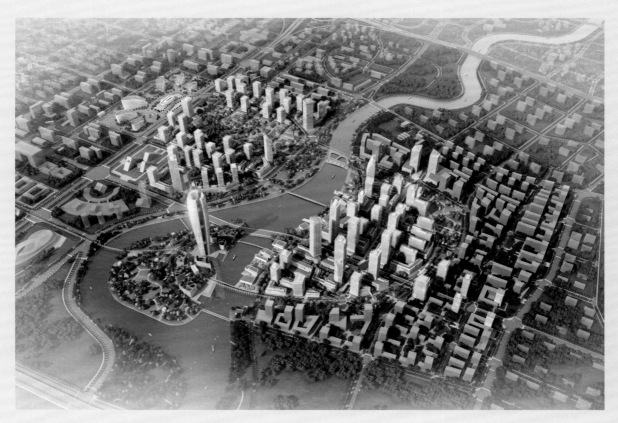

Chengdu Financial District as seen from the south-east, surrounded by Chengdu Hi-tech Industrial Development Zone

principles rather than urban design considerations, and create major obstacles to good place making. In this case, the main roads at the northern edge of the site, as well as those along the riverbank and across the island, have all been designed, and even built, before the plan for the financial district had been in place. On a more positive note, however, the urban design plan determined the design of most local roads – allowing for more flexible layouts, smaller road widths and more reasonable block sizes.

The western area

The western area is located directly opposite Paul Andreu's landmark complex (the group of elliptical buildings on the left of the plan), which establishes a strong symmetrical axis. Rather than continuing this axis, the masterplan seeks a more informal, flexible arrangement: a central leisure and entertainment area with low-rise buildings, narrow streets and small courtyards can accommodate the restaurants, bars and cafes, which are so often missing in typical mono-functional business districts. Likewise, the central park establishes a strong yet informal green

link in an east–west direction towards the river. Here the green link meets the riverside landscape belt and leads directly to a new pedestrian bridge across the river, which provides direct walking and cycling access to the eastern part of the CFD. It is indeed worth noting that the entire scheme contains more footbridges than road bridges – a decidedly unusual approach in car-obsessed China.

The eastern area

The eastern area will provide the majority of the new office space. In contrast to the conventional building typology in China, namely stand-alone office towers surrounded by corporate plazas and private green spaces, the scheme proposes to combine its towers with mixed-used podiums. The latter can accommodate a variety of uses vital for vibrant spaces, not least active commercial space at ground level. The podiums will also create a much better sense of enclosure and a more comfortable environment for pedestrians than free-standing towers. Hotels, serviced apartments and upmarket residential properties complete the mix of uses in the eastern area.

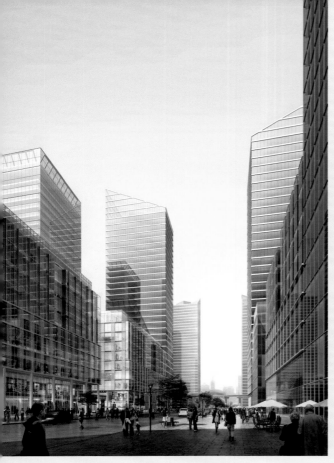

The main street in the eastern part of the site with wide sidewalks, a relatively narrow road space, mixed-use podiums and active ground levels with shops, cafes and restaurants

Chengdu citizens love to take their meals of incredibly spicy local cuisine on the streets or next to the water. The riverfront of the eastern area is therefore the perfect place for the locals to congregate at the various waterfront restaurants and bars. These will undoubtedly attract people at lunchtimes and in the evenings, thereby contributing to the goal of creating a vibrant 24-hour district rather than a monofunctional area that falls dead after office hours.

The island

The island in the middle of the Fuhe river is home to the International Financial Forum. Its centrepiece is a very tall hybrid tower with offices, hotel and serviced apartments. At the bottom of the tower, a major conference venue provides its services to the business community. The larger part of the island is otherwise kept as public green space, and is connected to the business areas by several footbridges and the elevated tram line.

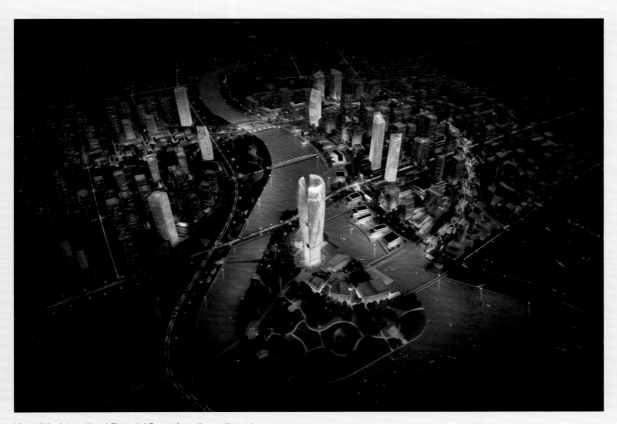

View of the International Financial Forum from the south-west, with the island and the `signature' tower at the centre

Evaluation

What sets this scheme apart from other business districts in China is its distinctive mix of uses with strong leisure, entertainment and residential components, as well as the strong connection to existing and proposed public transport options. The sustainable urban planning and design approach is therefore going well beyond the usual 'greenwashing' (showing cliched 'green' architecture and a couple of wind turbines in the background) to tackle sustainability at a fundamental planning level.

Unfortunately at the end of the second stage, the clients decided to go with a competing scheme which had shown more detailed architectural design and – more importantly – a taller landmark tower. This blurring of the lines between urban planning and urban design on one hand, and architecture on the other is not uncommon in China, often to the detriment of genuine urban design solutions. This is not the end of the line though: the plan will go through (many) further modifications and adjustments, and there will be further competitions for smaller parts of the site.

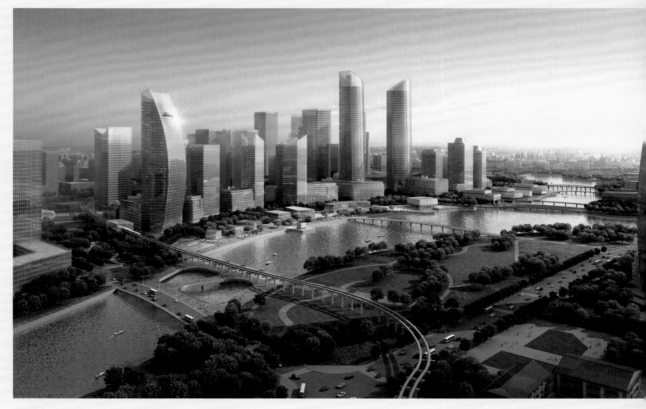

View from the western side towards the eastern bank of the river, which is lined with restaurants and bars

CASE STUDY 2

YINGKOU PENINSULA

This project is located 500 km north-east of Beijing in the third-tier city of Yingkou, formerly called Newchwang, one of the lesser-known British treaty ports.

China's north-east is known as the 'rust belt' due to the former dominance of heavy industries and coal mining, which are now in decline. Recent favourable government policies, however, have led to a strong economic resurgence. Yingkou is benefiting from the new Coastal Industrial Base immediately to the south of the city centre. In addition, along the coast substantial new port facilities and associated industries have taken shape in recent years. While Yingkou's economy has certainly improved, its public spaces and leisure options have not kept pace. The project described here may have a role in remedying the situation.

The site is located about 5 km to the west of the city centre, where Yingkou's mother river, the Liao, joins the Bohai bay. The peninsula is currently an underused wasteland with almost no vegetation, some fishponds, salt pans and coastal wetlands. A new cable-stayed bridge looms large over the site and has greatly improved access to this area.

The project consisted of distinct parts:
- The residential community (key design area), 57 ha in size
- The riverside commercial street
- The peninsula (extended design area), 287 ha in size

It falls broadly into two of the categories of typical projects outlined earlier: firstly, it is a conceptual design for a residential community on behalf of the developer who wishes to acquire the land from the local government. Secondly, the local authorities have asked the developer to provide a strategic planning framework for the wider area of the entire peninsula. As the scope of the work did not include

detailed urban or architectural design, all building designs shown are merely illustrative.

The project presented the designers with a number of conflicting interests and agendas: the local authority was looking for spectacular landmark projects to put Yingkou city on the map and to raise its profile. The developer wished to secure the land-use rights for the residential community, and in the long term to open up profitable development opportunities on the surrounding land. The general public hoped for an attractive public park and a public waterfront promenade as well as leisure, recreation and sports facilities. Finally, from the point of view of environmental protection any new development could be potentially harmful. The design proposal attempts to balance these conflicting agendas and to create a flexible and robust framework, which can be developed step by step.

Residential community

The residential area at the southern edge of the plan represents a fairly typical example of a contemporary Chinese housing project. One single developer is in charge of a very large land parcel. All dwellings – high-rises and town houses – are arranged in the typical fashion, inevitably facing south with only minor variations. A central green space with generous water bodies lies at the heart of the neighbourhood.

The density, considerable by western standards, is normal in China, and its Floor Area Ratio (FAR) of 1.9 is not even particularly high. However, low-density town houses and a substantial area of green spaces and water have to be balanced by high-rises to achieve the required density. A mixed-use complex with shops, restaurants, a cinema and high-rise apartments occupies the north-eastern corner of this area, facing the major access roads and the cable-stayed bridge, and connecting to the internal lake with waterfront restaurants and cafes.

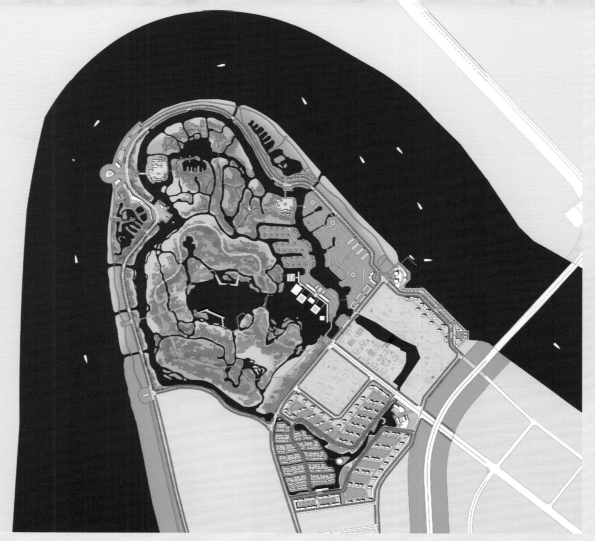

The initial masterplan outlining the conceptual development
framework for future development on the peninsula –
bottom: residential community; right: riverside development with
views to the new bridge; centre: retained and newly constructed
wetlands combined with leisure and tourism facilities

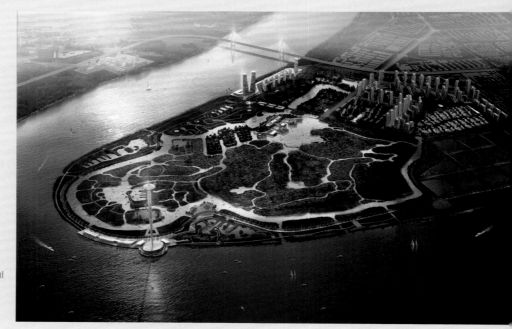

Bird's-eye view across the
peninsula, with the new cable-
stayed bridge, the riverside
development and the residential
community (background, from
left to right) and the public
waterfront (foreground)

Case study 2: Yingkou Peninsula ~ **CHINA**

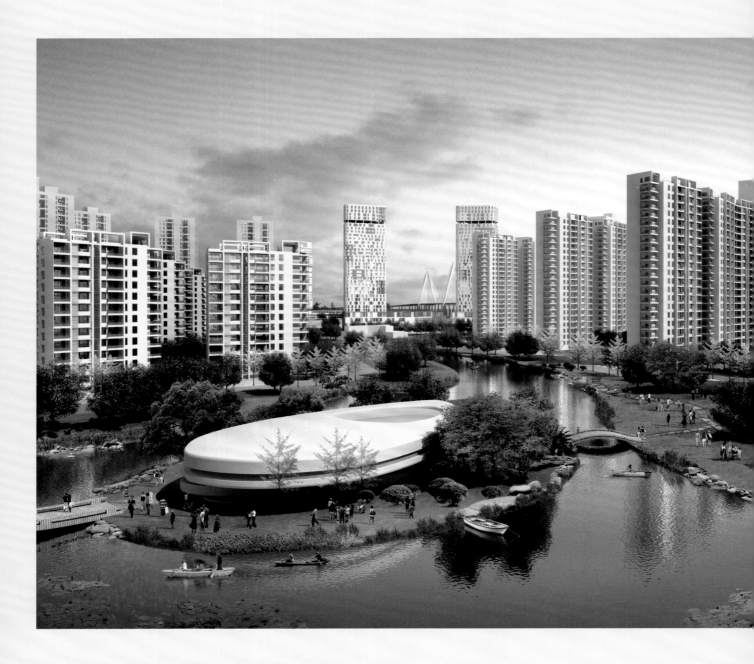

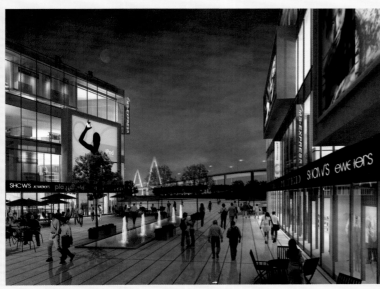

View from the pedestrian shopping street, which serves the residential community, towards the new cable-stayed bridge

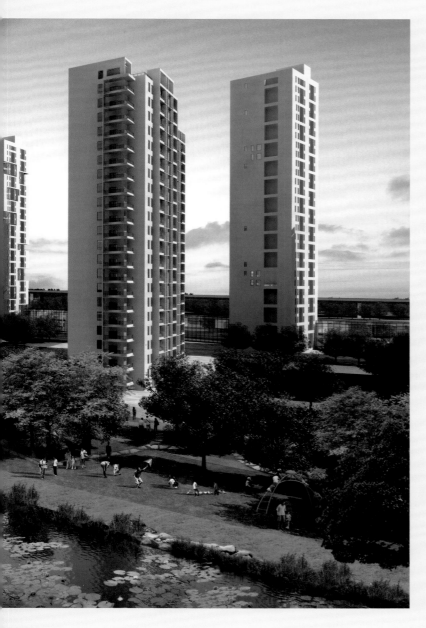

The riverside

At the north-eastern edge of the site, a diverse pedestrian-friendly riverfront destination is planned next to the new bridge. This area is highly visible for those arriving in Yingkou by car across the bridge. The design takes this opportunity to create an impressive new skyline along the river. At the same time, a pedestrian riverfront promenade lined with restaurants, cafes and bars offers spectacular views of the illuminated bridge at night-time. A public square surrounded by entertainment uses is at one end of the promenade, while a marina with a commercial complex and landmark twin towers is at the other end of this vibrant waterfront space.

The peninsula

Previous planning options treated the entire peninsula as an undefined, potentially privatised space with limited public access and few public facilities. There were also unspecified plans for a golf course, a theme park and gated housing. This created a dilemma: restricted public access would potentially limit the environmental impact on the

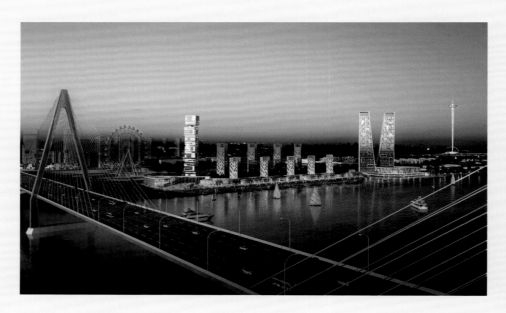

Yingkou's new gateway as seen when crossing the bridge – featuring a continuous pedestrian waterfront promenade lined with restaurants and bars

Case study 2: Yingkou Peninsula ~ **CHINA**

213

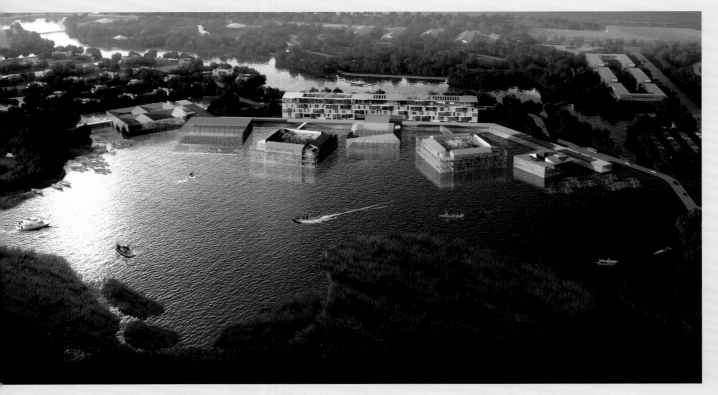

Bird's-eye view of the constructed wetland and the hotel, which features conference venues, restaurants and a spa all floating in the lake (all architecture for illustrative purposes only)

wetlands, but the wider public would not benefit from the project. In the end, the public interests prevailed and the design proposal makes the entire waterfront, along both the river and the seashore, publicly accessible. Consequently, a landscaped scenic road and a continuous promenade connect several attractions such as an equestrian centre, a fishing spot and various public spaces. The outstanding highlight will be the new television tower required by the local authority. Rather than leaving this tower as an isolated landmark, the design combines it with leisure uses, public spaces and a wetland visitor and interpretation centre. A constructed wetland landscape with a public park, a major hotel and a conference venue are proposed for the heart of the peninsula.

Evaluation

On the whole, the scheme succeeds in balancing the contradicting requirements:

- The existing wetlands have been retained and extensive constructed wetlands added
- The entire waterfront is open to the public with various attractions along the way, and the TV tower is integrated into the overall concept
- The riverfront creates an exciting new meeting place for the locals, yet satisfies the government's desire for an impressive skyline
- The residential neighbourhood will be highly attractive to the local market

In addition, the project identifies future development opportunities, yet limits the potential impact on natural areas.

As with most schemes in China, this project is likely to go through many rounds of modifications. As it stands, its greatest achievement lies in its insistence on both public access and environmental protection, and as such it will be a good base for further discussions and negotiations.

Conclusion

There is a perception in the west that foreign designers working in China can come up with the most ambitious and outrageous schemes, and get them built within months. In reality, planning and urban design are often parts of a long-winded and arduous process. For the time being, urban design remains a tool to create fiscal revenue for local governments, and profits for real-estate developers. To create great places and spaces for people, to make development environmentally friendly and more sustainable – these goals are not yet high on the agenda.

Urban design in China has come a long way in a very short time. To work as an urban designer there is doubtlessly exciting, yet challenging and frequently frustrating. But things are changing – and in China they tend to change fast.

A quick guide to
China

1 TYPES OF CLIENT

Local government, usually the local planning bureau

Private real-estate developers (local)

....

2 TYPES OF
PROJECT/WORK

Conceptual masterplans at various scales, from extremely large regional plans to more manageable local plans

New towns, large-scale residential communities, industrial parks, high-tech research-and-development (R&D) parks, office and retail developments, tourism developments, etc

....

3 APPROACH NEEDED
TO WORK IN COUNTRY

Local presence in China is preferable, at least with a small representative office

Partnership/joint venture with a local firm is possible, but not legally required

Foreign firms can only submit 'conceptual plans' and cannot sign-off legally binding plans (development control plans); for the latter type of work, they may need to cooperate with a local design institute

International competitions are a feasible way to win work in the country, but many developers may assign projects directly to one design firm

Attention must be paid to the exact wording of any contract, the exact list of deliverables and the detailed payment schedule

Appropriate due diligence should be carried out to establish whether or not a client is able and willing to pay

Foreign designers should insist on a sizeable initial down payment before any design work is started

....

4 LEGISLATION
THAT NEEDS TO BE
REFERRED TO

Chinese planning legislation

Existing regional and local plans, especially land-use plans and development-control plans

....

5 SPECIFIC TIPS
FOR SUCCESS

Reliable local staff with good knowledge of the local market, local business customs, tax regulations, etc is essential

Local Chinese planning laws, design standards and typologies need to be respected; success will not come from simply 'copying and pasting' a design solution from another country

Make an effort to understand the client's actual agenda: does the client already own the land and want to get a pragmatic, implementable design scheme, or do they require some lofty conceptual ideas to woo the local government?

Treat all representatives of the client – especially at senior level – with the utmost respect and give them 'face': for example, meetings with senior client representatives must by default be attended by equally senior staff from the designer's side

Clearly understand restrictions and obstacles affecting the design site (such as existing and planned roads, power lines, existing buildings, height limits, setback requirements and so on), and establish whether or not these must be incorporated into your plan or can be removed

Put some effort into the visual presentation of your project; elaborate masterplan drawings, detailed 3D renderings or even animated films might be required – hand sketches and Photoshop collages will often not do

Prepare to change, adjust and modify your scheme time and again – and occasionally to start again from scratch; therefore, your design fee should be sufficient to cover a potentially long-winded work process

....

6 USEFUL WEBSITES

Architectural Society of China: www.chinaasc.org

International Association for China Planning: www.chinaplanning.org

Urban Planning Society of China: www.planning.org.cn

....

SELECTED FACTS

1	area	9,596,960 km²
2	population	1,338,299,512
3	annual population growth (2009)	0.5%
4	urban population	45%
5	population density	139 p/km²
6	GDP	$5,878,629,246,677
7	GNI per capita	$4,260

Source: The World Bank (2010)

INDIA

Professor Christopher Benninger, *architect and urban planner*

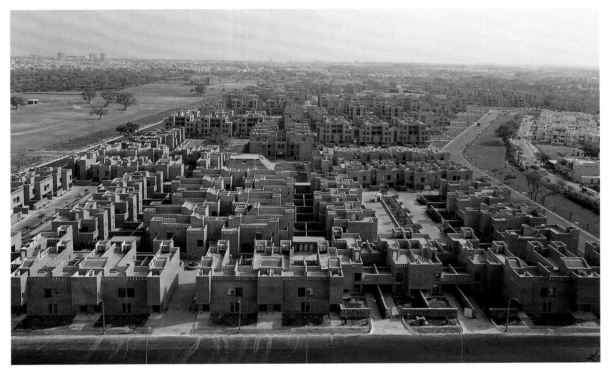

Asian Games Village in New Delhi by Raj Rewal

|NDIA is a federal republic comprising 35 states, seven of which are union territories ruled directly by the federal government. In addition there are about 550 districts. The federal government and the state assemblies share planning powers according to specific lists. Municipal authorities and districts are involved in the preparation of plans and development control.

Urban design in India

While the country can boast of a great tradition in place making, urban design has been a weak voice in modern India. The design of New Delhi by Sir Edwin Lutyens and Herbert Baker in the early 20th century, and Chandigarh by Le Corbusier, Jane Drew and Maxwell Fry after independence, created an awareness of civic design and the desire to integrate large architectural projects within the urban fabric. Major urban design initiatives in Madras, Bombay and Calcutta in the colonial era, along with the creation of 55 cantonments and hill stations, left an indelible mark on India's sense of urbanity.

Urban design was given further impetus by the 1962 Delhi Master Plan, which included 15 district centres and many community centres requiring design inputs. Subsequently, a number of institutional initiatives created a clear mandate for urban designers. The New Delhi Redevelopment Advisory Committee (NDRAC) was created in 1972 to review the proposed extension of the Connaught Place commercial area. In the same year the Housing and Urban Development Corporation (HUDCO) was created, channelling funds into large-scale low-income housing schemes and urban infrastructure. In 1973, the Delhi Urban Art Commission was established out of concern for the fate of Lutyens' Bungalow Zone. In 1978, in Ahmedabad, the Vastu-Shilpa Foundation was the first non-governmental organisation (NGO) mixing urban design research and consulting. The Indian National Trust for Art and Culture (INTACH), created in 1984, sponsored heritage-area studies and projects. In the same year, the Urban Design Research Institute was created in Mumbai (then, Bombay), carrying out studies of the Fort area and advocating solutions to alleviate metropolitan stresses. From 1987 on, Infrastructure Leasing and Financial Services Limited (IL&FS) invested into urban infrastructure, engaging urban designers in riverfront development and other projects.

Throughout the 1970s and 80s, urban development authorities emerged across India, spreading masterplanning and development planning concepts. Local authorities looked more carefully at their heritage and low-income settlements, and, more recently, at citywide environmental issues. All these activities enhanced an environment within which an urban design culture could emerge.

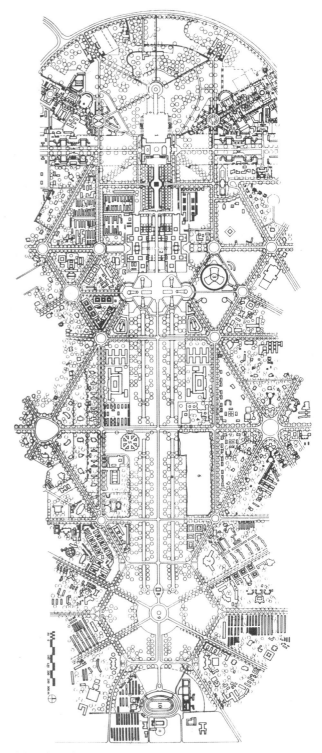

Lutyens' plan for New Delhi

In the years after independence, architects with no formal urban design training carried out major urban projects. Large extensions such as New Okhla Industrial Development Area (Noida) and Gurgaon, near Delhi, and the Back Bay Reclamation and Kurla-Bandra Complex in Mumbai were designed by government planners with architectural backgrounds. Later, after liberalisation, Special Economic Zones (SEZs) were conceived by Indian designers and New Urbanism gated towns by foreign consultants.

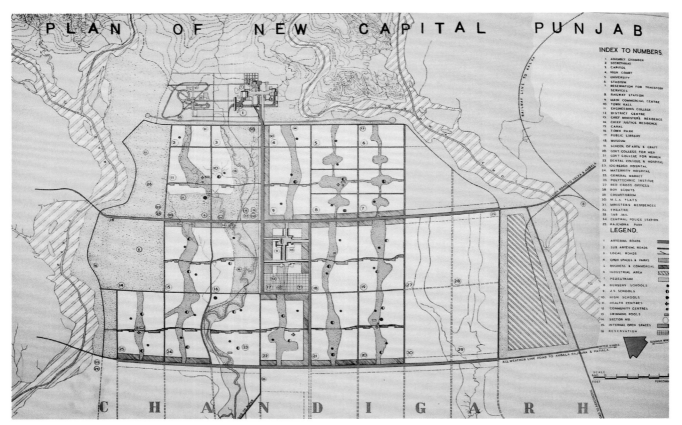

Le Corbusier's plan for Chandigarh

The Institute of Urban Designers, India (IUDI), established in 2007, defines urban design as

> The aesthetic, scientific and orderly development of land, buildings and their regulation, with the view to securing physical, economic and social efficiency, health and wellbeing of settlements, cities, regions, villages and the nation.

This definition leaves a very thin line between the professions of urban design and traditional planning.

There is no statutory mechanism to register either urban planners or urban designers, making the Council of Architecture (a statutory body under the Architects Regulation and Registration Act) the sole arbitrator of professional accreditation, and only the title of 'architect' is legally protected. The paucity of Indian urban designers engaged in the making of modern Indian cities is notable.

The urban scenario

The urban population and the infrastructure of the Indian subcontinent are expanding dramatically as a result of accelerated industrialisation and maturing financial institutions. Foreign investment, deregulation and economic growth are driving this transformation. The Indian Planning Commission envisions investment in urban infrastructure of about one trillion US dollars (£638,000 million) over the next decade.

These resources will be derived from revenue mobilisation, development charges and public–private joint-venture investments.

A concomitant migration to larger cities by young workers seeking employment in growth sectors (information technology, investment finance, professional services and management) is redefining the demographic landscape. About 55% of India's population is 24 years of age or younger. This is not only a 'midriff bulge' of middle- and upper-class aspiration, but also a dramatic increase in semi-skilled workers seeking blue-collar jobs in sectors like transport, maintenance, construction and manufacturing. With about 68% of its population residing in rural areas, the migration to cities of India's young will greatly inflate the sizes of urban agglomerations. The Mumbai metropolitan region alone doubled its population between 1992 and 2012. Projections indicate that the Indian urban population will increase from the present 320 million to 530 million (33% of the total) by 2021. This is about an eight and a half-fold increase from the total of 62 million urban dwellers (17% of the total) in 1951.

Changing lifestyles more than growth shall transform cities

More than a change in size, this is a dramatic change in lifestyles and aspirations: for instance, only 18% of the residents of Mumbai currently own their homes but expectations among new citizens include home ownership, and this is not limited to large conurbations.

At the dawn of deregulation in 1991, 97% of India's retail activity was in the informal sector. But as consumers demand branded goods and services, space is needed to accommodate these. New acquisition mechanisms and urban development schemes have led to the creation of large-scale gated residential communities, unaffordable to the vast majority. Private-education and healthcare companies have also grown dramatically, and need to be accommodated. Along with new metro lines and expressways, these projects are shaping India's urban patterns and visible landscapes.

Economic growth and unevenly distributed incomes have resulted in the disproportionate expansion of a middle class, whose aspirations mirror the fantasy

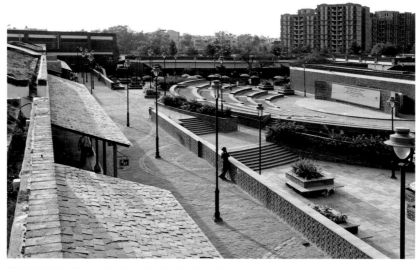

Delhi Haat, New Delhi crafts village by Pradeep Sachdeva

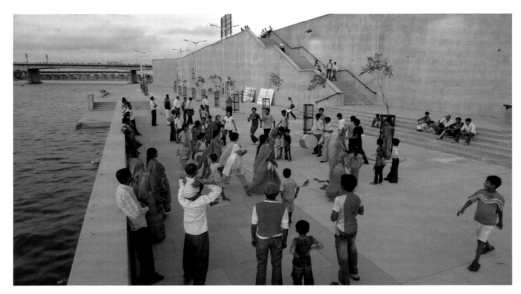

Ahmedabad: Sabarmati riverfront redevelopment project by Bimal Patel

images of emerging economies. To respond to these aspirations, a number of public projects have been developed such as the Delhi Haat crafts village and numerous recreation projects, the redevelopment of Ahmedabad's Sabarmati river, Mumbai's Marine Drive and many others. These have created breathing spaces for households residing in overcrowded environments. Such relatively small projects are carried out by Indian designers who are sensitive to traditions, employing traditional motifs and craftspeople, though drawing upon international models for global themes with an Indian ambiance. An outstanding example is the historic Jama Masjid precinct, combining facilities for humble bicycle-rickshaw pushers, conservation of historic structures, management of street activities and complex traffic, while accommodating several hundred hawkers.

Managing the transformation and designing its shape

The existing urban-development procedures are embedded within archaic statutory regulations, empowering bureaucrats born of a culture of control and regulation, rather than one that facilitates and encourages the vast energies of cities. The 1935 Model Town Planning Act, employing land pooling and an equitable mechanism for acquiring land for public roads, gardens and amenities, soon succumbed to lengthy court proceedings. Post-independence planning legislation emerged from western models where population projections and the resulting area requirements for roads and services produced supply-based land-use plans. Today, these planning prototypes are inadequate to meet the challenges ahead. From demographic data that never included 'illegal' slum dwellers, or properly estimated growth, a 'shelf of schemes' of required projects was portrayed as a blueprint for the future. Separate transportation studies underestimated the increase of private vehicular movement as well as the requirements for mass transit. These two-dimensional planning exercises employed land banking along with low densities, spreading out city growth in an inefficient manner. Traditional town planning itself became the cause of urban problems, rather than the solution.

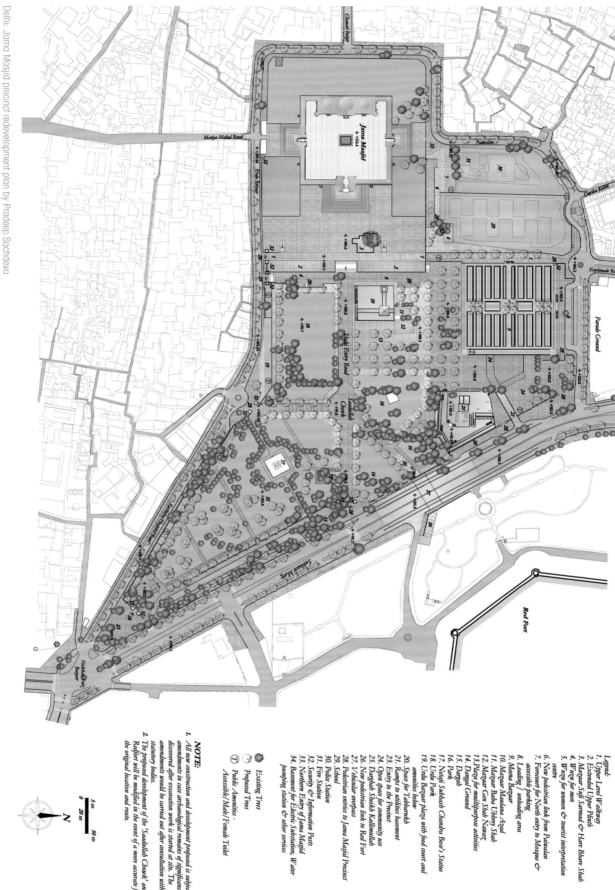

Delhi: Jama Masjid precinct redevelopment plan by Pradeep Sachdeva

Legend:
1. Upper Level Walkway
2. Extended Upper Plinth
3. Mazgar Sufi Sarmad & Hare Bhare Shah
4. Wtteq for men
5. Wtteq for women & tourist interpretation centre
6. New pedestrian link from Paiwalan
7. Forecourt for North entry to Mosque & accessible parking
8. Loading / unloading area
9. Meena Bazaar
10. Mazgar Maulana Azad
11. Mazgar Baba Ubirry Shah
12. Mazgar Gen Shah Nawaz
13. Plaza for multipurpose activities
14. Dargah Ground
15. Dargah
16. Park
17. Netaji Subhash Chandra Bose's Statue
18. Urdu Park
19. Urdu Bazaar plaza with food court and amenities below
20. Space for Tashbaneb
21. Ramps to utilities basement
22. Entry to the Precinct
23. Open space for community use
24. Darfteh Sheikh Kalimullah
25. New pedestrian link to Red Fort
26. Vehicular overpass
27. Pedestrian entries to Jama Masjid Precinct
28. School
29. Police Station
30. Fire Station
31. Security & Information Posts
32. Northern Entry of Jama Masjid
33. Basement for Electric Substation, Water pumping station & other services

● Existing Trees
● Proposed Trees
Ⓣ Public Amenities - Accessible/Male/Female Toilet

NOTE:
1. All new construction and development proposed is subject to amendments in case archaeological remains of significance are discovered after excavation work is started at site. The amendments would be carried out after consultation with all statutory bodies.
2. The proposed development of the 'Saadullah Chowk' and link to Redfort will be modified in the event of a more accurate finding of the original location and route.

The first Indian masterplan, the 1962 plan for New Delhi, cast a shadow over the nation by allowing low density: 35% plot coverage and large setbacks on all plot sides. This was the opposite of the ancient, dense and walkable urban fabric of India with shared walls, internal courtyards and large building footprints. It made cities spread horizontally, while their buildings grew vertically. It created isolated developments and redefined planning as the control of architects' designs through complex rules that varied from one land-use zone to another. Even in large urban schemes such as the United Breweries City in Bengaluru (formerly Bangalore) this system, conceived for suburban plots, shaped cities into islands of high-rise boxes, leaving no place for creative urban design.

Urban design education

Urban design, planning, management and public-finance skills are lacking from the profiles of development authorities. The education of urban designers is inadequate to fill this challenge!

Professor Ranjit Sabiki initiated the first Indian course in urban design in 1969 at the School of Planning and Architecture (SPA), New Delhi. Subsequently, courses started at the Centre for Environmental Planning and Technology (CEPT) in Ahmedabad and at the Jadavpur University in Kolkata (then, Calcutta). The number of urban design courses has recently increased to eight, with an output of 100 graduates per year. In comparison, 183 schools of architecture have about 35,000 degree candidates.

Twenty institutions offer postgraduate and undergraduate urban planning programmes. At CEPT in Ahmedabad, there are more than 220 candidates in a range of urban planning programmes but only 47 candidates in urban design, even with a twofold increase between 2010 and 2011. CEPT and SPA benefit from housing their urban planning and design courses on the same campus, enriching both disciplines. Their faculties are deeply involved in the nation's urban future: Professor KT Ravindran, for example, heads the Urban Art Commission and is a member of the Advisory Board of the United Nations Capitol Plan for the redevelopment of the UN Headquarters in New York.

Generally, urban design courses try to integrate the skills needed for large-scale architectural projects with the sensitivities and knowledge required to address more complex issues of city extensions, urban renewal and heritage conservation. While schools of urban planning offer a range of degrees in housing, infrastructure planning and urban management, urban design is mostly an architectural postgraduate option. But schools of architecture with urban design courses lack the critical mass of faculty in urban studies, finance and infrastructure design needed to provide a sound and multidisciplinary professional education.

The majority of the country's 600 qualified urban designers works in architectural practices. There are few posts for qualified urban designers within the nation's multilevel urban planning system. Central and state governments have been slow to recognise urban design qualifications, favouring traditional planning graduates for senior management posts. It is now imperative that the Government of India and individual state governments bring the words 'urban design' into their official lexicons, positions and placements.

New approaches to urban design

India's place-making ethos is grounded in a long tradition of colonial cities: after independence, urban models from railway and company towns, which developed the cantonment pattern, inspired the new democracy to create its own footprint in the form of Chandigarh and other subsequent state capitals. Similarly, new company towns growing across the country borrowed ideas from New Delhi, Chandigarh and colonial cantonments, whose influence on the urban fabric lasted long after independence.

But as wealth is being injected into the economy and consumerism into the working population, Indian society is distancing itself from its traditions. New urban forms that are part of this radical break with the past appear in many schemes. Unfortunately they all lack three-dimensional concepts of public space, and guidelines for place making and the articulation of urban landscapes. The resulting neighbourhoods are dull two-dimensional and mono-functional, laid out with inefficient setbacks and surrounded by inefficient roads. They have no identity, and lack arcades or urban spaces.

The heart of Mumbai shows examples of missed opportunities. The Back Bay Reclamation Project south of the high density Fort precinct, based on landfill, was built from the 1960s to the 1990s. The more recent Bandra-Kurla Complex in the centre of the metropolis, developed on swampland from the late 1980s to the present, is emerging as India's new financial centre. Both schemes suffer from the complete absence of urban design concepts, employing walled-off and gated layouts with large setbacks and low ground coverage. Similarly Mumbai's mill lands were parcelled without any overall urban design scheme or intention to preserve irreplaceable industrial heritage structures. The resulting high-rise structures are set apart one from another, each a screaming baby trying to grab attention through stylish facades, and surrounded by wasted open space, used for parking. There are no amenities for the public, be it gardens, arcades, squares or promenades, nor any of the many features that could have been inspired by the nearby Fort district. Moreover, these Mumbai projects are neither linked to public transport nor include adequate parking.

The Belapur Central Business District and Navi Mumbai, across the broad Thane creek bay to the east of Mumbai, are much grander schemes linked to the city by a rail bridge and a vehicular toll bridge. Areas near the new metro stops in central Navi Mumbai have exploded into unplanned commercial and amenities districts. Similarly to what happened in poorly conceived neighbourhoods based on foreign models in New Delhi, skyrocketing rents for offices pushed retail activities into unplanned urban villages and low-income neighbourhoods. While Indian traditions underpin work in heritage precincts and smaller projects, major schemes like this one copy imported models with little reference to Indian lifestyles, affordability, or place-making practices.

Pleasant exceptions are the Gujarat State Fertilizer Township near Vadodara and the Indian Fertilizer Corporation Township at Kalol, north of Ahmedabad, which employ Indian traditions of low-rise shared-wall courtyard and terrace houses, and meandering narrow streets. Similar schemes by Raj Rewal, such as the Asian Games Village in New Delhi, exhibit mature urban design strategies that hold the clues for further work. His mixed-use office and housing schemes, with

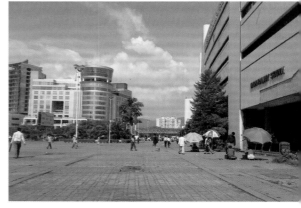

The Vashi Railway Station in Navi Mumbai

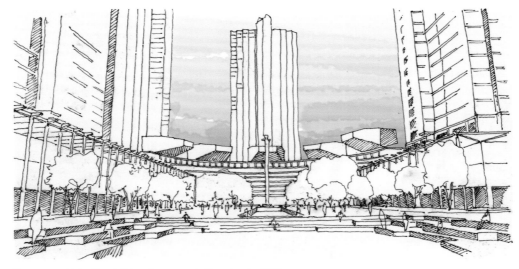

The proposed Azim Premji University campus in Bangalore by CCBA

landscape, leisure and cultural facilities and underground parking, are an excellent response to India's aspiring youth and emerging lifestyle.

The Delhi Metro Project, which will eventually extend to a length of 225 km, is covered by structures that have created 'no-man's land' areas. The authorities undertook no serious urban design studies to assess the metro's impact, or to utilise the potential of new, highly accessible areas that could have become major urban nodes with parks and arcaded shopping. Neither was the metro's layout used to generate a more efficient city structure, with new nodes and hubs. The multi-city Delhi–Mumbai Industrial Corridor is another missed opportunity, going the way of two-dimensional planning.

The involvement of urban designers in campus planning illustrates concepts from which city administrators and entrepreneurs could draw lessons. The Indian Institutes of Management (IIMs) at Ahmedabad and Bengaluru (then Bangalore), extensions to the IIMs in Ahmedabad and Kolkata, and the private Flame College in Pune and Azim Premji University in Bengaluru have cloistered pedestrian gardens within mixed-use dense clusters. With the exception of Louis Kahn's work at Ahmedabad, Indian architects have designed most of these academic campuses.

Where are the Indians?

The projects described hitherto might never be seen by the average inhabitant of India's cities. They may never ride on a metro train, nor shop in the malls or visit a multiplex. About 55% of India's urban population lives in under-serviced, unhygienic, overcrowded slums, most of which are unauthorised shanty towns within urban agglomerations. The masterplans prepared for the vast cities surrounding them ignore them. The inhabitants have no access to modern healthcare or minimum education, they will never see the parks and gardens we eulogise. The gates and guards at the new malls, multiplexes, airports and townships built by them would shoe them away before they'd get a whiff of the air conditioning. This 'other half' is really the majority of India's future and unless they are included within the planned urban scenario, economic disparity, social inequality, resentment and chaos will characterise the subcontinent's future.

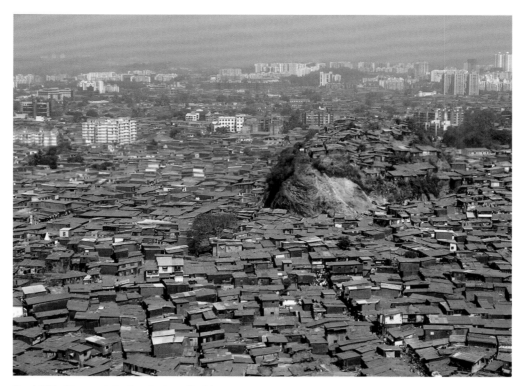

About 55% of the population lives in slums like this one

A recent analysis by the Monitor Group in Mumbai indicates that only 3% of the city's population could afford a shelter in the 'island city' of Mumbai. Another 6% would be able to afford accommodation within the western and eastern suburbs and the outlying suburbs of Navi Mumbai, Belapur Central Business District and Thane. And a further 8% may find affordable accommodation more than an hour's commute from the urban core. Thus, only 17% of the population of the Mumbai Metropolitan Region could ever imagine buying into the role of stakeholder through the acquisition of a home. There is considerable potential to create affordable shelter for the next lower 29% of the population through public–private ventures. Still, 54% of the urban population who earn less than $175 (£112) per month, would be left out of the system. But that too is a myth! They will find their way into shelters unimagined by market economies or middle-class professionals. This apparently irresolvable conundrum awaits the genius of future urban designers, who will unravel the true urban model of India's future.

Decades of urban poverty alleviation hint at solutions: the Slum Improvement Scheme, which provided basic services from the 1970s onwards; the Slum Redevelopment Schemes that operate in statutorily 'recognised slums'; the Busti Improvement Schemes of Kolkata; the 15,000 small-plot self-help Site and Services schemes in Chennai and the 'growing houses' in Hyderabad's Yusafguda incremental shelter scheme; pioneering low-income programmes by the Ahmedabad Study Action Group and Vikas' Centre for Development; the work of Society for Promotion of Area Resource Centres in Mumbai; along with Maharashtra Social Housing and Action League and Habitat and Associates in Pune – all stand out as pathfinders towards a possible humane urban future.

Faced with an irresolvable mushrooming of slums and the political might of slum dwellers, the Slum Rehabilitation Act in Maharashtra allows developers to rehouse them in free 25 m² multistorey units; all slum dwellers are thus rehoused on

25% of the built-up area, with the 75% additional built-up area available for luxury apartment towers. Though the scheme has practical benefits, extending free housing has retrogressive implications for the future: many of the small units are converted into migrants' hostels or sold to higher-income households, and the original slum dwellers disappear into the urban jungles. A similar institutional mechanism to improve living conditions is Regulation 33 of the Development Control Rules of Greater Mumbai, facilitating redevelopment proposals outside of recognised slums in old labour colonies and subdivided high-density urban neighbourhoods. Here too, the rehabilitation of dwellings allows for upmarket development on the remaining land.

These programmes are missed opportunities for the government to employ urban designers, social workers and capable city planners. The authorities should prepare appropriate urban design schemes prior to authorising such developments. The successful bidders would then implement the predesigned developments that had been reviewed by the households affected. Hope is promised by the Jawaharlal Nehru National Urban Renewal Mission, under which participation of stakeholders, monitoring of social infrastructure by responsible NGOs, and analysis of stress areas and services gaps will be implemented.

Finding the sustainable city

Indian architects, accustomed to designing low-energy buildings, have taken a keen interest in carbon emissions, toxic materials and air and water pollution, but investment in sustainability has been slow. The Centre for Development Studies and Activities at Pune pioneered studies in water management, biodiversity and environmental improvement of slums. The National Green Building Council promotes the American LEEDS rating system, and the Energy Research Institute (TERI) has innovated with more contextual norms for sustainable buildings, with their own TERI-Griha rating system. In 2003 after wide stakeholder debate and participation, the Royal Government of Bhutan approved the first urban 'green' plan of the subcontinent, which protects a number of areas under various headings covering more than half of the plan area. Waterways' edges are now protected and building controls take into account public-health considerations.

Depending on the project size, Environmental Impact Assessments and certifications are required by the ministry of environment, state governments, and district pollution boards. In 1996, the ministry published Urban Development Plan Formulation Implementation Guidelines that included rudimentary standards and procedures for environmental control. These applied standards of sustainability, depending on project typologies and functions. A National Mission on Sustainable Habitat now promotes citywide standards, better use of resources and sustainability at every level. However, vague standards are frequently arbitrarily applied to the private sector, leaving large sites vacant while ameliorative measures are being considered; if similar measures were applied across all government-administered schemes, they would close down all construction in India. Environmentalists working on an integrated approach to urban sustainability caution that in a rush to reduce emissions in a market-driven economy, costs should not be imposed on those least able to bear them.

In 2005, the Mumbai Metropolitan Regional Development Authority (MMRDA) was designated as Special Planning Authority for a 115 ha site in central Mumbai, to create a new transport hub and a cluster of tall buildings. In 2010, bids were invited for the development of this area, including an urban design proposal. The Abhishek Lodha Group, a private developer, won the tender, engaging Jay Berman of Pei Cobb Freed and Partners to prepare an urban design scheme. Berman's strategy was to demonstrate that thoughtful planning, strong urban design, consideration of environment and infrastructure could create a vigorous civic realm. This was the first time a foreign designer was engaged by a private developer to prepare a large-scale development in Mumbai.

The site lies at the centre of the Mumbai metropolitan region, to the east of the city's core. It has huge potential for rapid transformation due to its nascent transit and roadway connectivity, including a planned monorail line with an on-site station which would give it access to all parts of the metropolis.

The urban designers categorise their plan as exploratory, with an ambition to bring other stakeholders into the process. Their starting point was an analysis of the natural context and the site's connectivity, taking into account future traffic and transit infrastructure requirements. An open wetland abutting the site was separated from it by a mass-transit line and expressway. The team then looked at block structures and pedestrian networks in order to create a sense of place. Within this network, key areas for green spaces, recreation and gathering spaces, and cultural institutions were incorporated, to establish a vigorous civic realm. Systems responsive to local climate, ecology and hydrology were identified in order to celebrate these qualities in the new centre.

Based on a programme which proposed 85,000 residents, 290,000 workers and 50,000 visitors, the necessary built-up area could be estimated. Accordingly, roadways, sidewalks, playgrounds and parks were proposed, integrating landscape, infrastructure and buildings. All open spaces were to be accessible to the general public, breaking with gated-community concepts. On the basis of a plot ratio of four, 4,635,820 m^2 of floor space could be generated. The design included proposals for a second metro station and other infrastructure enhancements, and guidelines for developing 15 discrete land parcels. An analysis of Mumbai's urban fabric, including appropriate precinct sizes, image making, pedestrian movement patterns and building typologies, was the basis for establishing block sizes. Massing was studied and ownership patterns were analysed.

The proposal goes beyond the Development Plan of Mumbai to create a civic realm, integrating park and roadway systems, suggesting locations for important civic institutions, and incorporating iconic landscape and architecture. The intention is to create people-friendly street fronts, open building lobbies on to sidewalks, banish boundary walls, keep parking below ground and establish a range of spaces that can function at different neighbourhood and building scales. Green 'fingers' connect the interior open spaces with the adjoining wetland's open space. A podium covers the mass-transit line and expressway, which separate the site from natural open spaces and waterways, providing a pedestrian link to the latter. A number of boulevards, plazas, arcades and social gathering spaces are proposed. While the extension of street fronts into residential courts reflects indigenous street patterns, the scale of this project is new to India.

The project has four main characteristics. The first is its integration within the natural environment, employing sustainable measures for the

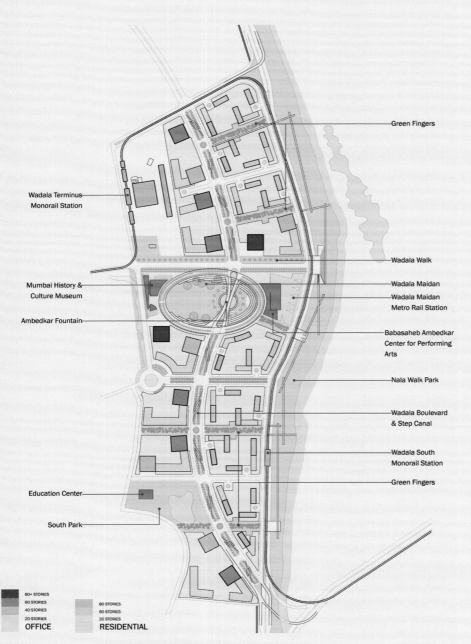

Green Fingers

Wadala Terminus
Monorail Station

Mumbai History &
Culture Museum

Ambedkar Fountain

Wadala Walk

Wadala Maidan

Wadala Maidan
Metro Rail Station

Babasaheb Ambedkar
Center for Performing
Arts

Nala Walk Park

Wadala Boulevard
& Step Canal

Wadala South
Monorail Station

Green Fingers

Education Center

South Park

80+ STORIES		80 STORIES
60 STORIES		60 STORIES
40 STORIES		20 STORIES
20 STORIES		
OFFICE		**RESIDENTIAL**

Wadala Metropolitan Centre, Mumbai: the master plan

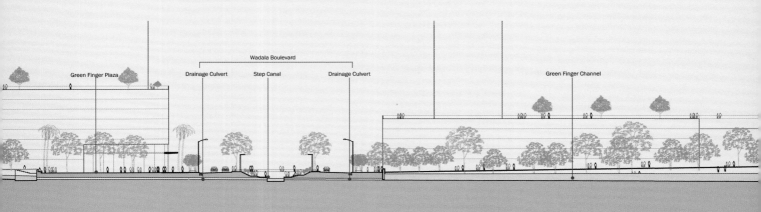

Green Finger Plaza

Wadala Boulevard

Drainage Culvert

Step Canal

Drainage Culvert

Green Finger Channel

Overview of the Wadala
proposed masterplan

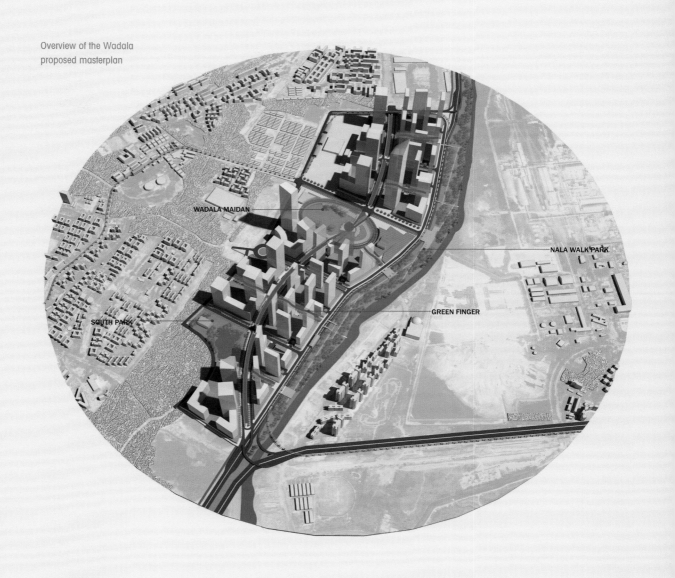

WADALA MAIDAN

NALA WALK PARK

GREEN FINGER

SOUTH PARK

Section through the proposed
Wadala Metropolitan Centre

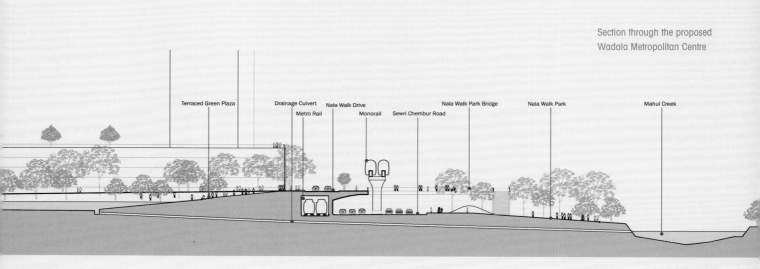

Terraced Green Plaza
Metro Rail
Drainage Culvert
Nala Walk Drive
Monorail
Sewri Chembur Road
Nala Walk Park Bridge
Nala Walk Park
Mahul Creek

Case study: Wadala Metropolitan Centre ~ **INDIA**

management, of water, solid waste, sewage and air conditioning. The second is linking the large site with arterial roads and the regional mass-transit system. The third is the creation of a sense of place and social integration through an extensive and well-conceived system of public spaces and pedestrian paths. The final one is the creation of a vibrant metropolitan centre enriched by cultural, civic, commercial and residential functions that are symbolic of Mumbai's creative role.

If completed, the Wadala Metropolitan Centre should provide the region with an accessible cultural, retail and entertainment hub. The problems encountered in earlier urban extensions should be overcome through ample parking, connectivity with mass transit, provision for retail and amenities, and a landscape pattern to make the large open spaces accessible and enjoyable to residents and visitors alike. However, both Mumbai's government planning agencies and private developers have a poor record on following through with such visionary schemes, and until firm commitments emerge this visionary idea remains just that!

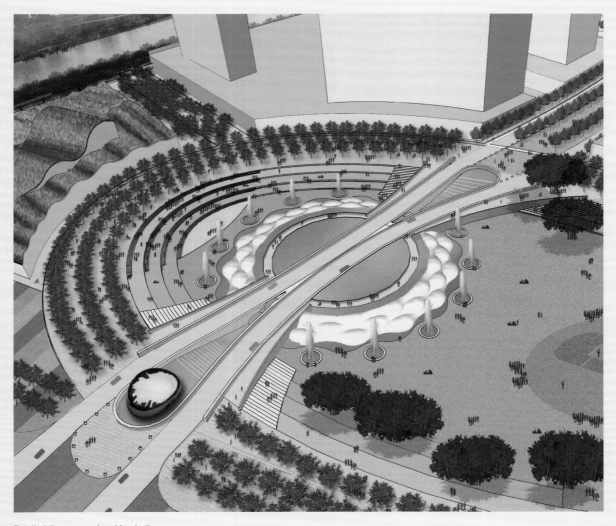

Detail of the proposed maidan in the
Wadala Metropolitan Centre

Conclusion:
the challenges for a possible tomorrow

India faces a huge challenge to create liveable, inclusive and sustainable cities, offering lively urban districts and convivial neighbourhoods to its citizens. Mobilising financial resources through a combination of public–private partnerships and cost savings and efficiencies is only part of this challenge.

The greater problem is the inability to conceptualise the urban conundrum of masses of low-income marginally educated workers who will make up the largest proportion of India's urban population. Their education, human-resource development, skills mobilisation and employment are the keys to India's survival and success. Unless the urban design and planning professions reinvent themselves to deal with the neglected poorest 60% of urban dwellers, this problem will not be resolved. Beautiful, cosy, pedestrian-friendly high-density human places will not be sufficient if they are only 'responsible luxury' for the upper 20% of the population. The challenge is to build liveable, sustainable and affordable habitats for lower-income groups.

The Indian Planning Commission, in analysing how to invest a trillion US dollars (£638,000 million) into urban infrastructure has divided the task into several categories. Among them are managing the economic environment to bring about inclusion and efficiency; enhancing the skills linked to rapid employment generation; decentralising decision-making; giving better access to information; employing technology and facilitating innovation; accelerating the development of sustainable transportation infrastructure; improving urban management; facilitating access to appropriate human-resources development; and improving preventive and curative healthcare.

This should be the basis for a new urban design charter and aggressive advocacy. For the first time, issues such as sustainability, liveability, transportation and urbanisation are being articulated specifically, with an understanding that all these achievements will emanate from India's urban centres where 65% of its wealth is generated!

A quick guide to
India

1 TYPES OF CLIENT

Urban development authorities

Municipal authorities

Universities

Urban development finance corporations, such as the Financial Services Limited Corporation

Private developers

International investment companies (not always successfully)

....

2 TYPES OF
PROJECT/WORK

Urban masterplans and urban extensions

Plans for transport infrastructure: ports, airports, terminals

Plans for industrial and university campuses and IT parks

Township layouts

Parks, river- and oceanfront developments

Main street redevelopment

....

3 APPROACH NEEDED
TO WORK IN COUNTRY

Open local offices in metropolitan hubs and market your services

Establish partnerships with better-connected local firms

Offer specialised expertise

Monitor web-based announcements of schemes

Well-known national firms are overextended and often seek partnerships to add capacity and capability

....

4 LEGISLATION
THAT NEEDS TO BE
REFERRED TO

States in India have opaque town-planning measures, metropolitan and regional planning acts, city-based development-control rules and formative fire regulations impinging on layouts. There are also new statutory measures and executive directives facilitating new town-development schemes, urban redevelopment and special economic zones

....

5	SPECIFIC TIPS FOR SUCCESS	Compliance with *vaastu* is a daunting obstacle: plans need to address these 'lucky and unlucky' orientations, relative locations, heights and positions of 'hot' and 'cold' activities, in auspicious and inauspicious zones
		Incentives are offered to facilitate the provision of social housing
		Across India, planning and architectural firms engage agencies specialising in development-control rules compliance and clearance procedures to navigate the byzantine bureaucracy and labyrinth of planning legislation

6	USEFUL WEBSITES	Institute of Urban Designers India: www.udesindia.org
		Planning Commission, Government of India: www.planningcommission.nic.in
		The Indian Institute of Architects: www.iia-india.org

SELECTED FACTS

1	area	3,287,590 km²
2	population	1,170,938,000
3	annual population growth	1.3%
4	urban population	30%
5	population density	356 p/km²
6	GDP	$1,727,111,096,363
7	GNI per capita	$1,330

Source: The World Bank (2010)

SECTION 4

THE
AMERICAS

ARGENTINA

Elba Rodriguez, *architect–planner*
Raquel Perahia, *architect–planner*

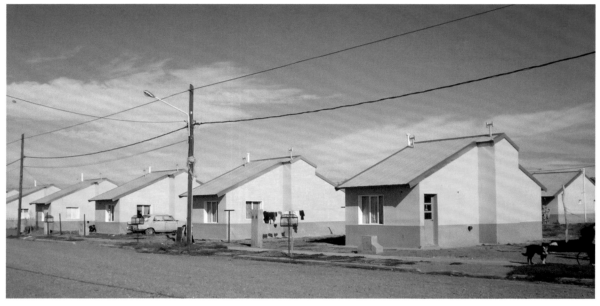

Public housing development in Sarmiento, province of Chubut

LOCATED at the far south of the American continent, Argentina borders Bolivia and Paraguay in the north, Brazil, Uruguay and the Atlantic ocean in the east, and Chile in the west. The mainland extends over 3,700 km from north to south, and as a result its climate varies from subtropical to subartic.

About a third of the country lies in humid zones and 30% of it includes forests and subtropical woodland; the remaining 600,000 km² are covered by the pampas, one of the most fertile plains in the world. It is here that 70% of the country's population lives, and where 80% of the agricultural and 85% of its industrial activities are located.

Argentina is a constitutional federal republic; the president and the congress are directly elected. The country is divided into 23 provinces plus the Federal District, which is Buenos Aires, the capital. The provinces and the city of Buenos Aires are autonomous states with their own constitution, political, economic and administrative powers.

The municipalities establish and implement land policies as well as social and economic ones at the local level. As such, they have responsibilities (delegated by the provincial constitutions) regarding the management of cities and the preparation of development plans. A municipality is generally created when a settlement reaches somewhere between 500 and 2,000 inhabitants. As a result, 82% of municipalities (1,700) have a population of less than 10,000, whilst 63 municipalities (0.03% of the total), with populations exceeding 100,000, comprise 60% of the country's total (2001 census).

The population distribution over the country as a whole is very unbalanced: one third of the total is located in the Buenos Aires Metropolitan Area (AMBA); two other cities, Córdoba and Rosario, follow with 1.3 million and 1.2 million inhabitants respectively; the third rank includes the other provincial capitals and a few tourist centres with populations of around 500,000 inhabitants each.

Buenos Aires Metropolitan Area covers 3,880 km² (including the city and 24 surrounding districts) and has a population of 13,416,067 inhabitants (2011 census). It is part of a wider area, the Metropolitan Region of Buenos Aires (the city plus 40 districts), covering 13,900 km² and with a population of 14,442,684 inhabitants (2011 census).

The scope of this chapter

As a result of the above-mentioned population concentration, this chapter deals mainly with the AMBA, the area with the most dynamic expansion but also with mobility and social tensions which have impacted not always successfully, on the process

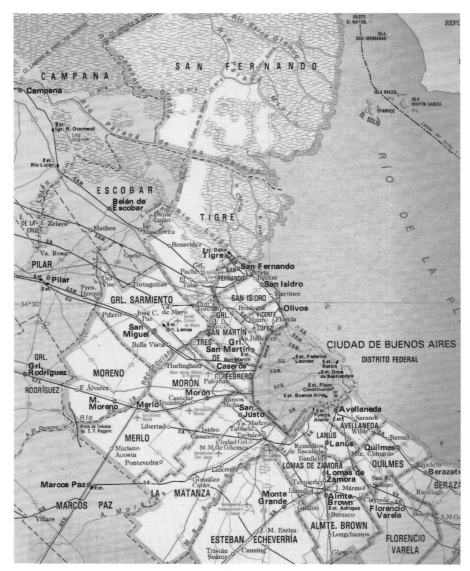

Buenos Aires Metropolitan Area covers several districts beyond the city of Buenos Aires

of urbanisation and on the environment. Two very different approaches to urban development are taken by the private and the public sectors respectively.

Cities in Argentina have always suffered from a housing deficit and a lack of basic infrastructure, in particular running water and sewers; only 60% of urban areas are connected to the sewerage system. That is why most public investment is directed to housing, whilst public space and other urban amenities are recognised as a necessary but rarely sufficient complement.

Private developments take a different approach, as they are directed at more affluent groups of the population which expect attractive designs that incorporate amenities such as large green areas and water features allowing for sport activities. Developers of these neighbourhoods apply devices which interpret the provincial legislation for 'country clubs' in a very non-traditional way.

Definitions: a conceptual approach

The term 'urban design' has been translated literally as *diseño urbano*, which in general terms means the organising of urban space in order to adapt its physical, socio-cultural, economic and historical characteristics to the current reality. However, because of the conservative character of academic curricula, urban design has remained more closely linked to the architectural 'object' than to its relationship with the urban environment. Urban design always was, and still is, an undefined area contested both by architects and planners. The latter, with their wider overview, have concentrated mainly on regulation and urban policy rather than the spatial dimension of the city. In some cases, they have worked on specialised urban districts such as industrial parks or conservation areas, which require a comprehensive approach and their own specific regulations.

Even the architect's professional body lists for the purpose of honoraria the design and construction of a building or a group of buildings and planning activities, but does not mention urban design. And yet such work can be found, particularly in the province of Buenos Aires: for instance, in housing developments where the design includes not just the individual buildings but an ensemble with public spaces that promote community interaction, and that respond well to the surrounding urban district.

Historical background

Argentine cities, like those throughout colonial Spain founded from the 15th century onwards, followed a pattern established by the Laws of the Indies: a grid layout with, at its centre, a civic square with the governor's house, the church and the *cabildo*, or town hall.

Towards the end of the 19th century, as the city of Buenos Aires was experiencing considerable urban expansion, another pattern was superimposed onto the original grid: some streets were widened and became avenues, and two major diagonals cut through the urban chequerboard. In 1894, the Avenida de Mayo was opened as a kind of institutional mall linking the government and the congress buildings. Also at the

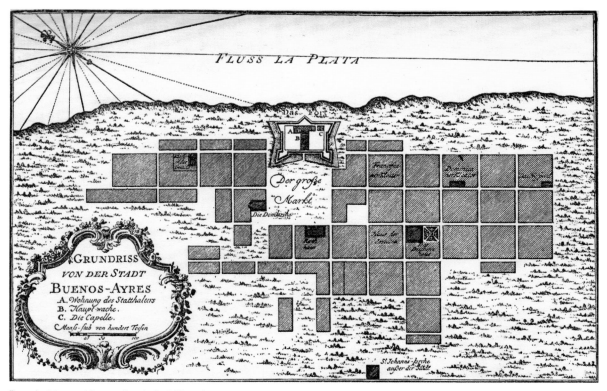

The colonial core of Buenos Aires in the 16th century

time, hygienist and City Beautiful ideas combined to provide the city with large open spaces. The French landscape designer Carlos Thays was invited to design the Tres de Febrero park, which continues to be the main 'green lung' of the city, and he followed this with a number of other smaller parks.

As the capital grew (at a very different rate than the rest of the country), its transport infrastructure was gradually developed – first with the opening in 1897 of a network of electrical tramways radiating from the city centre and later with the underground, inaugurated in 1913 and the first such line in Latin America. In 1913, the tramlines were removed from one of the main city-centre streets, Florida, so as to turn it into a pedestrian promenade, making it probably the first example of its kind in the world. It attracted the most glamorous shops of the continent (including Harrods department store), and in 1971 a new unified road surface was laid down from facade to facade.

At the end of the 19th century, new typologies for housing development had appeared, breaking with the monotony of the traditional grid, sometimes through the introduction of a private communal passageway cutting through the urban block. In other cases, the block was structured around a private but communal internal patio. Examples of these can be found throughout the city, but the current building regulations no longer allow for these typologies to be replicated.

In addition, numerous estates for workers and immigrants were built by a variety of institutions: the railway companies, the armed forces, specific industries, religious congregations, etc. Even today, these small houses are sought after as they are well designed and in quiet locations:

> Buenos Aires hides many … real microclimates of tiny blocks, narrow
> footpaths and streets named after birds, trees or writers … The 21st Century

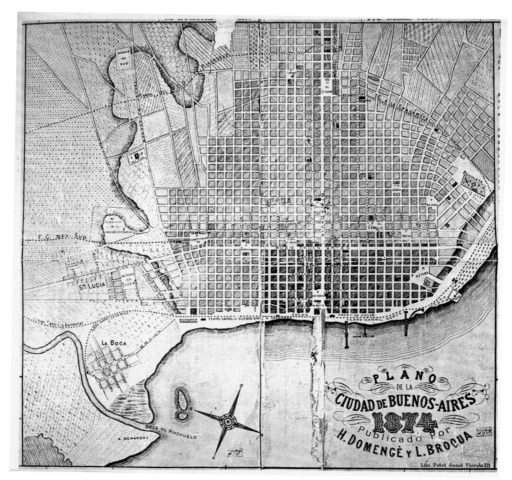

Buenos Aires at the end of the 19th century

SECCIONES CATASTRALES
ESCALA 1: 20000

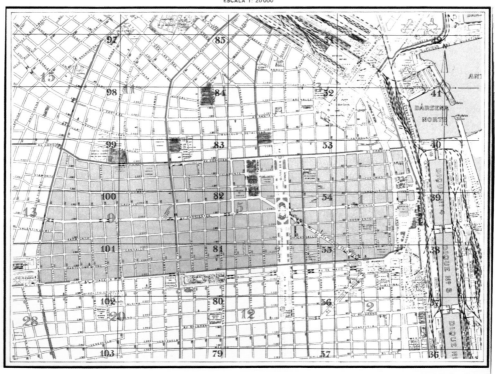

The central area of Buenos Aires with the diagonal avenues opened in the 1920s

has transformed them in fashionable neighbourhoods, ideal for those that search for calm in the middle of the city.

(Sanchez, N, Clarín, 12 September 2004)

During the first world war, the government also stimulated the construction of affordable neighbourhoods in order to improve conditions for thousands of families living in overcrowded tenements. In 1915, and following the Cheap Housing Act, a commission started building 'comfortable and hygienic' dwellings; the first of these neighbourhoods completed in 1921 comprises 161 small houses with 'a British appearance'. Thereafter, single-family houses on individual plots continued to be popular, even though from the 1970s onwards large social housing estates with apartment blocks were also built. About that time, and in response to the great shortage of housing and the increasing demand for it, a mass building programme took precedence over concerns of urban design. This might not have happened if an overall vision of buildings in their urban context had existed.

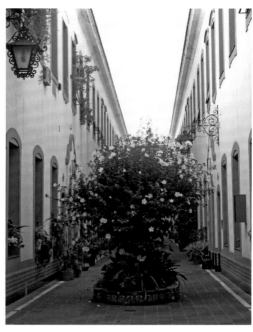

Pasaje Sarmiento: a passageway built in 1893 cutting through a street city block

The academic position of urban design

The national universities responsible for the education of professionals, wishing to widen the scope of architectural practice, include large-scale and complex projects in the latter years of the curriculum, but these still deal with buildings rather than the public realm, and do not help create a separate urban design specialism. As a result, the latter is functionally part of architectural professional practice but not formally a part of the academic concerns. As the universities widened and updated their curricula to respond to the evolving requirements and expectations of society, new academic fields developed, mainly at postgraduate level, such as urban and regional planning, landscape design, sustainability and conservation. These allowed professionals to collaborate in interdisciplinary teams, and to be better prepared to work on major urban schemes.

Early on, the University of Buenos Aires adopted the European tradition of the International Congress of Modern Architecture (CIAM) with an integrated approach that placed the architect–urbanist as the team leader – an image that has been maintained to this day, probably because of its all-embracing vision of the physical, environmental and social space. Postgraduate courses at this university cover specialisations that are complementary to urban design and are geared to professionals coming from a variety of backgrounds: engineers, architects, sociologists, archaeologists, etc. Examples of such courses are Preservation, Conservation and Reuse of the Built Heritage; Urban Landscape; and Environmental Urban Management (in collaboration with the Politécnico di Milano).

Urban design and legislation

Because of the country's federal constitution, legislation varies from province to province and also from one city to another. Regulations are supposedly adapted to the morphological and socio-cultural characteristics of each region, respecting the materials available and predominant local styles. In many cities – particularly the provincial capitals and other large cities – in addition to the standard building regulations, planning codes based on zoning regulate the character of new urban developments, covering the subdivision of land, land-use, building height, setbacks and plot ratios. They also establish standards for the public realm: street alignment, public spaces, squares, lighting, landscaping, etc. However, these documents are generic rather than based on analysis and an urban vision. The law does not oblige cities to prepare plans, although they are allowed to do so in order to organise their urban space according to their own local legislation. Municipalities either prepare these plans in-house or commission them from multidisciplinary teams of consultants.

In the case of large urban developments, some plans lay down special conditions that offer greater opportunities for urban design. They can apply as much to central areas as they can to conservation or the reuse of industrial districts. Special regulations also apply to social housing projects financed by the government: these cover their location, street layout and public spaces, the basic social amenities and general typologies for the dwellings.

Recently, the government has published a national strategic plan (Argentina 2016) with the objective of identifying priorities for investment in infrastructure and to provide a spatial framework for sustainable development. Equally, some provinces have physical development plans which should provide the framework for more local ones.

Current practice

From the 1990s onwards, urban development expanded strongly through both large private investment and the government's social housing plans. Since then, the main stakeholders in the financing, design and development of large urban design projects have tended to come from the private sector: real-estate investment companies, who commission teams of consultants from various disciplines (architecture, landscape, engineering, transport, etc). Occasionally, well-known and reputed urban designers are asked to be part of these teams in spite of the fact that their profession is not formally recognised. Increasingly, the investors are international agents who aim for a middle- or high-income clientele. Their aim is to maximise profits without much concern for local character, and they try to minimise the impact of existing regulations on their schemes. The subordination of the public sector is even apparent in public–private partnership schemes, where the private companies and the local authority are unequal partners and the latter tends to submit to the pressures of private capital. Private and public developments have their own specific morphological and typological characteristics.

Predominant types of private developments

Private-sector developments can be divided into four main categories:

1. Isolated buildings. In central areas and along the main traffic arteries the predominant typology is that of tall isolated buildings for the headquarters of leading enterprises, international hotels and retail or leisure complexes. The design of the building as 'object' predominates and the public realm is hardly a concern.

2. Large mixed-use developments in central areas or regenerated historic areas. The best known of this type is Puerto Madero, a public–private initiative that commenced some 20 years ago. Several distinct operations took place over the 170 ha of land available, resulting in high-rise office blocks aimed at headquarters of international corporations, luxury housing, hotels and a substantial amount of public and green spaces – all of which can compete in a global market in terms of design quality, materials and amenities.

   The buildings, designed by internationally reputed architectural firms and managed and marketed by local estate agents, have the advantage of being on large parcels of land that cannot be found elsewhere in the city centre. The area also has the advantage over other central districts of including a publicly accessible, though private, open space of a high quality of design and finishing, secure and well managed by the private–public Corporation of Puerto Madero. The model for this development seems to have been Canary Wharf in London's Isle of Dogs.

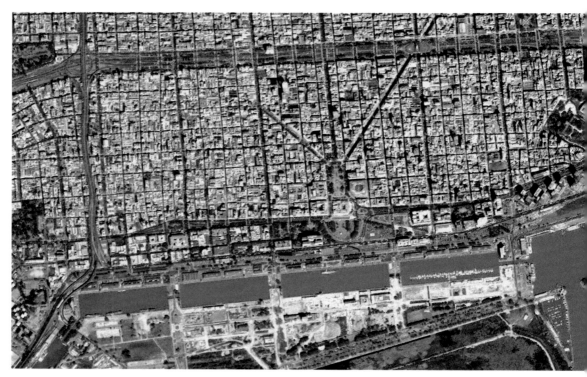

Aerial view of CBD shows the location of Puerto Madero near the city centre

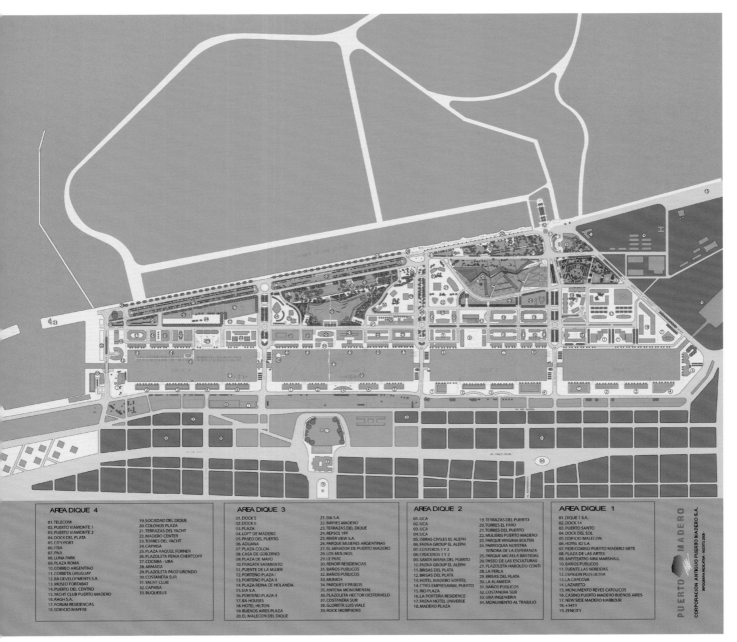

The new layout of the Puerto Madero district

3.   Within the Metropolitan Region of Buenos Aires, new and complex
     centralities with large shopping, recreation and service facilities have chosen
     to locate in the second or third outer ring of the metropolitan area, in order
     to maximise their accessibility and to be near the new private residential
     settlements described below. Helped by the improved accessibility provided
     by the motorway network and new distribution technologies, these large
     commercial developments establish themselves as the new centres for
     consumption and leisure. They have their own security services, and their
     customers are the residents of the new country clubs, polo clubs and gated
     communities. The large traffic flows generated by these developments
     influence the choice of location and the size of the land needed to
     accommodate circulation and parking. The developers' agents often search

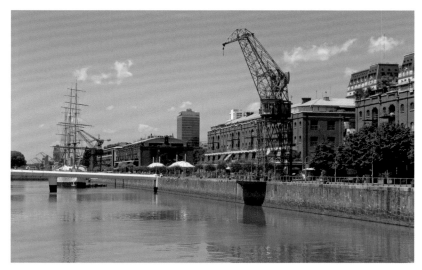

View of the renovated docks of Puerto Madero

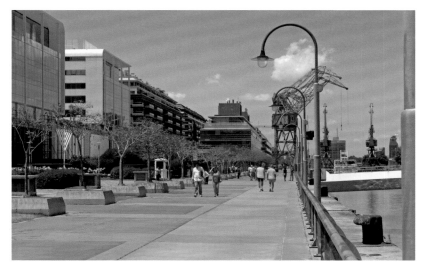

New developments along the quays in Puerto Madero

for the best peripheral locations, near the motorways and on rural or semi-rural land which can be purchased at low cost.

These 'New Centralities' compete with traditional commercial and leisure centres, which consequently lose customers and activities. Their design is similar to those in other countries, as they adopt imported models and international brands. In most cases they are built with foreign capital, and the same patterns and appearance can be found in all Argentina's large cities. As François Asher observed (Asher 2004, p. 60): 'The geometric centre is no longer the most accessible place, particularly for the car driving citizen.'

4. Private urban developments on the metropolitan edge. The expansion of suburban residential gated communities aimed at higher income groups, which choose them in search of a better quality of life, represent without doubt a new form of habitat that breaks with traditional urban forms. Their precursors first appeared in the 1970s as 'country clubs', aimed at providing second homes for the weekend and offering sports facilities.

For a number of reasons, this kind of development offers the most distinct type of urban design:

- The size of the schemes, the amount of land subdivided and urbanised but not always totally occupied, is in the order of 30,000 ha (about the size of the English city of Birmingham)
- The surprising continuity and permanence of these developments from around the 1990s to this day; they have even avoided the cyclic character of the construction and real-estate markets, with their peaks and troughs
- The common theme of these operations – housing and living – means that a variety of professions are involved in small, medium and large schemes, with considerable capital investments
- The local authorities of the peripheral districts have large areas of land where agricultural production is weak; they are therefore attracted by these urban schemes and are willing to lower their planning standards in order to accommodate the requirements of the investors
- The schemes end up being planned privately, according to regulations that respond to market forces instead of the weak or non-existing public plan

These gated communities – with a variety of labels from country clubs and marinas to 'urban villages' – are located mostly in a ring between 40 and 60 km around the capital. They are linked by the motorway network, rely on private cars and their own security services, and they spread the urban area in a fragmented way, with no connections to the existing morphology.

Part of the attraction of these developments for their customers is that retailers and educational establishments follow them. They also offer substantial open spaces, a quiet life closer to nature, easy commuting and easy shopping in retail malls reached by the motorways. They are a promising alternative to the increasingly stressful city life; they offer a high-quality infrastructure, well-kept public spaces, safety, status and a fairly transparent management with clear means of participation. These neighbourhoods are usually surrounded by a solid wall or a hedge; access is controlled, and the 'message' is clear: what is inside is private.

State-financed development of public housing

Benefiting from increasing tax revenues, and aiming to finally resolve the housing shortage affecting the weaker sectors of the population, the government decided in 2004 to increase the production of housing and, at the same time, generate employment and help to revive the construction industry.

The Federal Housing Plan I, initiated in June 2004, aimed to build 120,000 dwellings throughout the country. The Federal Housing Plan II, agreed with the provincial governments in August 2005, had the more ambitious aim of building 300,000 dwellings. Tenders are open to building firms putting forward proposals for land with a project, which in some cases includes urban design regulations. The land offered is sometimes of poor quality and presents difficulties for the provision of infrastructure and services, thus requiring major investments.

Many of the schemes built as a result of these housing programmes are scattered and poorly linked to the existing urban grids. The developers choose to build on cheap land without considering accessibility or physical characteristics. In addition, these developments are rarely designed with reference to a planning framework – and even when such a document exists, it is mostly ignored by the housing developers for whom the cost of land is their prime criterion. As a result, the development costs are high and the schemes end up in vulnerable and dysfunctional locations, ignoring any planning or urban design strategy.

The neighbourhoods thus financed by the plan are mostly of very low density – single houses on individual plots – and a repeated typology that does not answer adequately the functional, spatial or climatic issues of the locality. In most cases, the townscape is characterless and monotonous as a result of the repetitive design of these dwellings and the lack of differentiation between them. They are totally disconnected from the multifunctional and lively urban fabric of the traditional cities.

Environmental issues

A central government department with the status of a ministry, the National Environment Establishment, has responsibilities for environmental matters and publishes overall directives. But local authorities and the housing institutes are in charge of planning and building norms.

As early as the 1980s, environmental guidelines were published concerning housing or neighbourhood schemes financed by central government. They recommended ways of conserving energy by taking into account the natural characteristics of the site (land form, climate, tree coverage, etc) and thus improving the liveability of the scheme. In the private domain, environmental protection has only recently become a growing concern as its links with public health and comfort have been understood. As a result, building standards have been altered to take into account energy conservation in particular. To this effect, the province of Buenos Aires has pioneered changes in legislation. Examples of sustainable developments in the city of Buenos Aires are the Madero Office development, and the first Leadership in Energy and Environmental Design (LEED) certified public building in Latin America, a branch of the Banco Ciudad designed by a local firm in partnership with Norman Foster.

The treatment and design of public and private spaces in the gated communities described above have enhanced the natural characteristics of the areas and created good-quality habitats. Furthermore, some of these schemes have developed and applied new techniques that conserve energy and protect the environment. These include the use of recycled materials, solar-heating panels, the storage and use of rainwater, geothermic energy generation and water-saving measures.

On the other hand, the Architecture and Planning Professional Organisation has produced a manual of environmental good practice, Sustainability in Architecture, with recommendations on the choice of sites, density and the positioning of buildings in respect to topography and climate, water, energy, materials, etc.

CASE STUDY

TIGRE DISTRICT

The Tigre district in the outskirts of Buenos Aires has one of highest levels of development and the largest concentration of private residential urbanisations in the country. Its environmental characteristics and landscape are exceptional as it is located at the end of the Parana river delta, on lowlands subject to flooding that have been made safe and buildable through major private investment. The advantage of being near the

capital city, and with land adjacent to water, have accelerated the expansion of the area as it responds to the demands of the market.

From 1990 onwards, and as a result of public investment in motorways and in the public realm, new developments appeared on the improved land of the so-called 'new Tigre'. Two companies operating in this area: Nordelta with 1,600 ha of

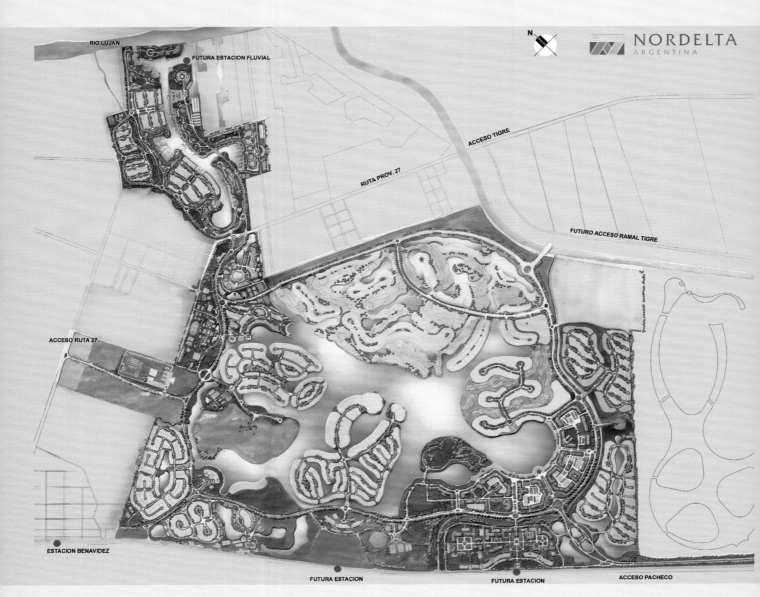

Nordelta, general plan

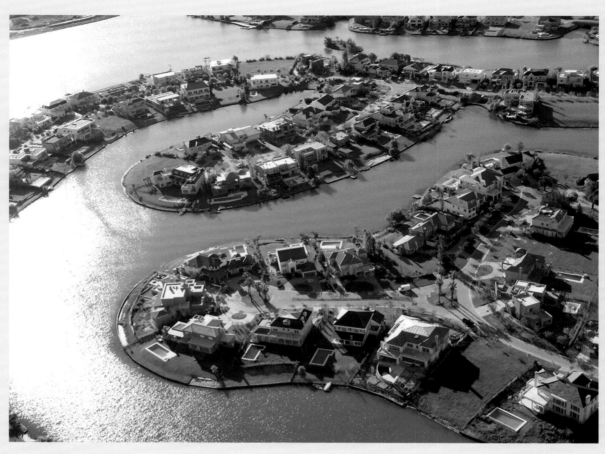

Nordelta, partial aerial view

land, has given its name to a new district; and Eidico, which deals with co-ownership schemes.

Nordelta is impressive because of its size and location. It includes educational facilities at all levels, retail centres, offices for high-end enterprises, marinas and docking facilities on the river Luján, and all amenities needed for a predicted population of between 80,000 and 120,000 inhabitants. The masterplan for what has been called the New City of Nordelta was prepared in 1990 by Ruben Pesci, a well-known and reputed architect–planner and founder of the Centre for Environmental Studies (CEPA), working in partnership with other local architects – Antonio Rossi and Omar Accattoli among them. The plan proposes the creation of 22 distinct neighbourhoods which will be developed and occupied in successive phases. At the centre of the area, where the lowlands have been filled and raised, the design has entirely modified the local environment and the topography.

The other firm, Eidico, makes clear its requirements in choosing the location for such a neighbourhood:
- Large rural parcels of land with few owners willing to convert them into residential development
- No informal occupants or subdivision of land
- Proximity to other large developments or other prestigious gated communities

This firm claims to 'recycle' the concept of cooperative housing by pooling the efforts of small investors in order to convert agricultural land into an equipped urban development. Legally, this is a form of trust in which Eidico is the administrator and the investors are the beneficiaries. The trust represents the interests of the client from the inception of the scheme until the buildings are delivered. This method of selling attracts a well-off clientele and guarantees the firm an early return on its capital. The buyers are attracted by short-term benefits and the possibility of getting access to urbanised land at a reasonable cost.

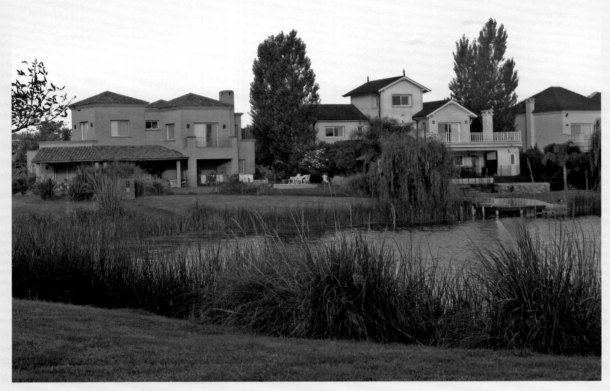

Nordelta, houses around one of the lakes

As the buildings have to be located on land elevated some 2 m above the existing ground level, the neighbourhoods are organised around small lakes that are created by soil movements. Densities are low and plots of land are about 800 m² in area, green spaces are abundant and well maintained, and residents can feel close to nature: looking at water and birds, undertaking water sports and other fitness activities.

A masterplan prepared for the whole development imposes certain standards for building heights, setbacks, materials, etc in order to give the ensemble some formal unity. Thereafter, each plot owner can commission an architect to design their home. Single-family houses are individually designed using different colours, materials, textures and technologies, though in accordance with standards established by the internal codes of the scheme. The projects are fairly imaginative and offer a range of urban patterns and spatial typologies. As a result of a constant inflow of capital the schemes succeed each other without discontinuity, and reasonable coherence is maintained overall.

Picturesque loops, cul-de-sacs and curves that reduce vehicular speed and increase the possibility of controlling passersby have replaced the traditional square grid of the open city. In addition to the wall surrounding the whole area and the strict control of access by non-residents, the curvilinear streets and restricted traffic all combine to emphasise the private and exclusive character of the neighbourhood

The variety of building forms; the positioning of the houses within a green space, with no fences between neighbours and no footpaths; and the high level of maintenance create a private–public environment of good landscape quality that attracts buyers and makes residents feel secure in an oasis far away from the fast, noisy and unsafe city.

More recently, the developers have started building two- or three-storey blocks of flats for those that prefer this kind of dwelling, or for buy-to-let investments.

Conclusions

Observing the main schemes completed in and around its large cities, one can conclude that urban design in Argentina is produced by a group of talented and well-informed professionals who rely on external influences for inspiration. Architects, planners and designers who are entrusted with such schemes, have access to other specialist professionals such as highway engineers or landscape architects. These teams normally design a group of buildings and its immediate surroundings, but are not concerned with its articulation within the wider urban context.

On the other hand, the historical schemes mentioned above and the government-financed housing developments of the 1930s did not establish a tradition or an accepted practice that could be replicated and adapted, in spite of the fact that these have always been recognised as good examples of urban design.

The most recent and numerous private urbanisations, the gated communities described above which enlarge the metropolitan outskirts, imitate foreign models marketed by specialised firms. Even when multidisciplinary teams with reputed and respected professionals at their helm are involved, the 'brand name' of the development and the marketing firms are of greater importance. New technologies that offer comfort and status, new morphologies, and residential typologies that reflect what is published in international magazines are introduced. The resulting townscape is not rooted in the place but corresponds to a globalised image, wherein what is artificial is seen as natural and is considered better than the existing landscape. It would seem that a sense of place, based on permanence, roots and appropriation by the inhabitants, has disappeared.

On the other hand, there is a lack of large-scale spatial planning and of a structure that would help the articulation between new neighbourhoods and the existing city. The urban area grows in a fragmented way, as new developments are completed without a masterplan or a method of incorporating them in their context.

As a result, no land is reserved to connect the neighbourhoods to one another or to the existing services. The in-between spaces of varying sizes have no planning controls and no infrastructure, and tend to attract illegal occupants who work for the residents of the adjacent gated communities but live in an environment of very poor quality.

The introduction of courses in urban design at university level is relatively recent (in the last 10 to 15 years), and their character varies according to the type of faculty they are attached to. However, the recognition of their value, whether formal or informal, is highly encouraging. Looking to the future of the profession, the inclusion of the urban environment in all its aspects – from the macro to the micro – among its concerns, would be welcome in order to improve the environmental quality and the quality of life of the population. To this end, postgraduate studies should make sure that at all levels 'the scheme' is placed within its immediate context (the block, the street, the neighbourhood), so that the architect–urbanist understands the impact of his/her work on the city. Therefore, postgraduate planning courses should not only be multidisciplinary but also specifically include urban design in their curricula. This would also ensure that professionals working for local authorities produce guidelines that would assist, rather than restrict, the work of their colleagues.

A quick guide to
Argentina

1 TYPES OF CLIENT

Municipalities (local authorities)

Private developers (local or international)

---

2 TYPES OF
PROJECT/WORK

Masterplan
- New communities
- Urban extensions

Very occasionally, design guidelines: mostly these are done in-house by local authorities, but a consultant may be asked to prepare the technical documentation

---

3 APPROACH NEEDED
TO WORK IN COUNTRY

Contact with local authorities, in particular the mayor or the person in charge of public works

International competitions, often with the involvement of the professional body (Sociedad Central de Arquitectos)

Direct negotiation with the client

Partnership with a local firm is highly recommended

---

4 LEGISLATION
THAT NEEDS TO BE
REFERRED TO

Cities' local plans

Design guidelines such as planning codes and building codes

Other requirements: in the case of new communities, the links with the existing road networks have to be checked and adhered to

---

5 SPECIFIC TIPS
FOR SUCCESS

A 'foreign' consultant is not going to be signing statutory documents; therefore, an Argentine professional qualification is not required

Patience is recommended in dealing with the bureaucracy and its unpredictability

---

6 USEFUL WEBSITES

Consejo Nacional de la Vivienda: www.cnvivienda.org.ar

Ministerio de Planificación Federal, Inversión Pública y Servicios: www.minplan.gov.ar

Sociedad Central de Arquitectos: www.socearq.org

1	area	2,766,890 km^2
2	population	40,412,376
3	annual population growth	0.9%
4	urban population	92%
5	population density	14.6 p/km^2
6	GDP	$368,711,957,358
7	GNI per capita	$8,620

Source: The World Bank (2010)

BRAZIL

Vicente del Rio, *professor of city and regional planning*

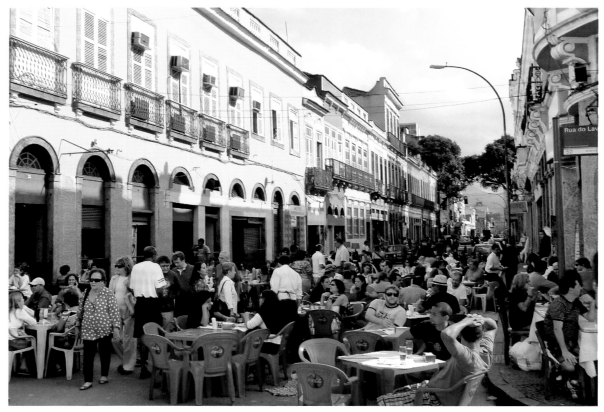

Bars in renovated historic buildings in Rio's Cultural Corridor extend their
functions into the streets, attracting shoppers to nearby commercial uses

BRAZIL is a democratic federal republic with a presidential system and three levels of governance: federal, state and municipal. All of these are autonomous and can approve legislation, but they have to be compatible with each other. There are 26 states plus the Federal District, and 5,560 municipalities.

Introduction

As is typical of a developing country, cities in Brazil are marked by historical and socio-economic inequalities, and by the long domination of the capitalist mode of production and market forces – now further accentuated by globalisation. Urban morphologies and cityscapes reveal strong dualities and a constant tension between opposite realms: global–local, private–public, and individual–collective. However, after Brazil's return to democracy in the late 1980s political forces forged a pact toward a new social order and a model of urban development for more just cities. During the last two decades, Brazil's political and economic advances have placed it in the international spotlight, and the evidence points to a new country in the making with undeniable advances in political representation, governance, social programmes and income distribution.

True to their early modernist origins, planning and urban design in Brazil are still strongly attached to ideals of equity, social justice, and a better quality of life in cities. They have long been incorporated into the public apparatus and their reach remains dependent on the public sector; as such, they are instrumental in Brazil's search for a new social and developmental agenda. Having originated in the domain of architecture in the late 1930s, neither planning nor urban design are recognised as disciplines or as stand-alone professions. They both remain very dependent on architecture, though at least planning can rely on a strong interdisciplinary network of postgraduate programmes. However, urban design in Brazil is mostly understood as part of the city planning process and, as such, it has been instrumental in reshaping places.

Over the last decade, numerous examples of cutting-edge research, programmes and projects in planning and urban design for better cities have emerged. This chapter deals with how contemporary Brazilian cities have been shaped, and discusses the major trends in Brazilian urban design, as a contribution to a better understanding of its role from an international perspective.[1]

A preface for contemporary urban design

In the last 20 years, Brazil has been successful in turning its politics and its economy around, and has become one of the world's top economic performers. However, the size and complexity of the urban question are huge, and cities still face a myriad of problems. In 2010, population exceeded 190 million, 84% of which lived in urban areas, and 15 cities had over one million inhabitants. Although the urban population's growth rate dropped over the last few decades, medium-sized cities are now growing at a much faster pace. In 2010 more that 11 million people lived in Sao Paulo, Brazil's largest city, and over 19 million in the Greater Sao Paulo region (covering an area of 7,943 km²). In the same year, over six million people lived in Rio, Brazil's second largest city, and over 11 million in the Greater Rio area.

Brazil's long-standing historical socio-economic disparities have generated cities of fragmented territories, worsened by new models imposed by globalisation. Although between 2000 and 2010 the population living in *favelas* decreased by 16%, 6 million people still live under such conditions. In Rio, although the population increased by less that 1% in the last decade, the amount of people living in *favelas* expanded by more that 2%, and they count for almost 20% of the city's residents. While 11% of people residing in the city of Sao Paulo are *favelados*, in the Greater Sao Paulo area their numbers increase to 25%. These figures expose only part of the problem: a much larger population lives in other types of substandard environments such as inner-city slums or illegal subdivisions far from the better-serviced city, and suffers from lack of public services such as piped water and sewage systems, decent public transport and easy access to schools, hospitals and jobs.

This sombre context for urban design started to change in the 1980s when the military dictatorship that had ruled since 1964 was ousted. Since returning to democracy, Brazil has made undeniable advances in political representation, governance, economic and social development, and – with the defeat of inflation – income distribution. The national debates leading up to the drafting of the 1988 national constitution exposed the need for urban reform, and moved away from the notion that urban problems resulted exclusively from demographics and uncontrolled growth. Cities' elitist management and socio-spatial models were regarded simultaneously as causes and consequences of disparities in income, access and power, which prevent social justice and the striving for democratic ideals. From this new angle, two major issues became central to the quest for better cities: social equity and democracy.

The constitution included chapters on urban and environmental policies, conceded sole control over urban development to municipalities, and mandated that urban development policies be approved by city councils as a local law and as masterplans for cities of over 20,000 residents. In terms of social justice in cities, the constitution conceded adverse possession for squatters who occupy no more than 250 m² of urban land and keep it as their residency for at least five years, thus stopping unrestricted evictions from *favelas*. It also conceded to cities the power to demand the utilisation of vacant urban land through compulsory development, the progressive increase of property taxes and compulsory purchase. The constitution recognised the city as a locus for the redistribution of wealth and for the reduction of social inequalities, and provided a legal platform for more specific national and local legislations.

In 2001, a national law regulated the constitutional mandates on urban policy and consolidated other pieces of legislation on urban development. Named *Estatuto da Cidade* (Statute of the City), it established a new legal–political paradigm in its mission to make cities more socially inclusive. It ratified the constitutional precept that urban property rights are subordinate to that property's social function, and extended the requirement for masterplans to all cities in metropolitan areas, in areas of interest for tourism and those affected by large projects. The statute set the deadline of October 2006 for these plans to be prepared (or revised) and approved by their legislatures, but two years later 1,700 such cities still had to comply.[2] Importantly for urban design, the statute introduced a series of progressive concepts for plan implementation and development control, including neighbourhood rights, public participation and participatory budgeting, public–private partnerships, transfer of development rights, adverse possession, special zoning for *favelas*, flexibility in real-estate taxation to discourage or encourage urban development, and the city's first option to buy any property (pre-emption right).

The ministry for cities, created in 2002 and divided into four secretariats (housing, urban programs, sanitation, and transportation and urban mobility), has the mission to propose and implement national policies and investment programmes, support masterplanning at the local level and invest in institutional enabling and training of local public officials. In 2003, the ministry summoned states, municipalities and major community groups to discuss a national urban development policy in national forums that included 320,000 participants whose elected representatives formed the National Council of the Cities.

Brazil's planning framework within the new democratic political framework (the Statute of the City), the ministry of the city's efforts, the evolving national policies and programmes and the strengthening of participatory processes in local planning have all started to impact on the shaping of Brazilian cities, and are major contributors for new types of urban design.

The trajectory of urban design

Urban design as a comprehensive set of actions started in Brazil in the early 1900s with a series of reforms in Rio de Janeiro. Trying to mark its place in the international scene and attract investments, the newly formed republic promoted a series of interventions in the capital including infrastructural works, expansions to the port and its accesses, and Haussmann-like renovations that were heavily influenced by French neo-classicism and the Beaux-Arts school.

In the late 1920s, Alfred Agache – one of the founders of the French Society of Urbanists – was invited to deliver talks in Rio, and later hired to prepare the city's first masterplan. The plan included the city's first socio-economic study, modern cartography, proposals for circulation and new suburbs, and design concepts including monumental plazas, pedestrian arcades, perimeter blocks with interior public plazas, and stepped setbacks. Agache moved his main practice to Rio de Janeiro and over the years was hired by several other Brazilian cities, such as Curitiba where his plan was superseded only in the mid-1960s.

Getulio Vargas' dictatorship (1930 to 1937) and his populist *Estado Novo* (New State; 1937 to 1945) pursued Brazil's modernisation through a series of social and economic reforms. In a quest for a new national identity, the state's vision of progress embraced modernism and planning, urban design, and architecture – particularly public housing. For instance, Vargas backed the construction of Goiania, the new capital for the state of Goiás, designed by modernist architect Attilio Correia Lima in the early 1930s. Goiana's modernity would serve Vargas as a symbolic gesture of

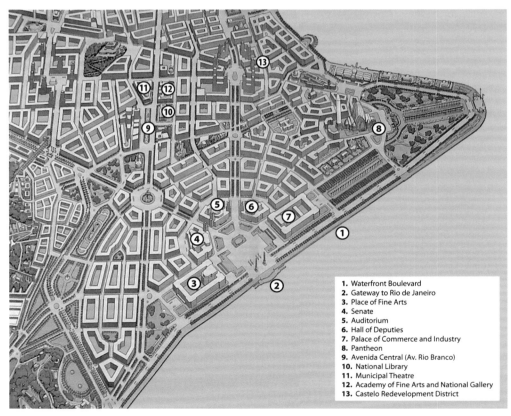

1. Waterfront Boulevard
2. Gateway to Rio de Janeiro
3. Place of Fine Arts
4. Senate
5. Auditorium
6. Hall of Deputies
7. Palace of Commerce and Industry
8. Pantheon
9. Avenida Central (Av. Rio Branco)
10. National Library
11. Municipal Theatre
12. Academy of Fine Arts and National Gallery
13. Castelo Redevelopment District

Urban design vision for the monumental centre,
from the 1930 Agache plan for Rio de Janeiro

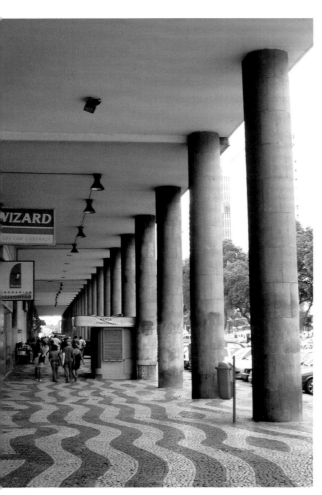

Galeria Getulio Vargas: one of the pedestrian
arcades that resulted from the legislation suggested
by Alfred Agache's plan for Rio de Janeiro

rupture with the old rural oligarchies and the establishment of a new industrial centre in the undeveloped interior of Brazil. Sao Paulo's 1930 Plano de Avenidas was also a break with tradition and sought to adapt the city to an ideal modern model for vehicular circulation, heavily influenced by North American planning.[3]

In the 1930s, planning departments were created in the major Brazilian cities, the first zoning laws were approved and several urbanists were appointed as mayors. Modernist projects spread out in the country as the movement's positivist ideals for development, social discipline, and order through design served the *Estado Novo* well. The clash between the Beaux-Arts tradition and upcoming modernism was evident in Rio de Janeiro and in Brazil's leading public architecture school. In 1931, immediately after being appointed as the school's new director, Lucio Costa – a leader among Brazilian modernists – hired other modernists as new faculty and changed the old curriculum with the full support of the students. Modernism would dominate debates in the first Brazilian Congress of Urbanism in 1941, and by the mid-1940s it would become Brazil's hegemonic design ideology.[4] The creation of the new capital, Brasilia, designed by Costa and inaugurated in 1960, marked the apex of Brazilian modernism, which continued to be the dominant ideology until the 1980s.

In the 1940s, urbanism became a subject within architecture and engineering programmes, and in the 1950s, still under French influence, the first graduate programmes in urbanism, for architects and engineers only, were established – along with the profession of *urbanista*. Under US and British influence, in the late 1960s the military government created a national planning system to support regional and urban development. By the 1970s, educational reforms resulted in the creation of MSc programmes in urban and regional planning, based on the University of Edinburgh model. Schools of architecture cancelled courses on urbanism and started teaching urban and regional planning, but at the same time – ironically – changed the nomenclature of their undergraduate diplomas from simply 'architect' to 'architect–urbanist', conferring a new professional status on all architects. Until the mid-1980s, these courses lost interest in physical design and turned instead to political economy and social sciences, reflecting the political climate of the time and societal worries. Architects working in planning 'unlearned' how to design, and were easily confused with social scientists.

The expression 'urban design' was introduced in Brazil in the late 1970s through a special course taught by David Gosling, from Sheffield University, as visiting professor at the University of Brasilia's school of architecture and urbanism. The expression started to catch on in the early 1980s when several architects came back from the UK and the US with degrees in urban design, including this author. In the late 1980s,

Benamy Turkienicz from the University of Brasilia spearheaded a series of national seminars on urban design, and their proceedings helped popularise urban design in architecture programmes. The first seminar had around 650 attendees and the second almost 1,500, both exceeding all expectations. There was much debate about whether the expression should even be adopted in Portuguese, due to its linguistic imprecision and in the face of the popularised terms *urbanismo* and *projeto urbano*.[5] However, urban design eventually found a niche for itself, helped by works of authors such as Lynch, Cullen, Alexander and Barnett. It was increasingly utilised in architecture programmes, by visiting faculty such as Brian Goodey, Amos Rapoport and David Gosling, by the proceedings of the national seminars and by the works of by Brazilian authors such as del Rio (1990).

Brazil´s return to democracy in the 1980s and debates around the urban question led to significant developments in the education of architects and planners. In 1994, a nationwide minimum curriculum for architect–urbanists was approved by the ministry of education; it includes mandatory classes in urban and regional planning, urban design, and landscape architecture. The urban question, and the planning and design of the city, became an inseparable part of architectural education in Brazil. At the same time, graduate programmes in urban and regional planning expanded and several started offering PhD programmes, although mostly in fields remote from urban design and physical planning.

Thus, educational programmes and professional niches in urban and regional planning, urbanism, and urban design coexist. This brief historical account helps one to understand the nature of urban design in Brazil, and why it has a wider foundation than is normally found in other countries. However, the architect is the professional more commonly involved with urban design simply because of the discipline's project-related implications. In the Brazilian context, urban design is seen as the conscious or unconscious process of shaping cities or parts of them, together with the various human and social operations that sustain and give them, i.e. the cities, meaning. Urban design is seen as multi-scale, interdisciplinary, procedural, public-oriented, participatory and socially inclusive.

Contemporary trends in Brazilian urban design

The new democracy was pivotal in overcoming the lack of political participation and in consolidating a new stage for new types of city building and urban design. Brasilia and its subversion of traditional urbanism lost its powerful symbolic hegemony, and different approaches to planning, urban design and architecture would henceforth compete with modernism. Local politics, public participation and the appreciation of context became important ingredients in the design process. Despite the historical social divide that still haunts Brazilian society, several cities have recently been investing in the quality of the public realm and in urban design. Groundbreaking and successful projects teach lessons in how urban design can be an important contributor to place making. However, besides the well-publicised innovations from Curitiba and a few recent accounts on specific projects, publications dealing specifically with the current state of urban design in Brazil are sparse. Current research and practice in different Brazilian cities can be found in publications by del Rio and Siembieda (2009) and del Rio (2010). Three trends in Brazilian urbanism seem to concentrate the most interesting lessons in urban design, and will be discussed in the following paragraphs[6] with reference to specific examples.

Late modernism

The positivist paradigm inherent in modernism still dominates most Brazilian planning, architecture and urban design, with convictions such as the belief that development is intrinsically good and represents a positive evolution, and that there is a rational order to things. By and large, cities are planned and public projects, zoning and regulatory codes are developed and implemented within a modernist frame of mind, encouraging the Corbusian model of 'towers in the green', single-use zoning and car-dependent design that previously generated disjointed districts, large distances between buildings, a landscape of highways and public areas that constitute a 'no man's land'. More than in any other Brazilian city, these problems are inherent in Brasilia.

Modernism and late modernism facilitate urban development processes that promote spatial segregation and segmentation, a 'formal versus informal city' dichotomy and exacerbate the dualities of the capitalist city. Much of the Brazilian urban landscape is being taken over by gated communities and controlled environments, with fencing around parks, plazas, shopping centres, business parks and even individual buildings in residential and local commercial streets. This phenomenon is particularly strong in areas with modernist spatial morphologies, which are more easily adapted to segregated social realms.

Late modernism represents the continuation of the model, partially adapted to local conditions and recognisant of some of its past mistakes. It still believes that if the government would only control the market and dictate development to fit an idealised model, then the results would guarantee the public good. The trend is mostly closed to public participation processes, and its planners and designers paternalistically decide what is good for the community.

The project for Palmas, the capital of the new state of Tocantins inaugurated in 1990, is an interesting example of late modernism.[7] In 1989, the first governor personally decided to hire Grupo Quatro Arquitetos Associados from Goiania, giving them less than a year to prepare the plan, a particularly short deadline given the surveying and environmental studies that had to be done. Like that of Brasilia, the

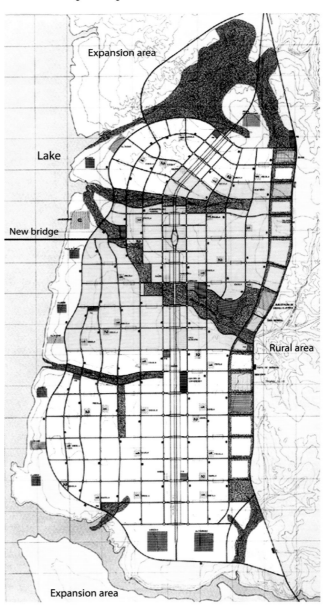

The linear open-grid masterplan concept for the new state capital city of Palmas, by Grupo Quatro Arquitetos

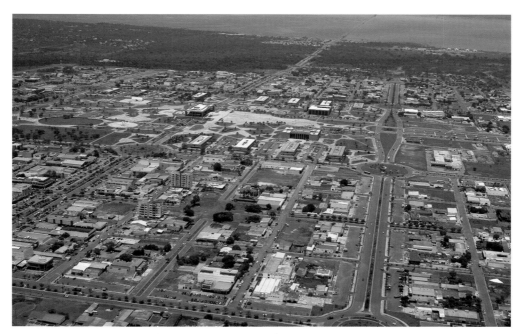

View of Palmas central area, showing the administrative centre
and, in the background, the bridge and the artificial lake

rationale behind the city's creation was that it would spur regional development. A
dam and an artificial lake were built, and a regional highway, a railway and an airport
connected the new city to the rest of the state. In 1996, Palmas had 86,116 residents;
in 2010, this number had jumped to 222,000. Between the last two national census
(2000 and 2010), while Brazil's yearly demographic growth rate was 1.17%, in Palmas
it reached an incredible 5.21%. In a backward region where everything remained to
be done, the city fulfilled its mission of generating a dynamic regional economy and
creating a new society in the midst of the Brazilian savannah.

   In their approach to the planning of the new city, designers Grupo Quatro Arquitetos were inspired by the examples of Brasilia and Milton Keynes: the major roads
generated a macro-grid and 42 ha sectors, within which private developers would be
granted flexibility in deciding the street grid and building arrangements. Originally
public spaces and facilities were linked by pedestrian walkways, and the residential blocks
were designed to spur a level of social integration among residents such that boundary walls between properties would not be needed. Utopia was trampled by reality, as the
state government acted as land developer and the openness of the original design induced
speculative development. Planning in Palmas was confused with the process of subdivid-
ing land and selling lots, which was constrained only by an obsolete zoning legislation.
Original land uses were changed, compromising city functions and the neighbourhood
scale of the original design concept. Avenues where bus lines were located turned into
dense commercial strips, and the wide modernist main boulevard divides the city in two,
speeds up traffic and makes crossing a nightmare. The town core, at the highest point of
an otherwise flat area, holds the governmental buildings isolated in the midst of a large
and barren plaza devoid of users out of office hours. However, the functionality of the
grid, the large open areas and parks, and the artificial beaches and amenities along the
lakefront make Palmas different from any other frontier town and help attract residents.

   The experience of Palmas demonstrates the difficulties of a centralised approach
to planning and urban design, which intensifies the gap between intentions and acts,

and public and private interests, and represents a lost opportunity to create a truly contemporary city, ecological and sustainable, as the original design concept envisaged. Palmas' problems are similar to those afflicting other large cities in Brazil: incomplete urban services and infrastructure, inefficient public transportation, disrespect of the zoning principles, great tracts of land left empty on fully serviced areas and a growing contingent of squatter settlements. However, in establishing a new administrative centre and attracting large numbers of governmental employees, entrepreneurs, developers, retail, services and thousands of families in search of opportunities, and in implementing new regional accessibilities, Palmas is undeniably a successful development effort with a clear impact on the whole region. Given Brazil's long love affair with modernism, it is no surprise that it continues to be a strong intellectual influence for the better – by bringing in the functionality and urbanisation much needed in developing areas – and for the worse – by facilitating spatial and social segregation.

Revitalisation

By the mid-1980s, most large cities in Brazil realised that they should direct planning and design efforts towards the redevelopment of their central areas. Deteriorating, underutilised and outdated buildings, vacancies, planning blight, antiquated zoning and regulations, and overambitious road projects were some of the problems that had to be faced. Most of these areas are intensely used by a white-collar population working in offices, as well as by the poorer sectors attracted by good public transportation and the informal economy. Central areas also showcase an important historic and cultural heritage that has to be respected. In the last three decades, several major Brazilian cities have implemented successful historical preservation and revitalisation projects, often with a cultural and recreational bias, some including waterfronts. Such examples can be found in Rio de Janeiro, Salvador, Sao Paulo, Recife, Porto Alegre, Fortaleza and Belem.

The most important of such projects is Rio de Janeiro's Cultural Corridor project, the first inner-city revitalisation programme in Brazil. Approved as a special local land-use regulation in 1982, it was the city's response to community groups and local entrepreneurs concerned with the fate of some of the most traditional places in the downtown and the displacement pressures from large economic groups. The project was conceived by architect Augusto Ivan Pinheiro at Rio de Janeiro's planning department, and during its first decade it was implemented by a special task force, whose work included the development of design guidelines, design

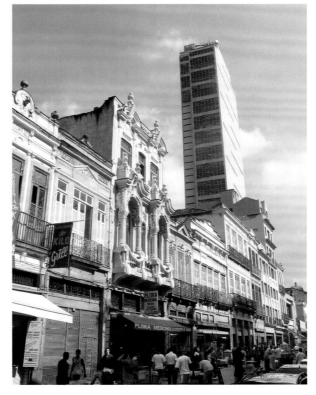

A street in the Cultural Corridor revitalisation area in downtown Rio de Janeiro showing protected historical buildings and popular commercial uses: the tower at the rear is an example of what the old land-use regulations permitted for the area

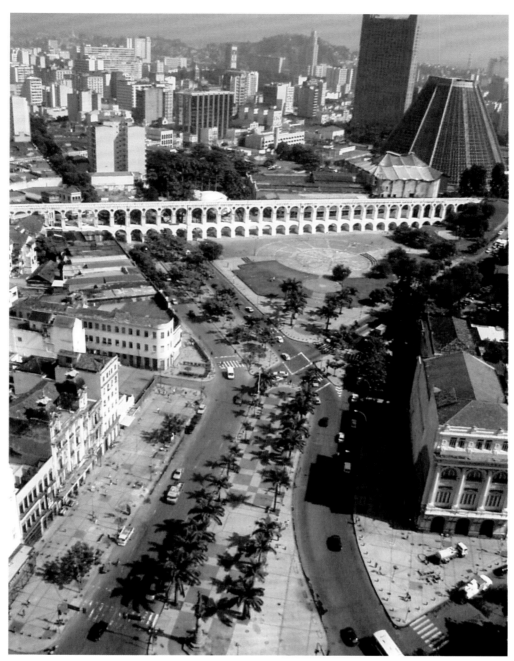

Renovated urban spaces support the nightlife in Lapa, Rio de Janeiro, its restaurants, dancing and show halls, and cultural centres; notice the plaza for public events and the old colonial aqueduct that now holds a tram line

support for stakeholders and a special approval process for granting building licenses and tax abatements. Now the area's management is carried out through the city's normal planning and building approvals system. The project covers an area of 1.3 million m², within which modernist zoning regulations were cancelled and special design guidelines now provide different levels of protection to more than 3,000 buildings – of which, 75% have been partially restored and around 900 totally renovated.

Guidelines at first covered only architectural design and were later expanded to encompass signage, facade colours and the interiors of the buildings declared to be of cultural or historic value. As architectural preservation alone would guarantee neither the survival nor the vitality of these historic areas, the Cultural Corridor protects traditional uses and supports complementary public actions such as educational campaigns, the renovation of public spaces, street beautification, cultural events, marketing and promotional material. Tax exemptions, and building incentives were set up to further encourage owners to preserve historic buildings and follow the guidelines. Having the McDonald's multinational fast-food chain comply with all the guidelines in renovating a building, for instance, was one of the early victories.

Renewal is well under way and traditional retail is alive: more than 25 new cultural centres, theatres and museums have been installed, mostly in renovated historic buildings; new shops, restaurants and places for simply socialising have been successful. Most of these are developed and managed either by public–private partnerships or entirely by private parties. Areas such as Lapa, a traditional bohemian sector which had deteriorated over the years, has recovered its cultural glamour and now attracts thousands who come for the new dance clubs and night-time activities. In 2002, the last modernist bastion fell when zoning changes in the central business district and in the Cultural Corridor permitted new residential buildings including hotels and studio apartments, the conversion of underutilised commercial buildings to residential use and reduced parking requirements. In 2006, the first private residential development replaced an abandoned brewery: a gated community of tower blocks with amenities for residents and retail on the ground floor along the major streets. Even the most optimistic were surprised: all 668 one- and two-bedroom apartments were sold on the first day, and the community is fully operational.

The Cultural Corridor project has been very successful in preserving old buildings and traditional inner-city commercial uses, in combining new and old, in attracting new uses and in renovating run-down areas. From the social point of view, it attracted different stakeholders and involved them in the decision-making process. From the economic point of view, it managed to maintain the diversity of land uses and the dynamics of the market. From the cultural point of view, it was fundamental in recuperating the symbolic and cultural role of the downtown city's past. The approach towards successfully integrating these aspects is neither nostalgic nor based on simplistic architectural protections. Rather, it relies on public–private partnerships and it is always looking for new opportunities to reconcile the need for preservation with the demand for development. This project has inspired several Brazilian cities in their quest for preserving historic architecture and revitalising central areas.

Social inclusion
The third urban design trend includes projects whose main mission is social inclusion, in contrast with models generated by globalisation. It reflects the efforts that started with democratisation and the notion of the city's social function, discussed above. Cities and communities realised that the quality of public spaces and services was fundamental to achieve full citizenship, diminish the gap between rich and poor, and establish a better image nationally and internationally. In this sense, public planning and urban design aim to reclaim the city as a pluralist environment and to extend social and cultural amenities to larger groups. These efforts are particularly clear in the well-known experiences of Curitiba,[8] but may also be seen in other cities through the renovation of public spaces and the upgrading of *favelas* and illegal subdivisions.

THE FAVELA BAIRRO PROJECTS IN RIO DE JANEIRO

The innovative Favela Bairro programme in Rio de Janeiro is an excellent example of urban design for social inclusion. For many years, *favelas* have been perceived negatively as places of marginality, particularly with the rise of organised drug trafficking or the self-appointed militia controlling these settlements, and there has been a consequent erosion of social capital. During the military era, the official approach to *favelas* was either to ignore them or to transfer their residents to housing projects far from the formal city and employment centres, thus adding to the population's problems. In 1994, the first democratically elected city government in Rio de Janeiro launched the Favela Bairro programme to upgrade *favelas* and integrate them into the fabric of the city through infrastructure and service improvements, turning them into *bairros* (neighbourhoods). Favela Bairro recognised the squatters' long-term social and capital investments, and the importance of *favelas* as distinct and valuable places for the communities. Physical improvements included the introduction of storm-drainage, sewage and drinking-water lines; public lighting; vehicular and pedestrian access; playgrounds; and recreation areas. Public services, such as rubbish collection and the installation of electricity meters, could then be implemented. Community development included educational and income-generation projects such as professional training, work cooperatives and employing residents in rubbish collection and reforestation. A few new buildings were provided by the programme, such as day-care centres, community buildings and housing for families evicted from their original homes by the projects.

The projects for Favela Bairro were developed by private firms hired through public competitions, and they targeted small and medium-sized *favelas* – the average population ranging from 500 to 2,500. Implemented by two consecutive city mayors, the programe included two public competitions organised through the Brazilian Institute of Architects for architectural firms in Rio de Janeiro. For both Favela Bairro I (1994) and Favela Bairro II (2000), participants had to explain their methodologies and develop concepts. Several local firms were hired as a result of the competitions, but more contracts were awarded through requests for proposals (RFP). The firms had the support of different city departments as well as its social workers, not only to help in developing the design solutions but also to run the complementary projects for community development. Favela Bairro's methodology was an essential ingredient of the

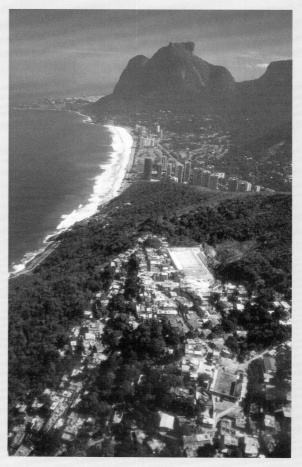

The Favela Bairro project for Vidigal, Rio de Janeiro, includes a sports and recreational complex at the top of the main community thoroughfare; project by Atelier Metropolitano – Jorge Mario Jauregui

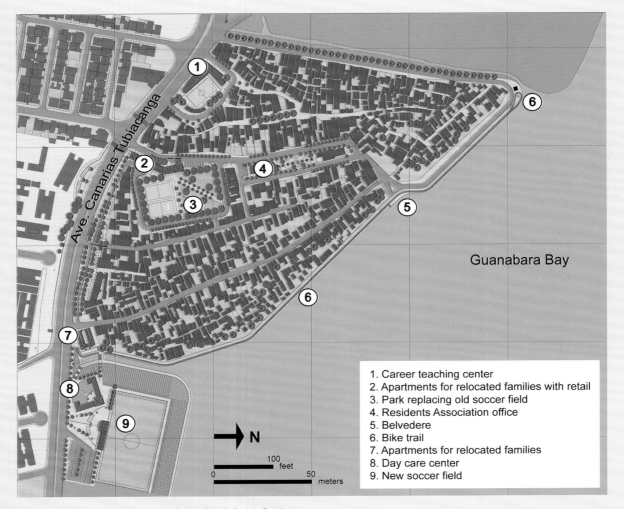

1. Career teaching center
2. Apartments for relocated families with retail
3. Park replacing old soccer field
4. Residents Association office
5. Belvedere
6. Bike trail
7. Apartments for relocated families
8. Day care center
9. New soccer field

Guanabara Bay

Ave. Canarias Tubiacanga

Illustrative site plan for the upgrading of Parque Royal, Projeto Favela Bairro, Rio de Janeiro: public facilities are located along the project's edges, integrating the community into the surrounding neighbourhood; project by Archi 5, Rio de Janeiro

process, not only because of the complex socio-cultural and spatial reality but also because at any given time it might engage dozens of simultaneous operations at various stages of execution.

The various projects included participatory processes, not only to engage the community in decision making and hiring their labour but most importantly to persuade local strongmen and drug lords. By 2003, the programme had served 168 communities and, according to the city, benefited 500,000 people, or 45% of the city's *favela* population. It is estimated that the total cost of the programme was around $600 million (£380 million).

In Favela Vidigal, a community of 9,900 people perching on slopes that overlook the ocean,

architect Jorge Jauregui and his team had to deal with a rugged topography and decided to make the main meandering access road the community 'spine', respecting the existing settlement patterns. Along this spine, and using the existing open spaces or through selective renovation, were located a series of parks and facilities such as two day-care centres, a building for a local theatre group and a community centre with computer rooms. The spine starts at the edge of the formal city, where a gateway plaza was placed on an empty city lot, and ends on a new belvedere at the top of the hill. There, the design took advantage of the flatter terrain and of an existing open space used by the community to place their Olympic Village: a soccer field, a multi-sports covered court and other facilities. In Favela Parque Royal, a community

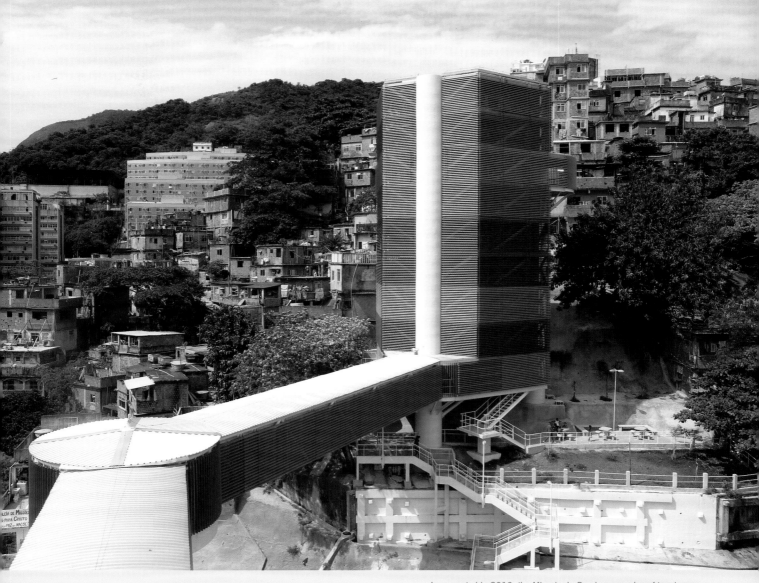

Inaugurated in 2010, the Mirante da Paz is a complex of two towers with elevators, stairs and bridges increasing accessibility to favelas Cantagalo and Pavão-Pavãozinhoin Ipanema, Rio de Janeiro: the observation decks on top of the towers quickly became popular spots for tourists; the complex includes community rooms and is directly connected to a subway station

of 4,146 residents bordered by the international airport and the Guanabara bay, architects Archi 5 decided to invest in improving the linkages between the community and the surrounding neighbourhood, as well as in increasing overall accessibility. The connectivity of the existing network of streets and alleyways was enhanced through minimal selective redevelopment, and a new street was built around the settlement and along the bay front, providing a bike lane, 'pocket' parks, and several vista points with seating. The project also included the careful insertion of a new park with sports fields, a day-care centre, an educational facility and new apartments

over retail for the few displaced families, all located along the periphery of the *favela* so as to also serve the surrounding and help in social integration.

Favela Barrio was a major success, it was recognised by the Inter-American Development Bank as its Project of the Year in 1998, and received the United Nations Habitat Prize. The communities gained better living conditions and access to infrastructure and public services, the sense of community improved and residents were encouraged to make further investments, particularly on their own houses (Duarte and Magalhaes 2009; del Rio et al 2011). By recognising demands from *favela* communities, the city fed and fortified notions of property, crystallising community ownership and fostering citizenship. Although, for political reasons, subsequent city administrations cancelled the brand Favela Bairro, the same methods and types of projects continued to be followed. However, it is important to note that the real problem afflicting *favelas* for the past 30 years has been their takeover by organised crime (drug traffic and/or militia) and the consequences: loss of community unity, of trust in the state, and of freedom of movement (Perlman 2010). Recently – undoubtedly in preparation for the 2014 World Cup and the 2016 Olympics

– Rio's government has been trying to 'reconquer' the territories of the *favelas* by coordinating the actions of the army and police, and by establishing 'Pacifying Police Units' and social programmes when they leave. So far, these actions have been successful and have received the full support of the communities affected (del Rio et al 2011). The city is expanding the scope of its interventions in some *favelas*, and together with such improvements in security and social services come urban design projects that improve accessibility – such as cable cars and elevators – and the conditions of public spaces and facilities.

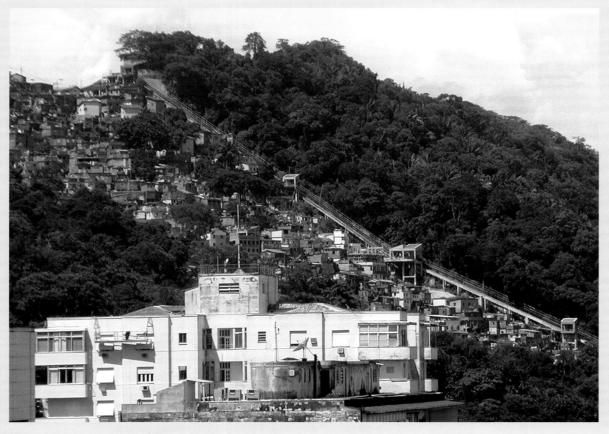

New modes of access are being built in several favelas, like this cable car built in 1998 at Favela Santa Marta, Rio de Janeiro

Conclusion

We noted how democratisation and the new legal–political framework in Brazil encourage more responsive modes of governance at the three levels of administration, as well as the search for efficient, pluralistic and just cities. Although urban design is far from being considered an item for national policy (as it is, for example, in the UK and New Zealand), local governments in Brazil increasingly utilise it as a tool to deliver more liveable, inclusive and responsive places. In contrast to the classic modernist paradigm – which relied on public sponsorship, centralised control and a rigid model of what a city should be – contemporary Brazilian urban design may be called postmodern, in that it relies more on public–private partnerships, community participation, critical cultural interpretations of the existing environment and on amalgamating different visions of quality in the construction of the public realm. It seems that in Brazil, urban design will continue to be regarded neither as a specific discipline nor a specific profession, but as a field of specialisation or postgraduate education. This has been an efficient way in which to fulfil the country's needs and to guarantee urban design's interdisciplinary agenda, while at the same time grounding it firmly within the physical–spatial tradition derived from the discipline of architecture.

A quick guide to
Brazil

1 TYPES OF CLIENT

Local, state and federal authorities

Public foundations and corporations

Private developer/landowner

....

2 TYPES OF
PROJECT/WORK

Masterplans (local and regional levels)

Land-use/zoning regulations

Infrastructure and transportation-related projects

Specific Plans
- Urban renewal
- New community
- Urban subdivisions
- Business parks
- University campuses
- Parks and waterfronts
- Slum/housing upgrading
- Public housing

....

3 APPROACH NEEDED
TO WORK IN COUNTRY

Open local office/local representation

Partnership with local firm

International competition/public bidding

Direct negotiation with client/developer or government

Professional licensing

....

4 LEGISLATION
THAT NEEDS TO BE
REFERRED TO

National constitution and state constitutions

City statute (national law)

National/state/local environmental laws

Specific sectorial requirements

State and city legislation

Municipal or city masterplan

Local land-use and zoning regulations

....

5	SPECIFIC TIPS FOR SUCCESS	Respect local professionals
		Awareness of national/regional/local political context
		Patience with maze of legislation and taxes: hire a good tax lawyer
		Get used to lower fees and smaller margins of profit
		Beware of private clients and do not expect public clients to pay promptly

6	USEFUL WEBSITES	Federação Nacional dos Arquitetos e Urbanistas (FNA): www.fna.org.br
		Instituto de Arquitetos do Brasil (IAB): www.iab.org.br
		Ministério do Planejamento, Orçamento e Gestão: www.planejamento.gov.br
		Ministry of the environment (MMA): www.mma.gov.br

SELECTED FACTS

1	area	8,511,965 km^2
2	population	194,946,470
3	annual population growth	0.9%
4	urban population	87%
5	population density	23 p/km^2
6	GDP	$2,087,889,553,822
7	GNI per capita	$9,390

Source: The World Bank (2010)

UNITED STATES

Howard Blackson, *urban designer*

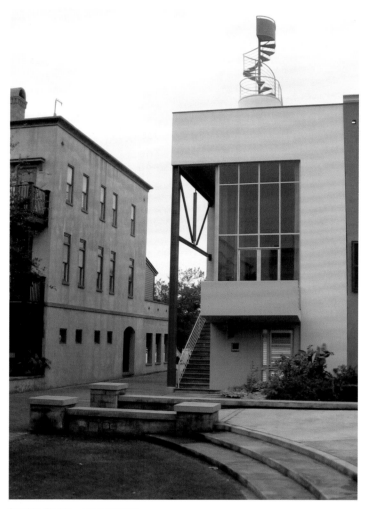

Seaside, Florida – Live/work lofts

THE UNITED STATES is a federal constitutional republic comprising 50 states plus the Federal District of Columbia with Washington, the capital. The federal government is composed of the congress (house of representatives and senate), the president and the courts. Each state in turn has a government structured in a similar fashion: a governor, two chambers and the courts. Each state can establish its own system of local government and most have a two-tier structure of counties and municipalities, though their size, responsibilities and exact form varies widely. The municipal authorities are responsible for planning. In some metropolitan areas, attempts have been made to create associations of local government, for instance to coordinate transportation plans, but these have rarely been successful.

Definitions

In the United States, urban design is seen as a relatively new addition to the design professions of architecture, landscape architecture and urban planning. Born at Harvard's Graduate School of Design (GSD) with the wave of German/European immigration at the beginning of the second world war, urban design was first developed as an academic tool in an attempt to conceptualise and solve the prolonged negative effects of the Industrial Revolution on urban areas. These imported European models, such as the towers-in-a-park formation of Le Corbusier's Radiant City, informed the coarse urban renewal policies of the 1950s. In turn, these provoked a nationwide citizen backlash leading to the rise of the historical preservation movement and the use of urban design to control the bulk, scale and intensity of new buildings.

Today, urban design is understood as a necessary, yet peripheral, discipline offered by most architecture, landscape architecture and urban planning firms. There are no professional registrations nor any legal liability for urban design. Therefore, as the legal risks are lower, most design firms are willing to offer and perform urban design services. However, there are very few firms specifically dedicated to urban design, and even fewer urban design departments within municipal planning and development services.

Despite not being a formally recognised discipline, urban design is understood to be important to the future redevelopment of underutilised single-use districts, such as dead shopping malls, redundant military installations and industrial sites. Recent changes in broad-ranging pluralistic policy planning processes have led to urban design plans being prepared across the nation in order to give three-dimensional physical form to regional, town and neighbourhood-scale plans. Innovative policies and guidelines backed by city or county authorities are now included in Comprehensive Plans, General Plans and Community Plans to ensure the general health, welfare and safety of local citizens. These are in turn implemented as Form-

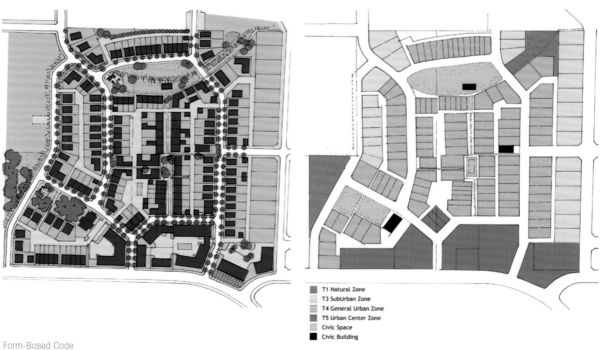

Form-Based Code

- T1 Natural Zone
- T3 SubUrban Zone
- T4 General Urban Zone
- T5 Urban Center Zone
- Civic Space
- Civic Building

Based Codes (FBC) or place-based planning, which prioritise sense of place over land use. These control the appearance of streetscapes and public spaces in concert with building types. Rather than regulating places by single land uses and related measurements, an FBC analyses and plans for particular street types ('Main Street', neighbourhood street, rural road), public spaces (green, square, plaza), and civic and private buildings, taking as a basis their character, context and place. Thus, cities such as Denver, Miami, Montgomery and El Paso have replaced their conventional zoning and subdivision ordinances with FBCs.

The rise of sustainability issues within the nation's consciousness has led to urban designers being in demand to achieve mixed-use, connected and walkable places in the existing urban context. And as a result of urban design work on redevelopment strategies and FBCs, and projects such as flagship developments, festival marketplaces or waterfront revitalisation, downtown areas throughout the nation are successfully being reinhabited. As development focuses on existing neighbourhoods, urban design is concerned with context-sensitive schemes, historic preservation and the identification of community character. In more rural greenfield areas, urban design is seen as a way to create new neighbourhoods, villages and town centres, as the antithesis to sprawling suburban subdivisions.

The professional place of urban design

For a variety of reasons, most importantly educational, a relatively small number of US practitioners are exclusively urban designers; most of them have been trained primarily as architects, landscape architects or urban planners, and they work in practices under the banner of these other professions.

Architects primarily practise urban design as site planners for private development projects, which today tend to be mostly residential. Engineers practising urban design tend to work mostly on large-scale infrastructure projects funded by the federal government. These include streetscape and thoroughfare improvements, and new road construction. Landscape architects practising urban design do so in support of these mostly private architectural and public engineering projects.

In the past few years, urban design work has moved away from large-scale private developments and municipal redevelopment projects towards smaller, block-scale infill projects in existing neighbourhoods. At the same time, urban designers are drafting larger policy and implementation codes for local authorities that wish to reinforce the character of existing neighbourhoods and define standards for new ones, in order to leverage value and compete for new businesses and residents.

Urban designers in the United States have no specific professional body, but they are organised and networked as a sub-chapter of the other licensed organisations representing design professionals: the American Institute of Architects (AIA), the American Society of Landscape Architects (ASLA), the American Institute of Certified Planners (AICP) and the American Society of Civil Engineers (ASCE). Other unlicensed design professional membership organisations are the American Planning Association (APA) and the Congress for the New Urbanism (CNU). In addition there are more local organisations, such as the Institute for Urban Design and the Van Alen Institute, both in New York City, which act as advocates and discussion forums.

The discipline

Currently, ten accredited universities and colleges offer specific degrees in urban design, most notably the University of California at Berkeley and Harvard University. This number is in stark contrast to the approximately 120 accredited architecture schools and the 300 non-accredited ones. In addition, there are 40 accredited urban planning schools and 100 non-accredited urban planning programmes, as well as 140 schools offering landscape architecture degrees. The conclusion is that, as an academic discipline, urban design has a fairly weak identity.

It follows that its body of research is also limited, though some important publications have been produced over the past century, marking the evolution of the discipline, mostly in relation to the primary profession of the author. This has also generated a healthy debate between academics and practitioners of urban design. The leading profession is easily identified, as architects emphasise buildings, landscape architects emphasise the unbuilt spaces, and planners the two-dimensional land use. Each of these three disciplines follows a distinct design methodology, as described below.

New Urbanism (NU), the current planning and urban design hegemony, was conceived by architects and applies a formal and typological approach to buildings and streets. New Urbanists focus on a building's orientation, configuration and function in relationship to its frontage, in different contexts such as main streets, neighbourhood streets, or rural roads. On the other hand, Harvard's GSD argues that landscape design rather than architecture is the appropriate discipline within which to conceive urban environments, and this view leads the emerging urban design methodology of Landscape Urbanism. The trend in urban planning is towards a Healthy Cities and Resilient Communities approach to urban design. With the continued threat of natural and human-made disasters – hurricanes, tsunamis, floods, droughts and oil spills – urban planners are beginning to take sustainability seriously and to respond with a sense of urgency missing until now from discussions about land use, and bringing more powerful people to the table. The current economic crisis has a similar impact, and strategies for fortifying communities' capacities for resilience coincide closely with those for making them, by definition, more economically and socially sustainable.

Over the past year, the most provocative urban design debates have taken place between Harvard's Landscape Urbanism leader, Charles Waldheim, and New Urbanism's most notable champion, Andres Duany, regarding who holds the urban design practice 'high ground'. These well-documented events have generated tremendous social-media content and multimedia dialogue, and have elevated the status of these two formerly subsidiary urban methodologies. While the debates focused on which methodology was more suburban than the other, they clearly assumed that the collective goal is an American urbanism, which in itself is a triumph for urban design. Both leaders focused on the shortcomings of the other's urban methodology: Duany accused Landscape Urbanism of using anti-city tools, such as undefined open spaces and ecological features. Waldheim criticised New Urbanism's work in greenfield areas as building a new suburbanism. The ongoing debate resonates with the design professions as it brings together concepts of architectural form, open space and urban planning's cultural complexities.

As a result of the recession, fewer examples of work by urban designers have been displayed in the nation's galleries and exhibition halls. One notable exception was the display of the work of San Diego architect Teddy Cruz at New York's

Museum of Modern Art. Titled Small Scale, Big Change: New Architectures of Social Engagement, the exhibition presented 11 projects on five continents that illustrated innovative architecture for poorly served communities. Teddy's work is closely aligned with the now-fading ideology known as Everyday Urbanism. This was a late 1990s' urban design methodology practised by the late John Chase, Margaret Crawford, and John Kaliski, authors of a book with the same title, and championed philosophically by Mike Davis in the USA and Richard Sennett in the UK. It focuses on the mundane, nondescript, temporary and unintentional vernacular within the mega-cityscape, and it continues to resonate with small-scale infill development in Los Angeles. It has been described as a non-utopian, informal approach that celebrates and builds on ordinary life 'with little pretence about the possibility of a perfectible, tidy, or ideal built environment'.

Legal status

While urban design has no statutory role and is not included in US legislation, municipal authorities have legal planning tools with which to protect the health, welfare and safety of their citizens through their 'police powers'. Land-use and zoning regulations lie within these powers if they are reasonably related to public welfare. The powers also provide a statutory framework for the related agencies, commissions and departments that implement them. State law outlines the legal authority of policy plans as well as regulatory zoning and subdivision ordinances. However, state governments rarely enforce these laws and therefore compliance must, in most cases, be sought through the common-law courts system.

As development tends to concentrate in urban areas, urban designers are increasingly involved in drafting policy and implementation regulations, including the already mentioned FBCs, for municipalities and counties. They are also commissioned by private developers to produce masterplans for specific projects, which are enforced through Development Agreements within a state's statutory framework.

Historical development

American urban design has a long history that starts with the colonial layouts of cities such as Philadelphia or Savannah. The geometrical grids on which they were based were easily adapted to the prairie landscapes, and became the model for all subsequent urban development in the US. In the late 19th and early 20th centuries, a few large cities such as Chicago and Washington, under the influence of French models, adopted the City Beautiful approach with grand diagonal avenues, plazas and monuments. The American Vitruvius: An Architect's Handbook of Civic Art by Warner Hegemann and Elbert Peets, originally published in 1922, marked a critical moment in the history of North American urbanism. This book illustrated the end of the City Beautiful movement, the final flowering of Renaissance-inspired urban design, and the rise of urban planning as a distinct professional discipline.

Meanwhile the internal combustion engine helped change an agrarian society into an urban one, and allowed individuals to travel increasingly longer distances.

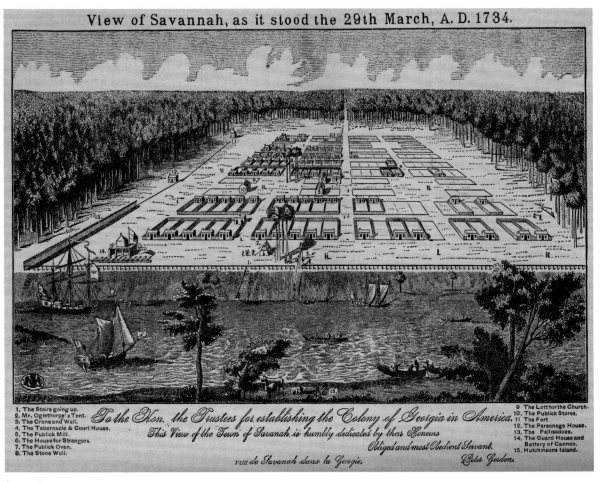

Savannah map

Most urban areas grew without much concern for the quality of the resulting public realm, and development was only regulated with fairly crude zoning documents. This led regional or city planners emerging from the established professions of architecture, landscape design or engineering, to attempt to redesign the way in which people lived.

Jose Luis Sert's 1942 essay Can our Cities Survive? led the Harvard school, and eventually the urban design profession, to claim that the city was filled with 'frightful ills' that necessitated an innovation-at-all-costs remedy. Sert's essay advocated anti-urban remedies in order to solve the city's inherent social ills. A mixture of influences, such as Le Corbusier's City of Tomorrow and the International Style, were intended to replace the blight of industrialisation and the fake ornamentation of Victorian architecture with a healthier, more equitable and agreeable city. Sert's modernist approach induced professionals towards applying mechanical planning and design principles to 20th-century social conditions. The resulting spatial separation of activities led to suburbanisation and sprawl.

During his term as Harvard GSD chairman, it was Sert who first used the expression 'urban design', and the term was also the title of an influential conference at Harvard in 1956 that brought together significant urban theorists, practitioners and writers such as Jane Jacobs, Lewis Mumford and Edmund Bacon. This once again marked a turning point in the practice of planning, architecture and urban design in the United States, as critiques of the modernist model led to the search for new

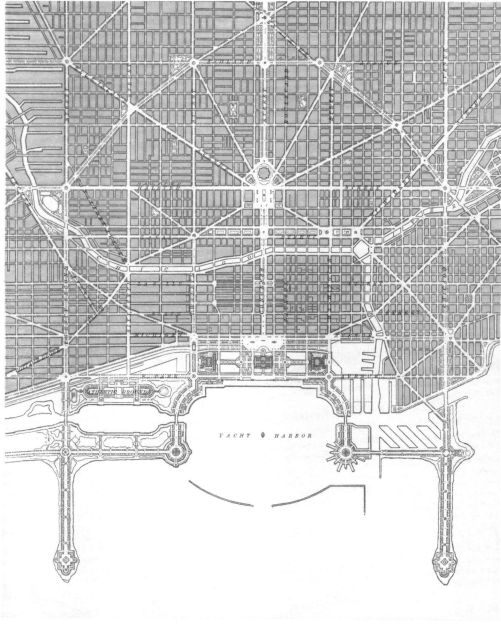

Chicago central area

approaches, even though suburbanisation continued unabated. In her 1961 seminal
The Death and Life of Great American Cities, Jane Jacobs attacked Sert's anti-urban
methodology as a series of unfortunate remedies. She successfully argued that his
approach led to unintended social ills, and she wrote about planning and designing at
the human scale in a way that resonates throughout the profession to this day. Together
with Kevin Lynch's The Image of the City, Jacobs' book became one of the fundamental
texts for urban design.

Influenced by these ideas, 20 years later, Seaside, a 32 ha resort town on the
Florida gulf coast, became another watershed in North American urban design.
Seaside, a neo-traditional development, was designed and coded by Andres Duany and
Elizabeth Plater-Zyberk as a self-contained, compact and connected neighbourhood,
in defiance of the excesses of suburban sprawl ubiquitous in contemporary North
America. Later, Plater-Zyberk, together with Peter Calthorpe and others, founded the

Congress for New Urbanism, and produced an influential series of books that defined their methodology, offering an alternative to suburban sprawl and the disinvestment in cities; they also outlined what an FBC should be.

Starting as an outsider movement critical of 20th-century planning, New Urbanism and its principles have very quickly become the new orthodoxy. It now has a proven set of tools to convey community-oriented plans into the 21st century. In the late 1990s, the federal government's Environmental Protection Agency's Smart Growth Office of Sustainable Communities incorporated the ideas and principles of the New Urbanism into its policy-reform work. In addition, the 'theological' rise of sustainability together with the recent great recession and oil instability are rapidly altering the understanding of urban design and development patterns in the United States. The collective approach to development has made the profession move away from suburban models towards more urban forms and densities. Social consciousness and attitudes have dramatically shifted in the direction of more walkable, mixed-use, compact and connected places, as promoted by New Urbanists.

Currently, advanced technology is once again giving people new ways of connecting and communicating. The results are expressed in the rise of social networks and access to data, information and mapping technology only available through computer technology. In this climate, urban design's value is rising as people understand the need to return to city centres and reinhabit existing neighbourhoods with increased densities and intensities. At the same time, this returning population requires well-designed and meaningful places that are loved in order to also be sustainable.

Finally, 30 years after Seaside, two important publications set today's normative approach to urban design: Donald Watson, Alan Plattus and Robert Shibley's Time-Saver Standards for Urban Design (McGraw-Hill, 2003); and the American Planning Association's Planning and Urban Design Standards (Wiley, 2006). These are the first major compendiums to encapsulate contemporary urban design standards and practices since the American Institute of Architects published Paul D Spreiregen's Urban Design: The Architecture of Towns and Cities in 1965. The switch in this 45-year period from one professional organisation (architecture) to the other (planning) as the urban design standard bearer is significant.

Current practice and concerns

The 21st-century's economic recession, or what urban theorist Richard Florida calls the Great Reset, bankrupted the majority of the private developers that until 2008 were the principal clients of urban designers. The US federal government's Transportation Investment Generating Economic Recovery (TIGER) grant programme, created from the stimulus package, shifted funding for Transit-Oriented Development (TOD) – a mixed-used residential development designed to maximise access to public transport – to local municipal projects. Regional metropolitan authorities are now major clients, replacing private developers hit by the recession.

Significantly, the majority of TIGER funds was awarded to areas with major investments in TOD, such as central Texas, central Utah and other streetcar systems throughout the nation. Salt Lake City, the site of the 2002 Winter Olympics, was allocated the largest TIGER II grant in order to build upon its existing Light Rail (TRAX) and Commuter Rail (Frontrunner) lines. Following central Texas' lead, cities throughout the country are being funded to prepare FBCs to implement and regulate mixed-use urban developments. As a result, regional plans such as Chicago Metropolis 2020, Portland 2040, Envision Central Texas, and Envision Utah have been funded and prepared by such prominent planner/urban designers as Peter Calthorpe and John Fregonese.

In an era when bridges fall, levies fail and states lease their toll roads to foreign-owned companies, Americans are realising the central importance of infrastructure, its impact on standards of living and quality of life, and on the prosperity or failure of entire places. Through the development of innovative planning and financial tools that facilitate growth, federal TIGER funding is attempting to lead the nation into the 21st century.

As Christopher Leinberger writes in The Option of Urbanism, 'Americans are voting with their feet to live in urban neighbourhoods', and our great recession has changed the market to focus on small-scale infill redevelopment in existing neighbourhoods. The consideration of increased density and traffic issues have therefore become essential, particularly if growth is to be achieved in a sustainable manner.

The development community is genuinely scared and looking for answers. As NIMBYs (devotees of the knee-jerk 'Not In My Back Yard' attitude to development) have for many years obstructed development effectively, city authorities and private developers have avoided engaging with them as a path of least resistance. However, with redevelopment of existing neighbourhoods often being a municipality's only hope for future revenue, NIMBYs simply cannot be avoided anymore and here urban designers can have a helpful role. Trained as generalists and with an understanding of a wide range of issues, they are well positioned to assist NIMBYs, municipal authorities and the development industry simultaneously, by offering not just design solutions but public facilitation, education, policy and regulatory tools. For worried neighbourhood groups, they can provide context-sensitive designs that reinforce the values of the existing area in connection to the new development. For municipalities and developers, they can offer opportunities to generate profits and tax revenues.

Fifty years after the publication of Jane Jacobs' book, her critics have reframed her legacy and blame her for the gentrification of Greenwich Village and the rise of NIMBYism. At the same time, they lament the loss of zeal on the part of New York City's former power broker Robert Moses (whom she attacked) and his authoritative, one-size-fits-all approach to public processes. The conundrum for urban designers is to reconcile the competing interests of NIMBYs wanting to preserve both land and their neighbourhoods, and the developers who want to profit from these, by showing that enhancing a place's quality can achieve both.

The current prolonged recession and the resulting scarcity of resources are reminiscent of the 1870-80s boom/bust period. This historical reference may give urban designers insights to develop innovative approaches to address the new phenomena of shrinking cities, such as Detroit and other rustbelt industrial conurbations, and at the same time take into account the rise of sustainability as a major issue. Once again, as generalists urban designers may be best equipped to provide solutions to such complex problems.

MISSION MERIDIAN VILLAGE, SOUTH PASADENA

Located in the historic Mission District of South Pasadena, this 0.67 ha half-block is an award-winning project noted for its context-sensitive redevelopment in a very contentious area. After years of neighbour- and community-led resistance to the Los Angeles Metropolitan Transit Agency (MTA) plans, the developer and designer were able to secure permission for 20,600 m² of building area, equivalent to 67 units (including 14 artist lofts), 465 m² of neighbourhood-serving retail (a cafe/market, a news stand and a bicycle shop for storage and maintenance). Two levels of underground parking that can accommodate 324 vehicles, to be used by commuters and local residents, are located across Meridian Street from the South Pasadena Gold Line Station.

South Pasadena is known for its quaint lifestyle and unrelenting desire to preserve its unique small-town feel, which has translated in the past into strong resistance to major community change. The city's fight against the Interstate 710 extension has been well documented, as has many residents' initial opposition to the Gold Line, the light rail which is part of the Los Angeles Metro system. Originally, the MTA had planned for the half-block to be a park-

and-ride facility, but faced vehement opposition from the surrounding neighbours living in a historic turn-of-the-century area of bungalows. Next, the MTA planned to develop the site using the existing zoning entitlement, which essentially allowed for garden apartments that would have increased the density five- or sixfold above that of the neighbouring area. Meridian Street consisted of commercial and attached buildings, while the less urban Mission Street had mostly single-family homes. The proposed garden-apartment alternative was met with equal opposition, as this typology was neither responsive to nor reflective of the neighbourhood character.

After 20 years of failing to find a development solution to this vacant half-block, a new team was assembled. It consisted of Stefanos Polyzoides of Moule Polyzoides Architects, a founder of New Urbanism, and Michael Dieden of Creative Housing Associates (CHA), who led a public–private partnership that included Lambert Development, the City of South Pasadena, the State of California and the MTA. This team took an innovative approach to public participation, entitlement and urban design strategies.

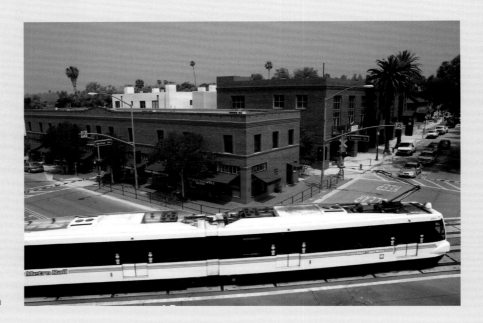

Mission Meridian

Importantly, an extensive public outreach programme was used to prove the merits of mixed-use complete and connected neighbourhoods. A public *charrette* was the main tool used to design the urban and architectural patterns. Working with the local neighbours and respecting the existing context, consensus was reached through the *charrette* to create a complex scheme that allowed for a transition from the more urban to the less urban neighbourhood. Whilst the existing zoning would only increase the density without providing any amenities, the proposal would also meet parking demands, allow for a mix of uses and increase the value of the surroundings.

The next important steps were the preparation of a Specific Plan, a Californian tool used to regulate zoning, and to develop a new FBC establishing design standards to implement the plan. The buildings nearer Meridian Street were to be more urban, with a mix of uses on the ground floor. Those fronting Mission Street were to be residential, ranging from attached units (two, four and six storeys) to single-family houses. The certainty offered by the standards set in the FBC helped to gain consensus and approval for this transit-oriented mixed-use development adjacent to the light-railway station.

In its effort to respond to the neighbourhood character, the project includes courtyard housing, single-family houses, duplexes and mixed-use lofts. These building types generate a streetscape that mediates between the commercial character of the existing neighbourhood centre and the residential scale of the Californian bungalows that surround it. The project fits easily with the traditional architecture of the area, which blends North American mercantile and arts-and-crafts influences, and is consistent with New Urbanist standards for walkable neighbourhoods. Following Jane Jacobs' advice, the buildings' living areas facing toward the street function as 'eyes on the street'. The varying typologies encourage occupants of different incomes to live in the same area. As a measure of its success, this innovative project built in 2005 is still holding its residential and commercial value in spite of the recession.

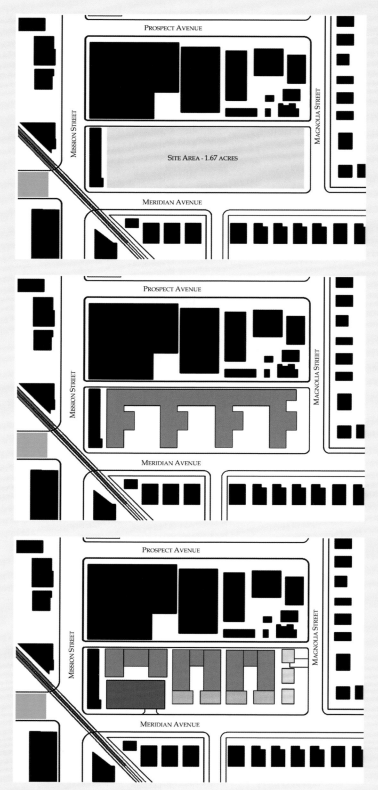

TOP: Mission site plan
MIDDLE: Mission site plan (conventional)
BOTTOM: Mission site plan (infill)

Critique and thoughts for the future

A large number of places in the United States show an unfortunate mixture of monotonous housing 'pods', supercentres, office parks and vacant commercial malls. If a more sustainable future is to be achieved, one that is less dependent on car access for every daily need, the relevance of these places rests upon their transformation in ways that improve the collective quality of life. However, most redevelopment practices are still based on the now-vilified urban-renewal approaches of the 1950s and 60s that devastated neighbourhoods on the pretext of slum clearance. The general public fears the redevelopment agencies responsible, and yet these continue to survive as the only tool the municipalities have to generate tax revenue and maintain infrastructure and general services. As a result of the current economic malaise, municipal authorities are broke and desperately need redevelopment taxes. The challenge is therefore to reverse the angst that redevelopment has caused among the public and which has given rise to so much opposition.

Another challenge for urban designers is how to assist the majority of planning departments which continue to use the same conventional land-use based tools that created the suburban blight to start with, and to offer them different methods. The same municipal authorities have separated responsibilities for place making by department: Public Works regulates streets, Park & Recreation regulates civic spaces, General Services builds civic buildings. As planning departments are being cut across the nation, code enforcement could be providing policy and regulations for future private development.

In a climate of austerity, urban designers are able to provide a new set of tools to help cities grow more strategically and sustainably. They can also ensure that new development contributes towards a sense of place that is socially, culturally and economically valuable. For example, FBCs adopted by cities such as Denver or Miami are an obvious planning tool that can stop suburban sprawl. Urban designers should ensure that similar methods are embraced by municipalities across the nation.

Since placeless-ness has affected citizens and the way in which they engage with each other, urban designers need to better explain their professional principles and foster an inclusive and localised public process built around the identification of character that will reduce the fear of redevelopment in urban and suburban areas. Urban design is well positioned to reinforce the value of local character and that elusive sense of place. The concepts of community and neighbourhood will help the nation through the changes required by the current challenges.

It will be our sense of community that will get our nation through the changes of peak oil, great recessions and the demand for sustainability. Through our internet-enabled smartphones and computers, we are more connected and linked to each other than ever before. For it is how we are linked, and able to subsequently connect physically, that will define our ability to endure and thrive as a culture into the 21st century.

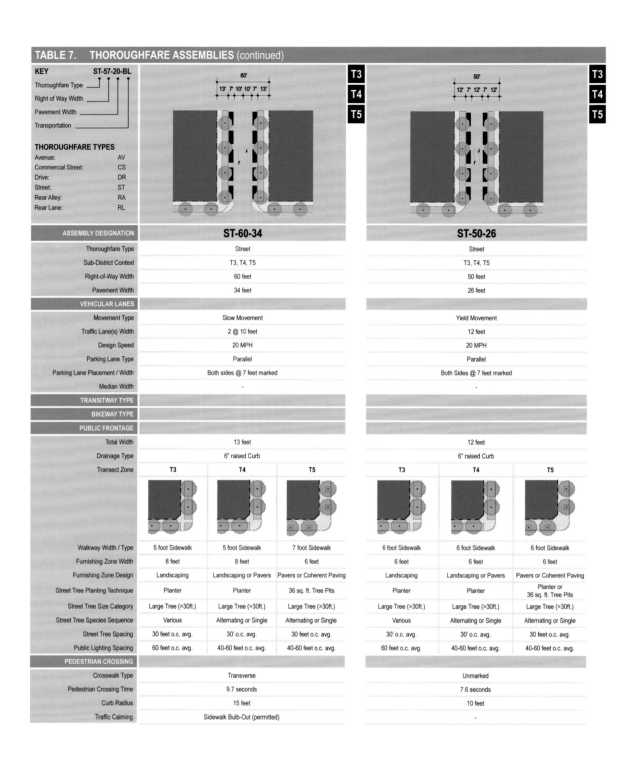

TABLE 7.   THOROUGHFARE ASSEMBLIES (continued)

KEY   ST-57-20-BL

Thoroughfare Type
Right of Way Width
Pavement Width
Transportation

THOROUGHFARE TYPES

Avenue:	AV
Commercial Street:	CS
Drive:	DR
Street:	ST
Rear Alley:	RA
Rear Lane:	RL

	T3		T3
	T4		T4
	T5		T5

ASSEMBLY DESIGNATION	ST-60-34			ST-50-26		
Thoroughfare Type	Street			Street		
Sub-District Context	T3, T4, T5			T3, T4, T5		
Right-of-Way Width	60 feet			50 feet		
Pavement Width	34 feet			26 feet		
VEHICULAR LANES						
Movement Type	Slow Movement			Yield Movement		
Traffic Lane(s) Width	2 @ 10 feet			12 feet		
Design Speed	20 MPH			20 MPH		
Parking Lane Type	Parallel			Parallel		
Parking Lane Placement / Width	Both sides @ 7 feet marked			Both Sides @ 7 feet marked		
Median Width	-			-		
TRANSITWAY TYPE						
BIKEWAY TYPE						
PUBLIC FRONTAGE						
Total Width	13 feet			12 feet		
Drainage Type	6" raised Curb			6" raised Curb		
Transect Zone	T3	T4	T5	T3	T4	T5
Walkway Width / Type	5 foot Sidewalk	5 foot Sidewalk	7 foot Sidewalk	6 foot Sidewalk	6 foot Sidewalk	6 foot Sidewalk
Furnishing Zone Width	8 feet	8 feet	6 feet	6 feet	6 feet	6 feet
Furnishing Zone Design	Landscaping	Landscaping or Pavers	Pavers or Coherent Paving	Landscaping	Landscaping or Pavers	Pavers or Coherent Paving
Street Tree Planting Technique	Planter	Planter	36 sq. ft. Tree Pits	Planter	Planter	Planter or 36 sq. ft. Tree Pits
Street Tree Size Category	Large Tree (>30ft.)	Large Tree (>30ft.)	Large Tree (>30ft.)	Large Tree (>30ft.)	Large Tree (>30ft.)	Large Tree (>30ft.)
Street Tree Species Sequence	Various	Alternating or Single	Alternating or Single	Various	Alternating or Single	Alternating or Single
Street Tree Spacing	30 feet o.c. avg.	30' o.c. avg.	30 feet o.c. avg.	30' o.c. avg.	30' o.c. avg.	30 feet o.c. avg.
Public Lighting Spacing	60 feet o.c. avg.	40-60 feet o.c. avg.	40-60 feet o.c. avg.	60 feet o.c. avg.	40-60 feet o.c. avg.	40-60 feet o.c. avg.
PEDESTRIAN CROSSING						
Crosswalk Type	Transverse			Unmarked		
Pedestrian Crossing Time	9.7 seconds			7.6 seconds		
Curb Radius	15 feet			10 feet		
Traffic Calming	Sidewalk Bulb-Out (permitted)			-		

Springville Utah, Two pages of the Westfields Village Centre Code:
Public realm: thoroughfare design standards (above)
Private realm: general to all sub-districts (facing page)

TABLE 14.   BUILDING TYPES (continued)

REARYARD

The placement of a building within the boundaries of its Lot to create a Rearyard, leaving the rear of the Lot as private space or available for dedicated parking in its commercial form. Common walls shared with adjacent buildings create a continuous Facade along the Frontage Line that steadily defines the public Thoroughfare in front of the building. Rear Elevations may be articulated for functional purposes.

Variants: Rowhouse, Apartment Building, Commercial Building, Office Building, Live-Work Building, Mixed-Use Building

GENERAL PLACEMENT

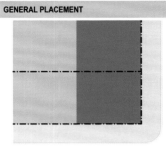

TYPE EXAMPLES	TRANSECT ZONE	T3	T4	T5
Rowhouse	**A. LOT OCCUPATION**			
	Lot Coverage	n/a	70% max.	80% max.
	Facade Buildout at Setback	n/a	60% min.	80% min.
	B. PRINCIPAL BUILDING SETBACKS			
	Primary Front Setback	n/a	10 ft. min. 15 ft max.	2 ft. min 15 ft max.
	Secondary Front Setback	n/a	10 ft. min 15 ft max.	2 ft. min. 15 ft. max.
	Side Setback	n/a	0 ft. min.	0 ft. min 24 ft. max.
	Rear Setback	n/a	3 ft. min.	3 ft. min.
	C. OUTBUILDING SETBACKS			
	Front Setback	n/a	setback + 20 ft min.	40 ft. max. from rear
	Side Setback	n/a	0 ft. or 3 ft. at corner	0 ft. or 3 ft. at corner
	Rear Setback	n/a	3 ft. min.	3 ft. min.
Apartment Building	**D. BUILDING HEIGHT (stories)**			
	Principal Building	n/a	3 max	5 max.
	Outbuilding	n/a	2 max.	2 max.
	E. ENCROACHMENTS			
	i. Setback Encroachments			
	Open Porch	n/a	80% max.	n/a
	Balcony and/or Bay Window	n/a	50% max.	100% max.
	Stoop, Lightwell, Terrace or Dooryard	n/a	100% max.	100% max.
	ii. Sidewalk Encroachments			
	Awning, Gallery, or Arcade	n/a	to within 2 ft. of curb	to within 2 ft. of curb
	iii. Encroachment Depths			
Commercial Building	Porch	n/a	8 ft. min.	n/a
	Gallery	n/a	10 ft. min.	10 ft. min.
	Arcade	n/a	n/a	12 ft. min.
	F. PARKING LOCATION			
	2nd Layer	n/a	not permitted	not permitted
	3rd Layer	n/a	permitted	permitted

A quick guide to
the United States

1 TYPES OF CLIENT

Federal government departments
- Housing and Urban Development (HUD)
- Department of Transportation (DOT)
- Environmental Protection Agency (EPA)
- Partnership for Sustainable Communities

State governments
- Office of State Architect
- Department of Transportation
- Sustainable communities
- Port districts

Local government
- Municipal Planning Agency (Transportation)
- City/county/joint-powers authorities

Private developers (local and international)

....

2 TYPES OF PROJECT/WORK

Municipal projects
- Policies: Visualisation Plans, Community and Neighbourhood Plans, Climate Action Plans
- Regulations: Form-Based Codes, Streetscape Masterplans, Redevelopment Masterplans

Private developer projects
- Masterplans for urban renewal, new communities, urban extensions
- Design guidelines

....

3 APPROACH NEEDED TO WORK IN COUNTRY

Local Business License

Urban design does not require state registration

State tax payments

Direct negotiation with client

....

4 LEGISLATION
THAT NEEDS TO BE
REFERRED TO

Regional Municipal Planning Organization (MPO) (or state-wide)
- Transportation Plans
- Action Plans
- Comprehensive Plans

Environmental Quality Acts (national and state)

Local Municipal Plans
- General/Comprehensive Plans
- Neighbourhood/Community Plans
- Zoning Ordinances
- Subdivision Ordinances
- Natural Resources Ordinances

Local Design Review Boards and Special Ordinances

5 SPECIFIC TIPS
FOR SUCCESS

Sustainability approaches are in great demand for all
planning and design efforts

6 USEFUL WEBSITES

American Institute of Architects (AIA): www.aia.org

American Planning Association (APA): www.planning.org

American Society of Landscape Architects (ASLA): www.asla.org

CNU Public Square: www.cnu.org

Institute for Urban Design: www.ifud.org

SELECTED FACTS

1	area	9,826,630 km^2
2	population	309,050,816
3	annual population growth	0.7%
4	urban population	82%
5	population density	31 p/km^2
6	GDP	$14,586,736,313,339
7	GNI per capita	$47,390

Source: The World Bank (2010)

SECTION 5

OCEANIA

AUSTRALIA

Mark Sheppard, *urban designer*

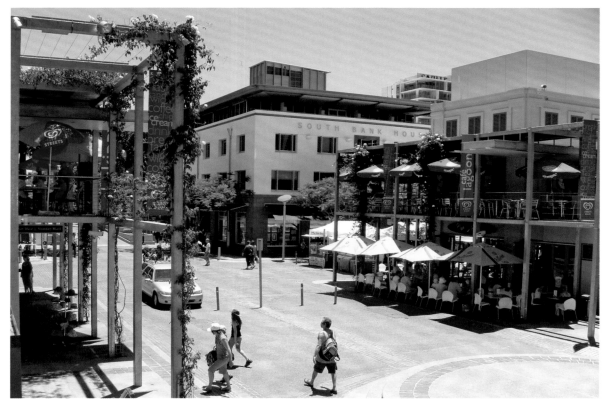

Brisbane Southbank – legacy of the World Expo 1988

AUSTRALIA is a developed, highly urbanised and comparatively prosperous nation. It is relatively sparsely populated in low-density towns and cities which hug its coastline. These urban centres, mainly developed in the last 150–200 years, are generally sprawling, car-dependent places dominated by detached houses. Current urban design challenges include retrofitting cities to improve their sustainability and resilience to a changing climate, while also accommodating escalating housing demand fuelled by population growth, falling household size and an ageing population.

Australia has a three-tiered system of government: a federal government, governments for each of its eight states and territories, and local councils.

Definitions

In Australia, urban design is generally taken to mean the three-dimensional design of parts of towns and cities. It usually refers to the overall arrangement of multi-building developments, policies and controls for the design of development in urban areas, and/ or the design of public spaces.

Good urban design is considered to be that which benefits the public interest by creating places that are well connected, enjoyable to be in, safe and visually appealing, and which reflect cultural values and local distinctiveness. It is also expected to contribute to broader planning objectives relating to environmental sustainability, social inclusion and economic prosperity.

The draft Australian Urban Design Protocol developed by heads of planning from state and territory governments, the federal government, the New Zealand Government and Australian Local Governments Association defines urban design as follows:

> Urban design concerns the physical arrangement, appearance and functioning of towns and cities, and their relationship to the natural environment. Good urban design supports the social, cultural, economic and environmental well-being of communities that live in cities and towns, or that are affected by them. Urban design is as concerned with the process of change as it is with the actual product of development.
>
> (Urban Design Forum Quarterly, issue 83, September 2008)

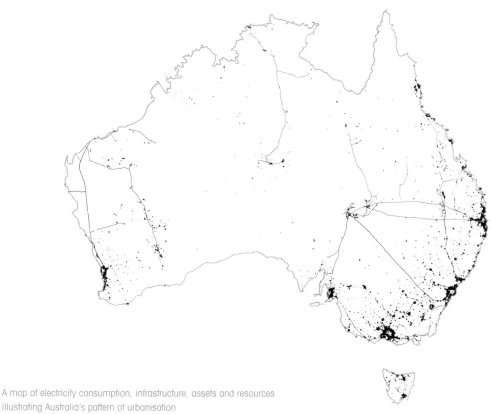

A map of electricity consumption, infrastructure, assets and resources illustrating Australia's pattern of urbanisation

The Urban Design Charter for the State of Victoria defines urban design as follows:

> Urban design is the practice of shaping human settlements to create practical, comfortable and delightful places for people to live and go about their daily lives. It is also about making well planned, logical connections between people, places and buildings.
>
> Urban design focuses on the public environment, which includes all places, regardless of ownership, that are open, available and inviting to public use.
>
> (www.dpcd.vic.gov.au/planning/urbandesign/
> urban-design-charter-for-victoria)

The professional place of urban design

In Australia, urban design is typically practised by specialist urban designers, architects, landscape architects and town planners. There is no formal registration of, or institute for, urban designers. However, there is a small number of informal groups that provide a network for the exchange of ideas on, and the promotion of, good urban design. These include:

- Urban Design Forum
- Urban Design Alliance of Queensland
- Australian Council for New Urbanism

The professional institutes of architects, landscape architects and town planners also promote good urban design. They all present annual awards for urban design at state and national level.

Urban design reached its apogee in Australia with the establishment of the prime minister's Urban Design Task Force in 1996. One legacy of this initiative is the annual Australia Award for Urban Design.

The discipline

Urban design is taught at postgraduate level in most major cities in Australia, leading to graduate certificates, diplomas and Master of Urban Design qualifications. These courses are generally provided by the architecture, landscape architecture or urban planning departments of universities, which also offer the elementary principles of urban design as part of their undergraduate degrees.

Australia's academic urban design programmes have led to the establishment of a body of original research. A recent example is a series of projects undertaken by staff and students at the University of Melbourne, focused on resolving the apparent conflict between the need for suburban intensification to create more sustainable and liveable cities and the desire for the protection and enhancement of local character.

Legal status

Each Australian state and territory has its own planning system, including legislation, policies, controls and processes.

The expression 'urban design' is rarely found in planning legislation in Australia, which tends to focus on environmental and land-use planning matters, planning instruments and development-approval processes. However, it is frequently emphasised in state and local plans and planning policies. Most state and territory governments also promote best-practice urban design through guidance documents.[1]

Historical development

Urban design did not come of age in Australia until the 1980s. Prior to that, with few exceptions, urban design was essentially a by-product of the work of surveyors, planners, architects and traffic engineers, rather than a specific area of expertise or a discipline in its own right.

The rise of urban design was triggered by a number of factors. From the late 1960s, the sterility and placelessness of mid-20th-century functionally driven street and building design drew mounting criticism. Outspoken architect Robin Boyd described postwar planning in scathing terms in his book, The Australian Ugliness:

> The plans which emerged from the various bureaucratic design departments promised to alleviate the worst tangles of traffic and industrial growth, but they were no help against ugliness. They did not pretend even to scratch the surface of the problems of the violent visual confusion of the streets of competitive architecture or the slightly psychopathic pioneering attitude to the landscape. The corrective plans had no artistic aspirations. They made no attempt to restore unity and dignity or to curb the self-advertising instincts of so many ill-trained or un-trained designers. The other type of town-planning, the art, the sort of design which aims for a delightful total environment, is very rare; but it is not unknown.

Boyd's criticisms paralleled the international rise of environmental concerns, heritage conservation and civic societies.

In the 1970s, increased overseas travel by city council bureaucrats and the advent of planners and architects with specialist urban design training from British and US universities brought a new awareness of both traditional urban design values and new urban design theories.

Urban design truly arrived as a recognised field in Australia in 1994, when Prime Minister Paul Keating established an Urban Design Task Force. This body was charged with reporting on the state of urban design in Australia and ultimately resulted in the annual Australia Award for Urban Design. To fully appreciate how remarkable this endorsement for urban design at the highest level was, it is necessary to understand the chequered history of urban design in Australia.

Permanent urban areas did not occur until British settlement in the late 18th century. Since then the design of towns and cities has experienced four distinct eras, whose primary influences can be characterised as: colonialism, idealism, modernism and place making. Each of these eras represented a pendulum swing between the importance attached to function and to delight.

The British brought a formula for town design, applied uniformly in their colonies the world over. Its defining feature was the orthogonal grid, adopted because of its efficiency. Sensitivity to place was limited to occasional twists of the alignment off due north in response to topography.

A unique set of dimensions gradually evolved for the components of these towns, which continues to characterise older urban areas in Australia today. Road widths were standardised at 20 or 30 m, generous by European measures. Minimum lot sizes were established, which led to Australia's continuing love affair with the 'quarter-acre block'. Front setbacks for residential buildings were set at 4 m, creating a New World suburban character.

The colonial towns were almost entirely designed to meet functional requirements, with no room for experiential aspirations. The only significant exception to this was the 'parkland towns', a distinctly Australian contribution to model town planning involving a frame of parkland around the urban core, demarcating it from surrounding suburbs.

In the late 19th century, Australian town planning entered a new idealistic phase, strongly influenced by the garden city and city beautiful movements. Whilst order and efficiency remained key objectives, this was overlaid by a desire for more attractive urban places.

The distinguishing characteristic of idealistic town plans in Australia was formal radial street patterns, offering the potential for decorous curved streets and boulevards focused on landmarks. The pinnacle of this era was the new city and national capital of Canberra, which resulted from an international competition. Conceived as a city in the landscape, the Walter Burley Griffin design was based on interlocking radial geometries rooted to major landforms.

By the 1920s, modernism's quest to define new ways of living had begun to introduce concepts such as the neighbourhood unit, land-use zoning, road hierarchies, and segregation of cars and pedestrians. Function took precedence again over beauty.

The mid-20th century was a low point in urban design in Australia, as its cities began to sprawl with little thought to place-specific design or visual appeal. The cul-de-sac emerged to become an icon of 20th-century suburban development, cemented by the long-running and widely exported Australian soap opera, Neighbours.

Australia was largely spared the excesses of large-scale modernist urban renewal projects such as those which assailed other cities around the world. However, the skylines of the larger metropolises are punctuated by clutches of 1960s public-housing towers set in unloved open space.

Ultimately, the failures of modernist planning and architecture led to the rise of urban design in Australia in the final decades of the 20th century. The creation of unique and attractive places re-emerged as an influential factor in the development and management of urban areas.

From the 1980s, Australia hosted a series of international events that led to major urban renewal projects, including the America's Cup in Fremantle, the World Expo in Brisbane and the Sydney Olympics. In these and other projects, the potential was recognised for post-industrial waterfront developments to be a key asset in the new age of competition between cities. This provided a high-profile canvas for the newly remembered practice of urban design.

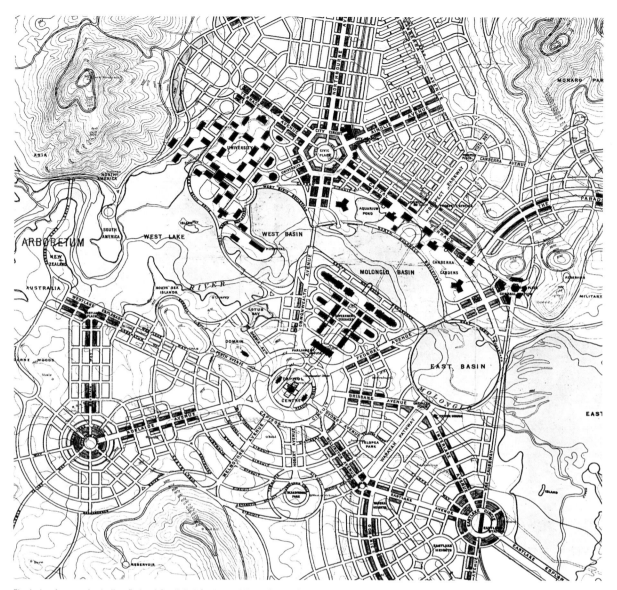

Final plan for new Australian Federal Capital at Canberra, Walter Burley Griffin –
pinnacle of the idealistic era of town and city design

At the same time, rising recognition of the importance of urban design led to programmes to improve the quality of the public realm within Australia's older city centres. These ranged from the incremental introduction of higher-quality footpaths, street trees and street furniture, to more significant interventions such as new public squares and the revitalisation of service lanes as intimate pedestrian links and spaces.

The 1980s also marked the beginning of a new phase of suburb design, primarily at the ever-expanding urban fringe. Improvements included better integration of local shops, schools and open space, a more sensitive response to nature, improved housing choice (including forms of medium-density accommodation such as row housing) and more pedestrian-friendly streets.

These innovations were triggered by a combination of private developers wanting to create a point of difference in the housing market, often borrowing ideas from the USA, and the imposition of higher environmental and development standards by authorities. They culminated in the emergence of comprehensively conceived masterplanned communities.

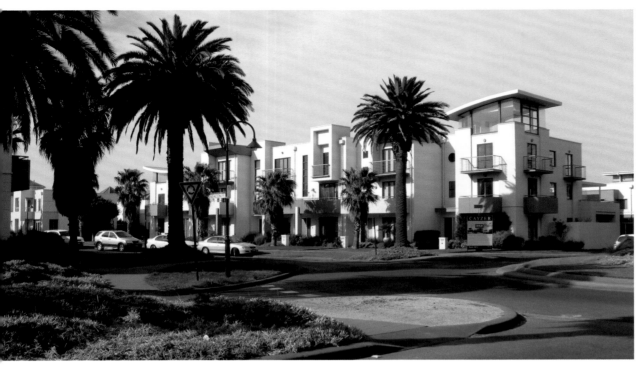

Beacon Cove – a 1990s masterplanned community

A companion advance of the 1990s was the introduction by state and local governments of guidelines to promote higher residential development standards. These established minimum benchmarks for residential amenity, streetscape character, energy-efficient siting and design, and public open space.[2] Over time, they have become entrenched as mandatory planning controls in most jurisdictions, although they are typically performance-based guidelines which provide flexibility in how their objectives can be achieved.

The New Urbanism movement, which emerged during this time, proved to be another important stimulus for improved urban design in new residential communities, particularly through its promotion of walkable neighbourhoods as a structuring device, interconnected streets, mixed use and good street frontages.

Urban design is now a well-entrenched consideration of planning, architecture and landscape architecture in Australia. This is reflected in the promotion of good urban design in state and local planning documents, policies that require specific urban design qualities to be considered in the assessment of planning applications, and controls that establish minimum standards.

Practice and concerns

Urban design work in Australia is mainly commissioned by state governments, local authorities and private developers. The federal government has been notably silent on urban planning and design, with rare exceptions.

Urban design work is undertaken by a wide range of different organisations, including state government and local authority planning departments;

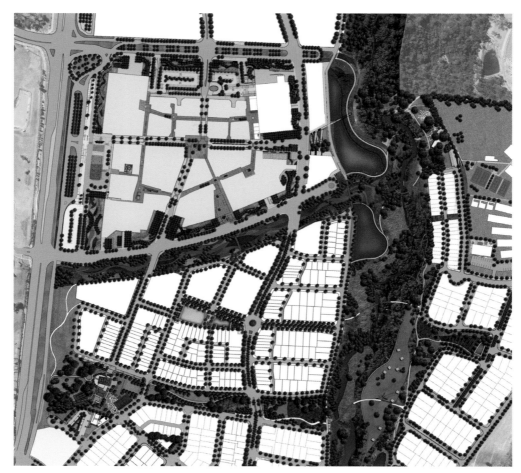

Rouse Hill, Sydney – a New Urbanist town centre

multidisciplinary consultancies that also offer architecture, town planning and/ or landscape architecture services; and a number of very small (one to two person) specialist urban design practices.

Current issues of concern to urban designers in Australia are summarised below:

- Australian cities and towns are dominated by relatively low-density suburbs (less than ten dwellings per hectare). Planners and urban designers have long recognised the need to intensify these suburbs to minimise urban sprawl and create more sustainable and liveable cities. However, there is significant community resistance to the change of character that goes with the introduction of denser housing. This position largely holds political sway, hindering the introduction of policies and controls to promote intensification. Urban designers in Australia's growing cities are seeking to address this by promoting the benefits of greater density and developing clever designs for medium-density housing that achieve higher densities in a form that fits comfortably with the prevailing low-density character.
- Australia is susceptible to extreme weather events – particularly bush fire, flooding and cyclones on a catastrophic scale. It is feared that climate change is increasing the frequency of such events, and will add sea-level rise into the bargain. Urban designers are typically included as key members of teams focused on the adaptation of towns and cities in response to these

events. This is seen as critical given the tendency for bureaucrats to choose quick practical solutions after traumatic events, relegating concerns about the quality of the public realm to the status of minor importance or an unaffordable luxury. Particular concerns include engineering solutions for sea-level rise or flood mitigation that may have significantly adverse impacts on the quality of adjoining streets and spaces.

- The dominance of the car during the second half of the 20th century, when Australia's cities experienced significant growth, has left a large proportion of their suburbs with a legacy of traffic-dominated and pedestrian-unfriendly streets. This problem includes convoluted and impermeable street networks, a lack of footpaths, streets lined by high fences, and limited landscaping. Urban designers are involved in the repair of these suburbs so that they are more inviting to pedestrians.

- Increasing road congestion in Australia's major cities has led to a massive increase in the use of bicycles for the daily commute to work (although it is still a very low proportion of journeys compared with many European countries). Urban designers have been at the vanguard of efforts to persuade the powerful roads lobby to release its stranglehold on the use of roads for cars and find more space for cycle lanes.

- Australia has belatedly realised that it must conserve its water resources. This has led to a new area of interest for urban designers: water-sensitive urban design. Collaboration between urban designers and hydraulic engineers has developed urban storm-water drainage systems that rely less on engineered solutions and instead use more natural techniques to retard and filter rainfall, at the same time creating valuable and distinctive recreational and education spaces for their communities.

- The increasing sprawl of Australia's major cities has obliterated valuable agricultural areas and pushed food production further from its customers, increasing the environmental costs of distribution. Urban designers are addressing this issue in urban renewal plans undertaken for government agencies, by investigating innovative ways for food to be produced within urban areas. This has become known as Food Sensitive Planning and Urban Design (FSPUD).

- Like many other countries, Australia has for some time promoted 'green' buildings through rating systems. However, a new development currently occupying urban designers is the creation of a tool for measuring the sustainability of whole urban areas. This will encompass social, economic and environmental sustainability, along with design excellence, and leadership and governance (www.gbca.org.au/green-star/green-star-communities).

- Despite its resurgence under Prime Minister Keating in the mid-1990s, the promotion of good urban design is still subject to the vagaries of local, state and federal politics in Australia. Therefore, a movement was begun in 2010 to establish a national organisation to promote good urban design using England's Commission for Architecture and the Built Environment (CABE) as a starting point. At the time of writing, widespread support for the Australian Urban Design Initiative (AUDI) has been garnered from across the country, although it is yet to be taken up by governments or an alternative funding body.

Urban design is playing a key part in ensuring that urban renewal projects in Australia are sustainable and liveable, and have a distinctive sense of place. A notable example of this is Claisebrook Village, a major urban renewal project in Perth, Western Australia.[3]

The Claisebrook Village project commenced in 1992, following the establishment of the East Perth Redevelopment Authority (EPRA). EPRA is a state government agency responsible for the redevelopment of underutilised inner urban land. EPRA's approach emphasises the importance of place making – the art of creating distinctive and enjoyable places that will attract people and investment.

At the time, Western Australia's largest urban renewal project, Claisebrook Village, is built on 137.5 ha of former industrial land along the Swan river immediately east of Perth's central business district (CBD). It involved extensive environmental rehabilitation, for which it has won awards.

The design of Claisebrook is based on the concept of an urban village. It contains a broad mix of uses, including 1,500 homes, employment space for 6,000 workers, shops, tertiary education and parks, creating opportunities to live close to work and facilities. The residential development takes the form of attached townhouses, low-rise apartment buildings and garage-top studios, providing a diverse range of housing opportunities, contributing to a socially balanced community and achieving a compactness that can support local services at a comfortable urban scale. EPRA has mandated the inclusion of approximately 10% social and affordable housing, a high proportion by Australian standards.

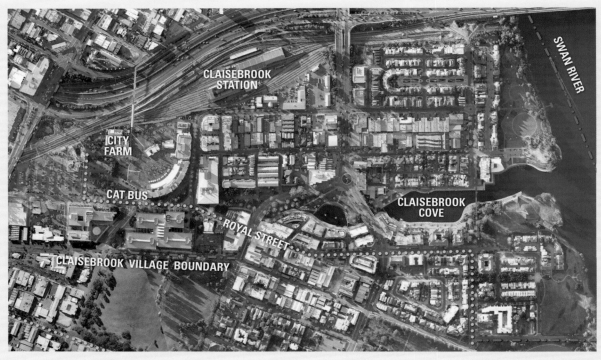

Caisebrook Village, Perth, aerial view

Non-motorised travel modes are encouraged through good pedestrian and cycle links, and the extension of the CBD's free and high-frequency Central Area Transit (CAT) bus system into the village. The CBD's street network has also been extended into the development in the form of a modified grid in order to ensure a well-connected, permeable and legible place. This is enhanced by the employment of a diverse range of street types, from narrow lanes to tree-lined boulevards, which add to the distinctiveness of each part of the development. The streets have been designed to create a low-speed environment, inviting to pedestrians and cyclists.

A key feature of the project is the level of public investment in the quality of the public realm, including attractive streetscapes and extensive parkland. The parkland engages the community through a wide range of passive and active recreation opportunities. A series of parks and water bodies runs centrally through the village, culminating in Claisebrook Cove which leads into the Swan river. The cove is animated by cafes, bars, restaurants and boating activity. This forms the centrepiece of the development and maximises access to waterside and waterborne recreation opportunities. Another linear park runs along the river's edge, connected across the cove by a

pedestrian and cycle bridge. Advance tree planting in the streets and parks created an instant and attractive character, which appealed to prospective residents and investors alike.

At the core of the village is a local retail and commercial centre focused on Royal Street. Rather than the sanitised and controlled enclosed shopping malls surrounded by a sea of car parking that characterise late 20th-century retail development in Australia, this is a street-based centre, focused on a genuinely public domain where social exchange is unconstrained. Shop-top apartments help to enliven the centre, while the design of the street creates an inviting pedestrian environment that coexists comfortably with the kerbside parking and slow-moving traffic necessary for the viability of small centres. A series of pedestrian plazas along the street provides focal points for the social life of the village.

Detailed design guidelines were prepared for each stage of the project in order to prescribe the overall form and detailed design of individual developments. Key aims of the guidelines were to promote a contemporary architectural character rather than superficial stylistic reference to historical design periods, and to achieve a coherent character for each part of the village while allowing freedom of design expression for individual buildings. This

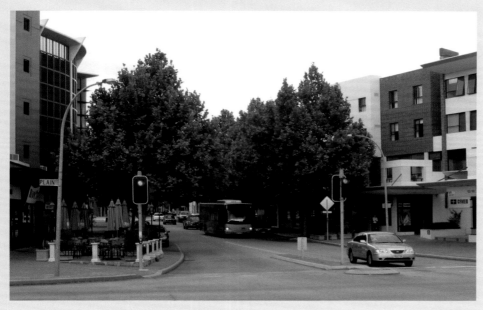

Street-based, mixed-use centre, Claisebrook Village, Perth

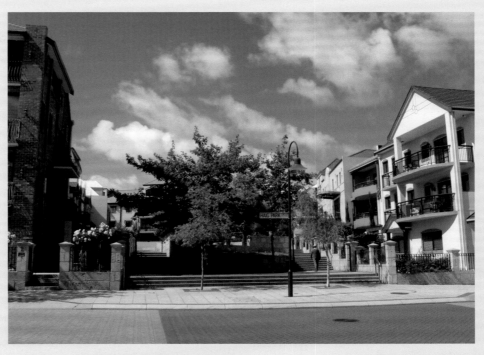

Compact housing forms and high-quality public realm,
Claisebrook Village, Perth

has largely been successful, with unity achieved through consistent scale and building typology along with a narrow palette of materials, and visual richness achieved through varied facade compositions and use of materials.

The site's indigenous heritage and industrial past has been recognised in the design of the project, through the restoration and refurbishment of a number of historic buildings and the expression of historic activities in public artworks. An art walk has been developed, using recycled materials from demolished buildings, which pays homage to the site's history.

The development also incorporates a community-run city farm, which promotes organic and sustainable food production practices, provides gardening and healthy cooking classes and hosts a farmers' market (www.perthcityfarm.org.au).

Claisebrook Village is a flag-bearer for urban design in Australia. Its vibrant mix of uses and high-quality and genuinely public streets and open spaces, structured around the site's natural setting and incorporating numerous detailed design features

rooted in its history, has resulted in a sustainable, liveable and distinctive place.

The project was initially funded by a combination of federal government money from the Building Better Cities Program and state government investment, totalling A$127 million (£86 million). It has since attracted A$685 million (£460 million) in private investment.

EPRA was the planning authority during the life of the project. Planning control has now largely returned to the City of Perth, with the remaining stages to be returned on completion. In addition to its environmental awards, Claisebrook Village has won three awards from the Urban Development Institute of Australia.

The future

Urban design has a relatively healthy profile in the creation of urban environments in Australia. Its importance is recognised in state and local government planning documents, in the assessment of planning applications, in the development of new infrastructure and in the redevelopment of ageing streets and spaces. The architecture, planning and landscape architecture institutes all confer urban design awards, and there is a national one sponsored jointly by them all. However, good urban design is not yet ubiquitous and it is constantly under threat from competing agendas.

The traditional city centres have fared best: blessed with a sound 19th-century structure, they have survived well the rigours of the 20th century to offer a robust framework for the continual evolution of the property market. At the same time, city bureaucrats' recognition of the importance of a high-quality public realm has led to the gradual development of more inviting streets and spaces, and the replacement of obsolete precincts with vibrant new places.

The rise of the conservation movement came just in time to save much of Australia's inner-urban Victorian-era neighbourhoods from destruction. Urban designers have played a key role in identifying ways in which these places can evolve to respond to contemporary needs while respecting their architectural heritage.

Less successful have been the larger urban renewal precincts at the fringes of Australia's city centres, whether waterfront redevelopments or the regeneration of redundant industrial areas. The urgent desire for economic renewal and a lack of experience among architects and planners in designing mid-rise environments has led in many cases to sterile monofunctional zones containing chaotic clusters of 'look-at-me' towers placed haphazardly in uninviting streets. Despite the relatively young age of some of these developments, there is already a recognised need to repair their poor-quality street environments and lack of diversity.

The middle-ring suburbs in Australia's larger cities, mainly built in the interwar and immediate postwar periods, have matured into much sought-after residential neighbourhoods due to their characterful architecture, mature landscape and, in many cases, relatively good local facilities and public-transport connections. However, they have also become a battleground as developers seek to introduce denser housing in response to its desirability and planning-policy support for urban consolidation, raising the ire of existing residents.

The reality is that these suburbs are environmentally, economically and socially unsustainable at their current densities, relying on the car for access to employment, shops and community facilities. To date, however, urban designers have been largely unsuccessful in overturning resistance to change in these areas.

The pressure for additional housing has led most of Australia's cities to expand their boundaries to accommodate new suburbs. At the same time, concern about housing affordability has led to the design of these suburbs being driven by cost-effectiveness as much as the creation of healthy and resilient communities with a unique identity.

In a return to the efficiency-driven layout of colonial townships, street networks designed to create a sense of place have been ruled out in favour of rigidly rectilinear grids, irrespective of local topography or features. In a continuation of modernist principles, local centres are being relegated to traffic-dominated main roads on the edge of the neighbourhood, resulting in sterile, car-dependent dormitory suburbs. And, in the final blow, the houses are allowed to take the form of deeply unsustainable

'McMansions' – eave-less boxes reliant on air conditioning and separated just enough to ensure unsustainable densities.

The desperate need for more affordable housing, and governments' unwillingness to invest in alternative solutions, has led to a misconception that, given the ability to build cheap suburbs, the housing industry will provide affordable housing. Not only have increasing house prices and transport costs demonstrated that this is folly, but in the meantime the opportunity to create genuinely attractive, vibrant, sustainable suburbs is being lost.

In short, urban design has come a long way in Australia in the last 30 years. It has made its mark, with successes to be proud of in the city centres and inner suburbs. It appears to be here to stay, with urban design issues frequently a subject of popular debate and widespread coverage in the media. Since the re-election of a Labor federal government, urban planning has even come back on to the national agenda with the creation of a Major Cities Unit, whose remit is to advise the government on issues of policy, planning and infrastructure that have an impact on Australia's cities and suburbs.

However, the big challenge of retrofitting Australia's low-density suburbs to be resilient in an uncertain low-carbon future has not yet been solved. Nor has the urban design community made itself heard loudly enough at the urban fringe, the last bastion of functionalist town design. This is Australian urban designers' final frontier.

A quick guide to
Australia

1 TYPES OF CLIENT

State governments

Local authorities

Private developers

Universities

....

2 TYPES OF PROJECT/WORK

Masterplans for urban extensions, urban renewal and streetscape renewal

Design policies and guidelines

Expert advice and evidence

....

3 APPROACH NEEDED TO WORK IN COUNTRY

Consultancies
* Respond to invitation to tender for public-sector work
* International competition
* Direct negotiation with private developers

Individuals
* Apply for visa
* Direct negotiation with potential employer – state or local government, or private consultancy

....

4 LEGISLATION THAT NEEDS TO BE REFERRED TO

State-wide strategic planning policies, planning controls and urban design guidance documents

Regional/metropolitan plans

Local planning scheme and guidelines

Creating Places for People – An Urban Design Protocol for Australian Cities (www.urbandesign.gov.au/)

....

5 SPECIFIC TIPS
FOR SUCCESS

Follow the advice in the above documents concerning mixed-use centres, increased densities, connected street networks, street-based public realm, response to context, etc

Climate-responsive approaches to design

Comprehensive community consultation

6 USEFUL WEBSITES

Australian Council for New Urbanism: www.acnu.org

Australian Institute of Architects: www.architecture.com.au

Planning Institute Australia (PIA): www.planning.org.au

Urban Design Alliance of Queensland: www.udal.org.au

Urban Design Forum: www.udf.org.au

SELECTED FACTS

1	area	7,686,850 km^2
2	population	22,328,800
3	annual population growth	1.7%
4	urban population	89%
5	population density	2.9 p/km^2
6	GDP (2009)	$924,843,128,521
7	GNI per capita (2009)	$43,590

Source: The World Bank (2010)

NEW ZEALAND

David Truscott, *urban designer, landscape architect and town planner*

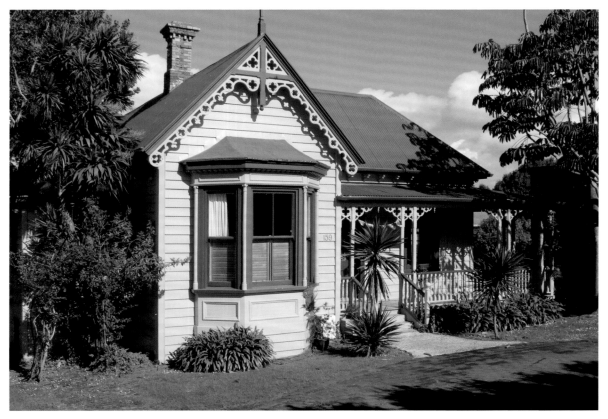

The suburban heritage reflects the abundance of local hardwoods

NEW ZEALAND has a constitutional monarchy, and is a parliamentary democracy. Wellington is its capital, where the central adminstration is based. The country is divided into 16 regions, which are mostly administered by regional and district/city authorities, while Auckland and four other regions have unitary authorties.

New Zealand is a highly urbanised, multicultural nation that celebrates its south Pacific and European heritage. Settlements developed from the mid-19th century onwards, generally beside natural harbours around the country's two main islands. The population distribution increasingly favours the upper North Island, with almost a third of the country's inhabitants now living in one city there – Auckland.

The country enjoys a clean 'green' image overseas, with some cities scoring highly in international quality-of-life studies (eg Mercer's). These green credentials do not, however, reflect its urban character. It has one of the world's highest per capita car-ownership rates, and a legacy of low-density, car-oriented urban development with inadequate investment in public transport. This poses a major challenge for New Zealand's urban future.

Nevertheless, significant progress has been made on several fronts over the last decade. Urban design principles now pervade professional thinking in the conception and regulation of much of the country's development, and the notion of 'good urban design' is even used in real-estate agents' details. A milestone in this journey was the Ministry for the Environment's publication of the New Zealand Urban Design Protocol in 2005.

Definition

In the protocol, urban design is defined as follows:

> The design of buildings, places, spaces and networks that make up our towns and cities, and the ways people use them. It ranges in scale from a metropolitan region, city and town down to a street, public space or even a single building. Urban design is concerned not just with appearances and built form, but with the environmental, economic, social and cultural consequences of design. It is an approach that draws together many different sectors and professions, and it includes both the process of decision-making as well as the outcomes of design.

Reflecting the regulatory context, the protocol definition covers aspects traditionally seen as urban planning, so that urban design addresses how the built form and public spaces of towns and cities look, work and change, and how they might be improved.

The professional place of urban design

Practitioners in New Zealand include specialist urban designers and others from a range of associated professions. Whilst urban designers do not have a separate professional institute, the Urban Design Forum was established in 2002 to foster and promote good urban design in New Zealand. This is a countrywide organisation sponsored and supported by the national institutes for architects, landscape architects, planners, surveyors and professional engineers, but open to all professionals and others interested in creating better towns and cities. Of the 606 members in March 2011, 255 declared a professional affiliation as follows:

- 42% planners
- 18% architects
- 16% surveyors
- 11% landscape architects
- 7% engineers
- 5% lawyers

The discipline

New Zealand's postgraduate urban design course was launched in 2005 at the University of Auckland. Enrolment comprises a balance mainly of architects, landscape architects and planners. An additional postgraduate course is under consideration at Auckland's Unitec.

Professional programmes in architecture, landscape architecture and surveying at various centres provide taught and studio courses in aspects of urban design as core subjects. Although design teaching is not required for course accreditation at the country's five planning schools, an urban design specialism is offered in the University of Auckland's Bachelor degree in Planning (Bplan).

Sustainability drives most of the country's diverse urban design research. This is predominantly Auckland-based, and topics include building design, settlement form, transport, energy and low-impact development. Publications include A Deeper Shade of Green (Bernhardt 2008), which explores sustainable building design for New Zealand.

Legal status

Urban design is not the subject of specific legislation in New Zealand. The Resource Management Act 1991 (RMA) provides the regulatory regime, and this enables authorities to control the adverse environmental effects of building and other activities. Rules that specify various standards and terms to be complied with can be adopted as part of each council's district plan, and urban design outcomes reflect these rules. The rules have the force of law.

Adoption of a district plan, or any subsequent plan change, involves a lengthy consultative process. A plan change is normally council-initiated, but it may be sought privately, with the costs being borne by the initiator, and can result in changes to development rules and zoning that may strengthen or relax controls.

Commercial and other zones are designated in each council's district plan and, typically, zone rules and general rules are applied to them. Some proposals constitute permitted activities, and are allowed as of right. Others requiring consent under the RMA, termed 'resource consent', are evaluated for their degree of infringement of each of the rules. The environmental effects are assessed using criteria listed in the plan and against the plan's policies and objectives.

In commercial zones, the rules might include a plot ratio, maximum building height, minimum service area, parking requirements, a street verandah requirement, noise limits and a minimum retail-frontage glazing ratio. The district plan rules vary; in Auckland's central area, for instance, the plot-ratio allowance offers a floor-space bonus where a community benefit is derived, such as through-site links, plazas or public art.

Within designated zones, development on the urban periphery involves a two-stage consent process. For land subdivision, rules establish density and specify road design and other standards. The subsequent development would typically be controlled by zone rules governing, for example, boundary setbacks, maximum site coverage, maximum height and height in relation to boundary. In effect, these rules prescribe a conceptual envelope, within which development is a permitted activity. Consent would be required for infringement of a rule, with assessment often limited to this single aspect of the proposal.

The rules prescribe minimum standards and compliance requirements rather than preferred outcomes. Generally, district plan rules do not cover building aesthetics, so that apart from some heritage and commercial areas where inappropriate development is a particular concern, the appearance of buildings does not require resource consent.

Most major urban centres and some towns are now covered by urban design policies. Increasingly, structure plans are required for new higher-density greenfield development and comprehensive urban design criteria apply, with no 'as of right' development. Some councils have also adopted district plan rules to enable design control for existing built areas, and notably for commercial centres. For example, Wellington City Council's policy review in 2005 recognised that the regulations engendered a mindset driven by compliance with the rules, and that this needed to be changed. A statutory design guide was adopted for the central area to encourage contextual design and to enable the council to control outcomes.

Historical development

The signing of the treaty of Waitangi by Maori chiefs and representatives of the British crown on 6 February 1840 cleared the way for new settlers. Where the crown acquired Maori land, the British system of land ownership and property rights was introduced. Settlement plans, often prepared in the UK and inspired more by practicality than townscape vision, generally prescribed a grid of streets and a rectilinear definition to land ownership. This imposed pattern was largely unrelated to the character of the landscape. The road network was not always adjusted to respond to topography and landscape features, and Dunedin's Baldwin Street, the steepest road in the world, is one result of this. Other parts of Dunedin's street grid proved to be unbuildable.

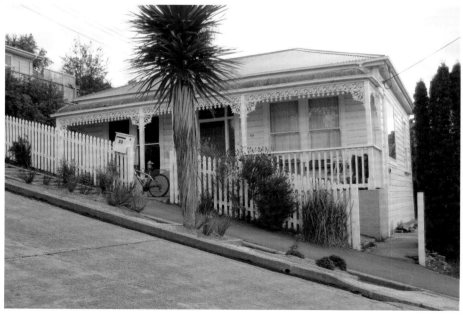

Dunedin: Baldwin Street has a 35% gradient

Urban growth took off in the late 19th century, and peripheral expansion throughout the 20th century cemented the essentially low-density character of New Zealand's towns and cities. Growing environmental regulation during the latter half of the 20th century culminated in a radical overhaul in 1991. Replacing the former town and country planning legislation, the RMA promoted the sustainable management of natural and physical resources and, as an attempt to install a less prescriptive regime, the RMA's primary focus was on the protection of the country's natural landscapes. Minimal reference to the built environment in the RMA suggests that urban areas were presumed to require limited regulation once sustainable management principles and standards had been established.

However, by the end of the decade there were concerns that the RMA was not delivering a good-quality urban environment. Following a review, the Ministry for the Environment published People, Places, Spaces: A Design Guide for Urban New Zealand in 2002. In this, it recognised that 'we have not given much thought to the design of our towns and cities'. The document also acknowledged that the existing legal tools for managing urban areas 'have generally not focused on the interrelated issues thrown up by urban design'. The ministry called for a comprehensive approach to creating sustainable development, and encouraged developers to find solutions that succeed socially as well as economically. In addition, the Local Government Act, introduced in the same year, promoted sustainability while facilitating long-term strategic planning and the funding of public projects.

In association with its Sustainable Cities programme, the ministry launched the New Zealand Urban Design Protocol three years later, calling for 'a significant step up in the quality of urban design in New Zealand and a change in the way we think about our towns and cities'. Importantly, the protocol was to be part of a broader and more radical project designed to promote action.

Organisations in the development sector – central- and local-government agencies, professional institutes, educational institutions, consultants, community groups and Maori authorities, as well as property developers and investors – were invited to commit to improving the quality of urban design. In becoming a signatory of the protocol, each organisation is required to appoint an Urban Design Champion to promote the agenda with their own action programme. Signatories receive a monthly ministry e-newsletter, Urban Leader.

The ministry released a raft of publications to support the protocol, including The Value of Urban Design (2005), The Urban Design Toolkit (2009), Summary of Urban Design Research, The Urban Design Action Pack, (2005) Review of Urban Design Case Law (2008) and Urban Design Case Studies (2008). An annual national urban design award was instigated, and 2005 was declared the Year of the Built Environment.

The protocol has attracted considerable support. By 20 April 2011, there were 183 signatories from the full range of organisations and this is indicative of wider approval. The ministry is regarded by most signatories as having been instrumental in increasing knowledge and awareness of urban design throughout the sector.

A National Policy Statement on Urban Design was proposed in 2008, but following the change of government not proceeded with. The protocol remains in place although a loss of momentum is evident, with environmental issues now given less priority and road building favoured over public transport infrastructure investment. The initiative for further progress in urban design has largely passed to local authorities.

Practice and concerns

Private developers and business are the main clients of urban designers. Consultants are also commissioned by local authorities for promotional and design services, for specialist policy advice and to adjudicate in consent hearings and environment court appeals.

A useful, if incomplete, picture of consultants offering urban design services is shown by the list of protocol signatories. There are 83 practices listed, and this includes the national multi-profession firms and many of the country's large design consultancies. Landscape architects, planners, engineers and surveyors are included, but architects are the most numerous. A total of 15% of the signatories are represented as being specialist urban design practices.

Over 30 councils are signatories, and this includes the metropolitan and most other urban authorities. While councils had a limited urban design capability in 2006, the situation has now improved and more planners receive design training. Surveys have revealed 'a significant change in attitudes' towards urban design within councils. Many have recruited urban design staff and have their own promotional initiatives. For example, Hamilton City Council's CityScope projected a vision supported by its design guide, Vista, and the setting up of an urban design panel.

Ten councils currently have an urban design panel, and some more than one, operating either as an in-house design clinic or as an external technical advisory team with members nominated by professional institutes.

The protocol highlighted the concern that the consent process did not engender a strong sense of place in new developments. The flexible application of zoning rules aimed, for example, at concentrating suburban development around district centres, and the adoption of urban design guidelines are addressing this and achieving a more sensitive integration with the landscape and local ecology.

A history of seismic activity is also a concern. This has resulted in rare but devastating damage, and sadly in loss of life. The 1931 Napier earthquake was followed by the inspired decision to rebuild most of the town in the art deco style. The 2010 and 2011 Christchurch earthquakes, along with several thousand aftershocks, have also resulted in a significant loss of buildings. Following extensive consultation, the community's vision is to rebuild central Christchurch as a low- to medium-rise 'city in a garden', embracing sustainable design principles.

Across the country, low development densities have historically satisfied the 'quarter acre dream' and a desire for generous space standards. These have also allowed better integration with the natural environment, particularly on the urban edge where, in some areas, zone rules require large properties that allow a self-sufficient lifestyle, known an 'lifestyle blocks'. While the low-density pattern of detached buildings offers the benefit of allowing future adaptation or rebuilding to accord with sustainable design principles, the transport implications of such a dispersed urban form constitute a significant issue.

Public transport and urban intensification around public transport nodes are high on the agenda of the proposed Auckland Spatial Plan, with the council's ambition to be the world's 'most liveable' city. A recent imaginative proposal to semi-pedestrianise several city-centre arteries is a sign of change, but with urban motorways and car-park buildings currently under construction the degraded environment of vehicle-dominated public spaces will remain a concern for some time.

CASE STUDY

BRITOMART AND THE AUCKLAND WATERFRONT

The city of Auckland developed on the isthmus between two sizeable natural harbours – the Waitemata and the larger Manukau to the south. From its founding in 1840, Auckland has grown to a city of over 1.4 million people, exceeding the combined populations of the next largest five urban centres in the country, and projections point to 2.4 million by 2040. Much of Auckland's history is bound up with a northern waterfront area called Britomart.

Britomart today borders the central business district. The rejuvenation of the Britomart precinct is currently underway, together with other projects along the waterfront. The city centre's connection with the harbour has largely been denied by the growth of the port, and the current vision is aimed at restoring this.

The area is historically significant: following the signing of the Treaty of Waitangi, Ngati Whatua o Orakei, the local Maori, sought an alliance and offered the Governor, William Hobson, 3,000 acres, which Hobson proposed would be the colony's

capital. Land at Horotiu Bay (Commercial Bay) was chosen for the settlement, and on 16 September 1840 the flag was raised on the adjacent clifftop, soon to be named Point Britomart.

A plan for the settlement was prepared by the Surveyor-General Felton Mathew in order to facilitate government land sales. Where this plan was implemented, a geometrical street grid was generally followed with the main streets aligned towards the harbour along the valleys and ridges.

Auckland's trading economy took off. By 1883, Point Britomart had been levelled and the material used in an extensive waterfront reclamation, allowing expansion of the port and railway construction into the centre. The rail terminus was later relocated, and after 1945 increasing car ownership accelerated a decline in public transport. This issue was recognised by 1973, when a light rail system linking to a new underground station at Britomart was first proposed.

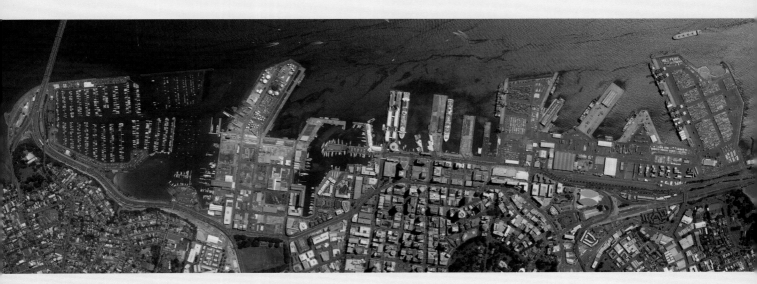

Waterfront Auckland's remit relates to the 1840 shoreline

The Britomart project

In 1995, Auckland City Council proposed an underground five-storey transport interchange accommodating bus and rail services, and 2,900 car-parking spaces on the 5.2 ha Britomart site. This was to be funded by high-rise development of up to 150 m in height. The highly contentious plan was abandoned and, following public consultation and a design competition, a revised 'Waitamata Waterfront (Britomart) Project' was approved in 1999. The new approach was intended to create a welcoming gateway to the city centre while integrating the proposed transport interchange with renewal that retained the area's established character.

An award-winning conversion of the scheduled former Central Post Office provided a travel centre and concourse serving the new underground rail terminus. The complex project management was a notable aspect of its success.

On completion in 2003, the council sold the land and leased the area's heritage buildings to a selected international development consortium for the above-ground project. This was subject to urban design guidelines and additional district plan provisions for the Britomart precinct that became operative in 2004. The plan specified design control of the external appearance of all new and altered buildings.

The precinct's 12 scheduled heritage buildings, along with five more deemed worthy of retention, are located in perimeter blocks facing the surrounding streets. These buildings exert a strong streetscape character and provide the framework for the area's renewal. This is the country's largest heritage restoration project to date and the district plan requires that building renovations be subject to individual conservation plans in addition to the general heritage controls.

About half of the precinct was available for new development, and design assessment criteria specify that 'buildings should combine to produce an urban form characterised by public squares, streets and lanes, with the "perimeter block" form of urban development of a human scale' (Auckland City Council 2004). Taller buildings are permitted inside the precinct along the central pedestrian priority link between two new public squares.

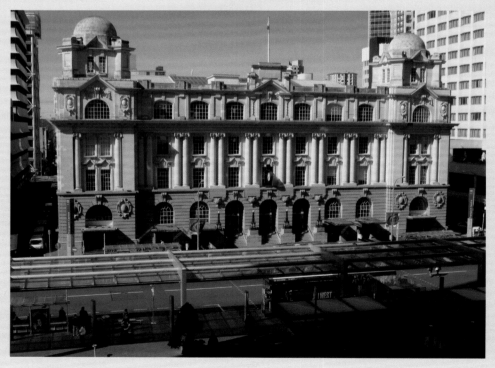

The Britomart Travel Centre is the hub for rail, bus and ferry services

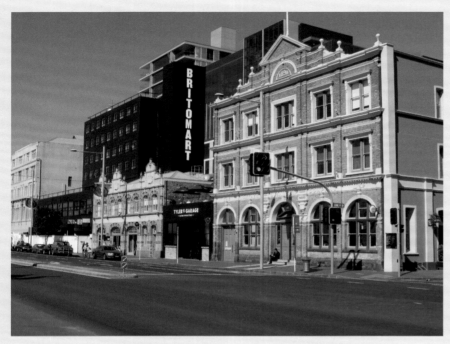

The proposed Seafarers redevelopment has a heritage context

A number of district plan rules were modified for the precinct. Notably, height controls were adjusted to ensure that new development reflected the more modest scale of the heritage buildings. The permitted site intensity was also set lower. Frontage design rules, specifying retail activity and allowing colonnades in lieu of verandahs, were added.

The Seafarers site, within a perimeter block facing the harbour, was identified in the district plan as an opportunity for a significant new building. The block includes five older structures, of which three are scheduled, and the new building was meant to complement this context in scale and detail.

A building over 30 m taller than permitted by the rules has been proposed for the site. It was granted resource consent by independent commissioners. Appeals against the consent decision are outstanding, including one by Auckland Council, as the effect of the building would be dominant. The developers have also initiated a district plan modification that is intended to change the site's development rules so that, for example, the permitted building height would be raised by approximately 30 m to match the general harbour edge control. The modification also increases the

floor area allowance for all of the block, and would permit the agglomeration of each site's allowance in the block to facilitate the taller development on part of it. It is also proposed that publicly accessible areas within the new building – including lobbies and areas giving harbour views, such as restaurants – would be excluded from the floor-space calculation. Additional design criteria are included, which would offer contextual reference in the building's lower frontage, while the upper floor's appearance would be differentiated and the adjoining heritage building acknowledged with a setback. The rules applying to the site will be clarified by the resource consent appeal decision which may result from the current appeal mediation or, if that proves unsuccessful, from a determination by the environment court.

As intended, the public transport investment has triggered the area's regeneration and much of the restoration and new building is completed and occupied, including several award-winning heritage projects. The strategy of promoting the use of public transport has also succeeded: a capacity threshold on the rail system could be reached several years earlier than anticipated, and plans to extend the network and create a central underground rail loop have considerable local support.

The Britomart project can be seen as the first phase of Auckland's waterfront revitalisation, and progress on other areas will reinforce Britomart's commercial success.

Waterfront Auckland

The Auckland Waterfront Vision 2040, published in 2005 by the former city and regional councils, envisaged the redevelopment of the western waterfront with the port's consolidation at the eastern end. Occupying 82 ha of operational land, the port has consents to expand its eastern area to 115 ha by new reclamation, in order to provide for the likely growth of the country's container hub. The rationalisation has released 70 ha of waterfront land, characterised by basins and wharves with marine industries including a fishing fleet and associated fish market, super-yacht refitting and one of the largest marinas in the southern hemisphere. The area's recreational and commercial potential was highlighted by the 2000 and 2003 America's Cup regattas. Hosting the 2011 Rugby World Cup has similarly provided a catalyst, and the completed waterfront projects are the result of investment to support this.

Progress is the result of several years' preparation and organisational restructuring. In 2010, the amalgamation of the region's eight local authorities to form the unitary Auckland Council also established the Waterfront Auckland (WA) development agency, charged with implementing the waterfront vision. It operates as a non-profit public-benefit entity, with a board of directors comprising predominantly consultant professionals. WA's remit is essentially to combine the realisation

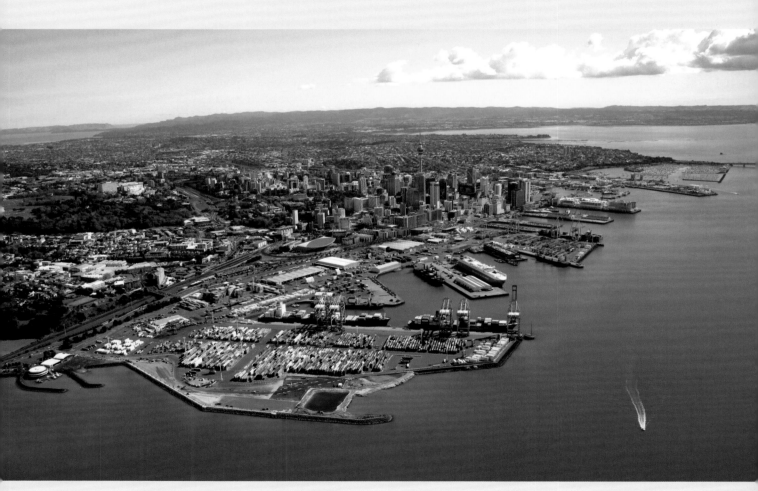

The Port: consolidation is releasing the western waterfront for development

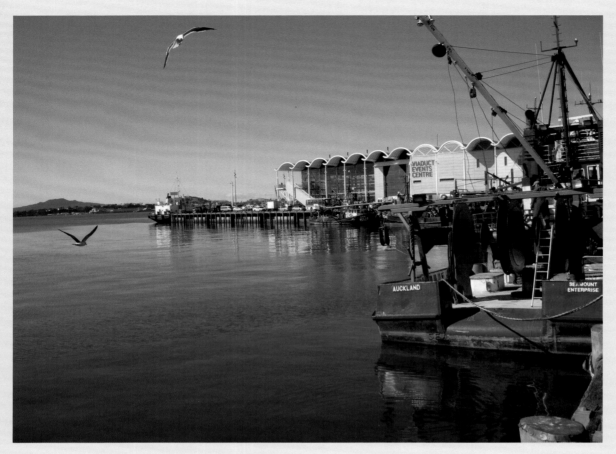

An award-wining venue – a key feature of the project's first stage

of the waterfront's development potential with the creation of a successful public realm. Termed a Council Controlled Organisation, WA is a developer with extensive holdings of publicly owned land. It also has responsibility for preparing the Waterfront Plan, which outlines a 30-year vision for all of the reclaimed land north of the 1840s' shoreline.

Making attractive public spaces and a focus on events are promoted as key elements in the strategy. The plan also notes the resonance of the area's history, so that retaining established marine activity and reusing port-related heritage structures maintains an authentic quality that enriches the waterfront's distinctive workaday character.

Following publication of an Urban Design Framework for the largest area, the Wynyard Quarter, the draft Waterfront Masterplan was released in 2009 to give spatial definition to the vision. In this plan, precincts are designated and

themes identified in order to underpin the logic of a development morphology. Axial spaces connecting the precincts to the city centre intersect at the Wynyard Quarter, where they generate a pattern of development sites.

The development proposals will be subject of a WA-initiated district plan modification scheduled to follow the 2011 Waterfront Plan public consultation. In this process, rules for each development block will be set and these will subsequently be incorporated in the city's new Unitary District Plan.

WA has established a Technical Advisory Group (TAG) that parallels the Council's Urban Design Panel, with a similar Place TAG for place making and events. There is a nominated talent pool of over 20 Australasian architectural firms available for use by developers. Design and sustainability guidelines have been prepared in order to ensure high public space standards.

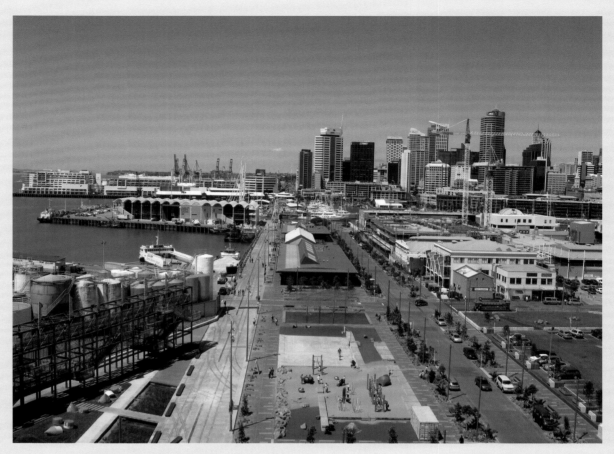

The waterfront axis — a defining component of the new urban structure

The recent completion of Jellicoe Street defined the waterfront axis, a key structural component of the plan. Movement along this axis offers a dramatic spatial experience, with a new lifting bridge linking plazas and muliple venues for marine and other events with Britomart in the east. Two retained 35 m high silo structures form a western axial landmark in the Wynyard Quarter. Silo park, screened from a future redevelopment zone by a gantry intended to support vegetation, features a wetland designed to collect and filter surface-water run-off.

The community has been quick to embrace this pedestrian-friendly environment, and popular expectations bode well for later phases. Ultimately, the project will have extended the city centre by remodelling a large area of industrial land, and provided new social destinations. The Wynyard Quarter is expected to accommodate about 5,000 residents and 15,000 employees in a new sustainable residential and commercial community.

As existing leases permit, blocks will be released for development subject to urban design guidelines and district plan rules. An innovation precinct utilising the character of the existing buildings has now been mooted as a core theme, although its method of achievement remains unclear. The development as a

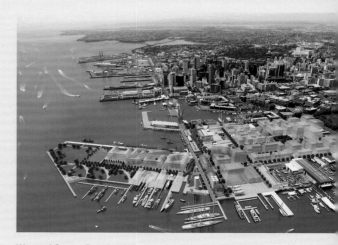

Wynyard Quarter Framework — an exploration of the area's potential

Case study: Britomart and the Auckland waterfront ~ **NEW ZEALAND**

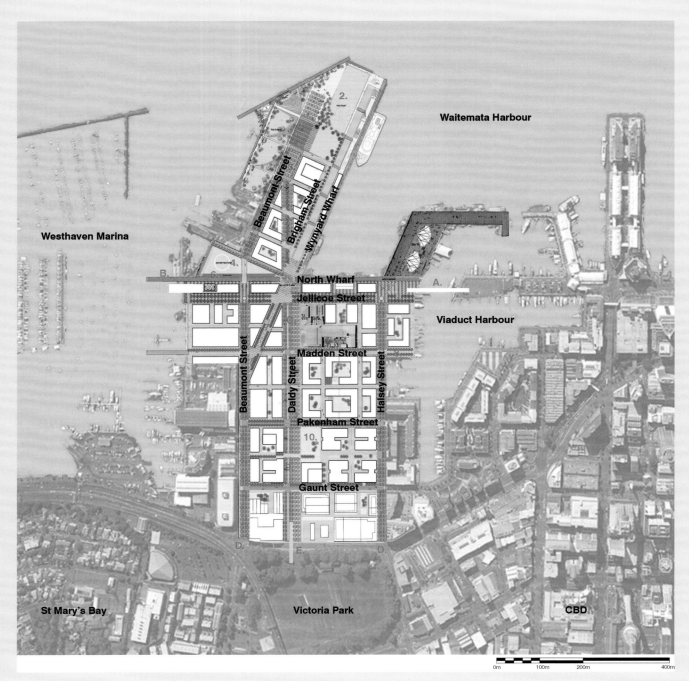

Wynyard Quarter – indicative site plan

whole will take decades to complete, and it remains to be seen whether the management strategy will be sustained over such an extended time frame. Nevertheless, adopting the model of a largely autonomous development agency to implement the waterfront vision is an important component of the strategy. An uncoordinated disposal of the surplus public land would have been likely to have seen regeneration with a different commercial focus, with a less-favourable outcome for the community.

The case study highlights the potential of partnership and the mutual benefit in combining the strengths of public- and private-sector organisations in order to ensure community support and the delivery of appropriate and viable development that works socially as well as economically. Although government-agency-led projects are rare in New Zealand, there are other opportunities at a scale where this approach would be productive.

Critique

Historically New Zealanders have preferred low-density urban living, and distance has commonly been used in regulations, for example through minimum plot sizes, to mitigate the adverse effects of building on the amenity of others and on the environment. A more sustainable urban future requires new thinking, and the previous government endeavoured to progress this.

The Urban Design Protocol has been a catalyst in promoting better urban design and planning. Akin to initiating a popular movement, the intention was to raise awareness of the value of urban design across New Zealand. The protocol invited the development sector to make a commitment to change, but as it does not have legal status the strategy fundamentally was based on persuasion.

The results have been mixed. Many organisations in the development sector have become signatories to the protocol. Progress in the education sector and in local government is particularly notable, but the commitment has been less positive among developers and property investors. Despite the ministry's ambition of enlisting them there are only 13 signatories in this category, and two have since ceased trading. National retail property companies are not represented, and resistance to the introduction of an urban design code in Auckland's north shore points to opposition rather than support from these companies.

Nevertheless, the last five years have seen a growing focus on improving urban design standards, and the potential for a better urban experience is more widely appreciated. City-centre improvements in Wellington and along Auckland's waterfront, for example, represent significant progress, and the projected rebuilding of central Christchurch has also elevated that city's urban future for debate.

The existing dispersed and largely detached building stock may in time offer scope for rebuilding or adapting to embrace sustainable design principles, but this does not offer a model for the pattern of greenfield development where both sustainable design and transport issues require attention. The move towards more intensive urban densities in new and rezoned areas has required new amenity safeguards, and urban design policy and design controls have been the response. Although this amounts to a return to a more prescriptive regime, the concern for improvement renders the matter one of finding a way forward within the current legal framework. However, a history of litigation suggests that this will not be straightforward.

Ultimately the issue is one of popular attitudes. Progress is being made with urban infrastructure investment and in the creation of attractive city-centre environments. While an alternative lifestyle may displace the love affair with the car for some, the suburban paradise will remain the aspiration of many.

A quick guide to
New Zealand

1 TYPES OF CLIENT

Mainly the local property sector, often with established links with Australian companies

Increasing interest from Asian investors, notably from China

....

2 TYPES OF PROJECT/WORK

Urban intensification and growth in Auckland, and the rebuilding of central Christchurch provide the country's main development opportunities in 2012

....

3 APPROACH NEEDED TO WORK IN COUNTRY

Overseas practitioners tend to associate with New Zealand practices in order to meet compliance requirements of New Zealand's Building Code and the Resource Management Act

Major projects may be the subject of international competitions

....

4 LEGISLATION THAT NEEDS TO BE REFERRED TO

The Resource Management Act 1991

Local policy requirements and district rules, and in some cases an urban design code, can be found online at the appropriate local authority website

Specific design guidance should also be available online

Councils have a planning and building helpdesk for general enquiries

....

5 SPECIFIC TIPS FOR SUCCESS

Projects that do not accord with District Plan provisions may be subject to a lengthy consultative process, reflecting New Zealand's diverse cultural traditions and pioneering history

....

6 USEFUL WEBSITES

Canterbury Earthquake Recovery Authority: www.cera.govt.nz

New Zealand Institute of Architects: www.nzia.co.nz

New Zealand Institute of Landscape Architects: www.nzila.co.nz

New Zealand Planning Institute: www.planning.org.nz

Property Council of New Zealand: www.propertynz.co.nz

For District Plan policy and district rules, see local authority websites,
eg: www.aucklandcouncil.govt.nz, and for national policy, see www.mfe.govt.nz

....

1	area	269,000 km²
2	population	4,367,800
3	annual population growth	1.2%
4	urban population	87%
5	population density	17 p/km²
6	GDP (2009)	$126,679,321,012
7	GNI per capita (2009)	$28,770

Source: The World Bank (2010)

Conclusion

The idea for this book originated from the question of how urban design was defined and practised in different parts of the world. Contributors from 18 different countries in five continents were asked to explain what they understood by urban design, to give a description of it as both an academic discipline and a professional practice, and to indicate how, if at all, it had evolved in their country over the years. Through a series of case studies, some of the principal current issues would be highlighted. A template was sent to all contributors, and they were asked to follow this while adapting it to the specifics of their country. Though this survey cannot claim to cover the whole world, it gives a reasonably representative panorama of the global situation of the profession.

Perhaps not surprisingly, the results have not been quite as predicted: the chapters ended being substantially different from each other, even though the general information is always available and the activities performed by urban designers in each of the countries comes clearly through. But because the historical, geographical, social, economic and political contexts are very different, urban design does not mean the same thing everywhere – nor does it operate in the same way.

Terminology and definitions

The first issue that created a certain amount of confusion was the expression 'urban design' itself and its translation into different languages. For many, and particularly for the Romance languages, it translates as 'urbanism', an accepted term that corresponds to a recognised profession in a majority of countries. However, the confusion didn't stop there: qualified architects in France, and many other countries that based their education on the French Beaux-Arts tradition, are automatically also qualified urbanists, as encapsulated by the phrase *architecte–urbaniste*. Elsewhere, an urbanist is a town planner and may, as they do in Britain, belong to a different professional body and follow a different education. Alternatively, as appears to be the case in the Netherlands, anyone involved in the design of the built environment is an 'urban designer'.

The confusion is not only the result of translation; even in the English-speaking word, there is not necessarily a unique interpretation of the role of the urban design profession. Only New Zealand and Australia, and to a certain extent South Africa, have definitions of urban design very close to the British one – perhaps not surprising in view of the frequent professional interchanges between these countries. In the US, on the other hand, the role of the urban designer seems much broader than in Britain.

(facing page)
The Covent Garden piazza, an early
example of public realm enhancement

Even taking 'urbanist' as the direct equivalent of 'urban designer' – and not everyone would agree about this – the question remains: what are the tasks performed by such a professional? The chapter on Sweden opens by posing a series of questions about the scale of intervention, concerns and stakeholders, and it does not have easy answers. For many, the word 'design' implies drawing (*dessin* means drawing in French) and representation in three dimensions, and the urban designer is seen as someone who produces an 'urban composition' in the Beaux-Arts tradition or its contemporary equivalent: the iconic project, as is still mostly the case in Morocco for example; yet, more than a few urban designers are mainly involved in coordination, management, regulation, commissioning or negotiation, and only rarely in drawing. Thierry Vilmin, in the chapter on France, uses *aménageur* as one equivalent of urban designer, whilst accepting that there are at least two types of these: one that manages and the other that conceives; the outcome, a *projet urbain*, an urban project, is probably a meaning shared by most. Similarly, Katja Stille divides the German profession of *Stadtplanung*, or city planning, into those that create (design) and those that manage (plan).

Since this is the reality, the authors of the 18 chapters have been left to describe urban design on the basis of their interpretation and their context. The result is a varied panorama of urban design, sometimes confusing, perhaps, but illuminating at the same time. In the absence of a universal definition or protected label, urban design is what practitioners make of it.

Historical development

The history of urban design over the past century helps explain its professional position and the way in which it is practised today. Parallel, but also contrasting, trends evolved, rooted in culture, system of governance and social structures. Going further back in history also throws light on why the past century saw the emergence of a distinct discipline called urban design. This is not the place to develop the history of cities, something that has been very well done by other authors – Lewis Mumford and Spiro Kostoff, for example. However, a few basic elements are worth mentioning because of their permanence.

Cities have always had economic, social, political and technical functions. They also always represented power, either that of the rulers or of those forces in conflict with them. They had to deal with practical matters on the one hand – defence, public order, movement, exchange, health and liveability, etc – and with image on the other. Consequently, engineers (or their historical equivalent) were responsible for the layout and building of cities well before the architectural profession emerged, and until very recently they continued to be the dominant profession: the Netherlands relied on engineers to protect it from the sea and extend its land; the Catalan Cerdà, responsible for the extension of Barcelona and most importantly for the first text on urbanism (General Theory of Urbanisation, 1867) was a civil engineer; and Baron Haussmann employed engineers to achieve the transformation of Paris in the second half of the 19th century. The quality of design and the public realm in many historic cities that are admired today are the result of 'engineering design'. The fact that architects in countries like Germany have Ing. (short for Ingenieur) still in their title is a relic of their historical role.

In parallel, rulers used the design of cities to show their power to both their own citizens and the rest of the world; the 16th-century transformation of Rome by Pope Sixtus V, and Louis XIV's Versailles are perhaps the best known historic examples, but there are many others and they are not limited to Europe. Colonial powers from very early times also used the settlements that they created to express their domination over the colonised, either through the defensive character of the urban area (the Roman *castrum*) or through the contrasting morphologies of the 'native' – mostly organic – and the 'imperial' – mostly geometric – districts, as is the case in Lutyens' plan for New Delhi and Prost's for Casablanca. Here, architects were employed to beautify the cities and give them a distinctive (European) image.

In the second half of the 19th century, the two traditions collaborated in the transformation of urban areas. The hygienists' public-health influences and the rapid development of new forms of transport gave a continuing role to engineers. At the same time, the rise of an industrial bourgeoisie and international competition required the embellishment of cities for their inhabitants, and here the architects, particularly those formed in the French Beaux-Arts tradition, dominated. The results can be seen in Chicago, Buenos Aires, Cairo and Madrid. In a modified form, the current efforts made by countries such as Argentina, Dubai, Morocco and China to 'brand' new neighbourhoods are a continuation of this phenomenon. In parallel, reactions against this formality developed into the garden city movement and Picturesque designs influenced by the work of Camilo Sitte. Schemes inspired by these movements were also exported from Europe to other countries, as is shown by the Cairo suburbs of Helipolis and Maadi.

None of the historical professionals above would have been called urban designers. They retained their label of architects, engineers or, exceptionally, landscape designers, but they all had a vision of the city with all its complexities.

In the early 20th century, the modern movement reacted against the past and mostly against the city itself, the place where all the ills resulting from the Industrial Revolution were deemed to be concentrated. Traditional morphologies were seen as not just irrelevant but damaging. Architects now saw their mission as one of creating something new and different, wherein the 'object' was more important than the urban realm; they believed that they had scientific justifications to group urban activities in separate zones and to express functions through the design of individual and isolated buildings. And here the domination of the architectural profession was total; it was held that they were the ones who could, through design, resolve the problems of urban society, and they added urbanism to their professional title. Engineers were there purely to resolve technical problems, and transport-related ones in particular, but the professions grew increasingly apart and developed distinct methods and vocabularies. Landscape architects were simply there to complement the work of architects.

The effects of these modernist ideas were not properly felt until after the second world war, resulting in two different urban typologies, both giving prominence to the building-object and neglecting public space. From Australia to Sweden, France to Egypt, and from Brazil to the Czech Republic, large modernist-inspired developments resulted in districts of 'towers in the park', alien to the local traditions. At the same time, the anti-city attitudes combined with the segregation of functions and the surge in car ownership resulted in the development of sprawling suburbs in most countries – though Australia, New Zealand and the US seem to have been particularly fond of them. Italy, on the other hand, maintained a stronger urban tradition for a longer time than other nations.

Soon, the problems resulting from both typologies led to critics and reactions, best expressed in the works of Jane Jacobs, Ian Nairn, Kevin Lynch and Gordon Cullen. The renewal of interest in urban space and urban morphology, the increased concern for the protection of heritage as well as the need to face new social problems required a search for different approaches. Urban planners, increasingly seen as a separate profession, tried to find more scientific solutions; engineers sought to resolve transport problems in isolation from land-use planners; some architects indulged in even more utopian imagery – creating ever-larger objects – with little communication with other professionals.

The French expression of *composition urbaine*, which perhaps translates best as 'civic design', reflects this attitude. The advantage that architects continued to have over other professionals was their three-dimensional perception, but at the same time the diminishing value of the isolated architectural object and the increasing complexity of the urban environment forced them to either collaborate with others or develop new skills. The Brazilian project for Palmas is a good example of late modernism, wherein utopian ideas could not be implemented as expected but some successes were achieved.

As the introduction showed, this is the point at which urban design emerged as a discipline in Britain, following a similar movement in the US. At first, most of the people involved were architect–planners that had qualified in both professions and could bridge the gap between them. The length of the studies required limited the numbers able to follow this route, and therefore courses emerged, mostly in Britain and the US, aimed at either architects or planners wanting to specialise in urban design.

Gradually, the need for different skills led to urban designers becoming distinct from their core professions, mostly by widening their interests and becoming a 'bridge' between disciplines: planners learning more about design, architects taking an interest in the public realm beyond their sites. To this day in most Anglo-Saxon countries and those influenced by them (this includes the Netherlands, Sweden, India, New Zealand, Australia and Argentina), urban designers have started out by being architects, planners or landscape architects, and the work they do tends to be close to their original discipline but with a more holistic approach. As commissions have increased, so has the demand for courses, for research and for information about good practice.

For a variety of reasons, change in other countries has been slower; architects there are still the dominant profession, with the label of urbanist attached to their name. Previous chapters have shown that power and the city are closely linked: how cities grow, where developments take place what they represent affects the choice of professionals and their education. Hence, the position of the urban design profession in China, Egypt, Argentina or Dubai is different from that in the Netherlands, Italy, Australia or Spain.

Education and professional affiliation

The precise terminology used to define urban design is less important than determining how its practitioners acquire their knowledge and their skills, and what their professional affiliations are. Undoubtedly, in the majority of countries urban design is seen as an integral part, or a specialisation of, architecture. As mentioned above, frequently a diploma in architecture automatically allows the word urbanist to be attached to it. Juan Luis de las Rivas, writing in the chapter on Spain, regrets this and sees it as the result of the monopoly held by the architecture 'corps'. A similar situation seems to exist in the Czech Republic. But in some countries, specialist postgraduate courses are offered not just to architects but to graduates with other backgrounds, from planning to social sciences: examples are found in Argentina, the Netherlands, Italy and India. In the past 20 years Brazil seems to have taken a particularly proactive approach, requiring specific subjects to be included in the architecture curriculum that give professionals a wider view and more involvement with the social reality of the country.

Landscape architects and town planners are the other two professions most frequently associated with urban design. Town planning can be a profession independent from architecture, as is the case in Britain and the US, with specific academic courses which include a variable – but often limited – level of design. Currently in the United States, two competing and opposing movements – New Urbanism and Landscape Urbanism; one based on architecture, and the other on landscape architecture – are each claiming to have the correct approach to urban design and the 'moral high ground' on environmental issues. This doesn't seem to be a mere academic argument, as practices from both professional backgrounds are competing for jobs. In a more limited number of cases, civil engineers – once a dominant force in the design of cities – can also become urban designers through postgraduate specialisation. Moreover, in Germany and the Czech Republic for instance, the professional titles of architects and planners include the word 'engineer', more for historical than practical reasons.

In the end, what matters is that the skills acquired correspond to those required in the particular situation. The lack of courses specifically dedicated to urban design, or the dominance of architecture (or any other profession), may not necessarily be a problem as long as practitioners can go beyond their first discipline and operate as well-rounded urban designers.

Nowhere outside of Britain is there a legal definition of urban design or a mention of it in official documents. Neither are there official professional bodies that register urban designers exclusively. On the other hand, loose associations of such practitioners, similar to the Urban Design Group in Britain, exist in a number of countries (Australia, New Zealand, South Africa and India). Urbanism, however, has a legal status in many countries; France, for instance, has an official *Code de l'Urbanisme* and a governmental accrediting organisation for urbanists. The lack of a body that protects and controls the profession may limit its status, but at the same time it gives practitioners greater independence: in the US, the fact that there is no liability involved in the work of the urban designer is attractive to clients; in Argentina there is no fixed fee scale for such work, which may make urban designers easier to employ than members of more structured professions. Another possible advantage is that urban designers are frequently seen as generalists, capable of coordinating the work of others and of having an overall view of projects that goes well beyond pure design. This is the case in Britain, and it appears to be also in a wide variety of countries such as Brazil, South Africa, the Netherlands or China. Finally, reputed engineering, architectural or landscape practices can offer urban design services by employing practitioners that have acquired more than one specialism without needing to register with a separate professional entity.

One consequence of this is that graduates from countries where the offer of urban design courses is very limited or non-existent (Morocco, Dubai, South Africa, China) travel to those that offer a wider range of them, in order to acquire their specialisation.

At the same time, international firms with urban design work draw their staff from a limited pool, whose 'occupants' may find themselves moving from a job in Germany to one in China, or from India to Argentina.

As specialist courses in urban design are still limited, there is also a paucity of academic research in the subject – though it has expanded lately, as is shown by the number of books being published and the growing number of peer-reviewed journals, at least in the Anglo-Saxon world. The US and Britain seem to dominate the field, at least as far as publications that specifically have urban design as their subject (or their title) are concerned.

Practice

Another way of understanding who are the urban designers, and what their competences are, is to consider the outcome of their work: as was mentioned in the case of France, this outcome is an 'urban project'. Although this again varies somewhat from one country to the other, producing masterplans seems to be a common denominator. The scale and the purpose of this kind of document ranges from large new cities, as is the case in China, to new urban extensions in Argentina, Morocco or Germany, to urban regeneration schemes in the Netherlands, New Zealand and the Czech Republic, to smaller remedial schemes in Spain or South Africa. All these scales and these kinds of urban projects coexist in most countries, but examples chosen by contributors to this book indicate that a particular type of work seems to them to be representative of the current role of urban designers in their country.

A masterplan can also be interpreted in more than one way. In some cases it is mostly a three-dimensional expression of planning policy. The process is creative and the outcome at least partly visual, emphasising the design aspects of the practice: case studies in China, Spain, the Czech Republic or Australia show the results of such a process. In other cases masterplanning can be mostly regulatory, and the outcome may be codes or guidelines, such as the Form-Based Codes in the US or the B-Plan in Germany and its equivalent in the Netherlands. Frequently the two types of activities coexist.

Furthermore, there is a significant split in the type of clients that commission work from urban designers, and their motivations. On the one hand there is a strong demand for gated estates, not just for residential developments but also for other activities such as retail or leisure. This phenomenon is apparent in countries as different as Argentina, where whole districts are gated: Brazil, China, India, Egypt and Dubai – the latter being an extreme case, since all its projects appear to be gated. In most cases, these are private schemes commissioned by international consortia from international consultants and aimed at a wealthy clientele – frequently international themselves. Urban designers – who do not necessarily have a connection with the place – will be employed to design schemes that are attractive for this clientele; therefore standards of landscape, public realm, environmental quality and amenities will be high, but the layouts will often break with the traditional urban morphology of the area, densities will be low (though not in the case of China), no social housing will be included and cars will dominate. Like their clients, the schemes have an international character and as a result there can be great similarities between such projects in totally different locations; the masterplans for New Giza in Egypt and

Nordelta in Argentina are symptomatic of this phenomenon. In these cases, an additional role for the designer has been to provide the 'brand' for the project, the image being as important as the layout itself. In some cases it is the name of the designer that provides the brand, hence the frequent appointment of 'archistars' to carry out such work.

One of the consequences of this kind of scheme is an increasing physical, social and economic segregation of populations; Noha Nasser believes that in the case of Egypt this is directly connected with urban design practice (even though it may have a very long history). The fact that these developments ignore the majority of the population leads Christopher Benninger to ask 'where are the Indians?' in the case of his adopted country, and this question could be transposed to a number of other countries. Uncomfortable with this situation, urban designers have responded in at least two different ways. In some countries, they have joined forces with local authorities to push for more open developments, even though these may still be aimed at an upmarket clientele. The role of urban designers seem to have been important in achieving a more integrated pattern in the case of Wadala in India and in some of the recent developments in Casablanca, in Morocco. In both cases, local firms of architects or urban designers tend to be in charge of the projects, even though international consultants may be employed as well.

Nevertheless, the contrast between these new districts and the rest of the cities of which they are a part has led to a totally different professional posture, whereby the urban designer also plays a social function, is employed by the local authority or a community group, and produces a very different type of work to that of the aforementioned 'archistars'. The most interesting examples, where the projects comprise instruments of social change whilst maintaining the traditional morphology, are the transformation of *favelas* in Brazil and the creation of a safe urban park out of a crime hotspot in South Africa. In these cases, the urban designers were local and worked with the local community without compromising the quality of their work. As is mentioned in the case of Morocco, urban design in the developing world ends up operating at three levels: the large international projects aimed at an elite, the urban renewal and urban extension schemes for the local middle classes and the neglected shanty towns for which there are no clients willing to finance projects.

Elsewhere, urban designers may be preparing masterplans for new urban extensions (as in the case Riedeberg in Germany or Bretigny in France), working on urban regeneration schemes aimed at incorporating former industrial or infrastructure land into the rest of the city, or to remedy the ills of massive social housing schemes of the 1960s and 70s. For instance, in the Czech Republic urban designers are working on humanising the housing estates built during the Soviet era, through infill development and the incorporation of amenities. In Spain, on the other hand, landscape is a strong element of regeneration schemes and has resulted in a number of new open spaces in cities like Barcelona and Madrid. Other regeneration schemes are taking place in Argentina (Puerto Madero), Sweden (Bo01), Italy (Portello) and New Zealand (Auckland's Waterfront). In Rotterdam in the Netherlands, the explicit aim is to increase the competitiveness of the city by working at various scales: a large urban vision document and a series of smaller local interventions to take place over some 20 years. Equally, the regeneration of Malmö is part of an effort at rebranding the city. In all these cases, the urban designers are playing a key role not just through their schemes and the production of documents, but by coordinating the work of various professionals and creating a link between local authorities, developers and the communities involved. They are mediators that interpret abstract policy concepts through images that non-professionals can understand; this role is emphasised in the cases of Germany, the Netherlands and the US.

In a number of countries, a dual system of commissioning work can complicate the position of urban designers. What is sometimes seen as a banal type of project involving the regeneration of poorer areas of town or as the more routine development, is given to local firms who will have to deal with slow local bureaucracies and will be paid local fees. At the same time, international consultants are being given the larger, more glamorous and better paid commissions which tend to bypass local controls, or at least take less time to be approved and implemented: examples of this duality are mentioned in Morocco and Argentina, but it appears to occur elsewhere. In other words, the division in employment of urban designers reflects those in the wider society. However, it would be wrong to generalise and to suggest that advanced economies commission one type of work and developing or emerging countries another. The pattern is more complicated than that, and in many countries the different kinds of schemes coexist.

Masterplanning work is rarely the main source of income for an architectural–urban design firm; on the contrary, it can be seen as a loss leader that may bring other more profitable work. This is more or less institutionalised in the case of France, where the firms in charge of the masterplan for an area are also given one or more sites on which to design and build, in order to increase their fees as well as to test the masterplan. The situation in China is more complex, as the international urban design consultants working there seem to be commissioned almost exclusively to give a glamorous image to a new scheme, often one of a very large scale, in order to 'sell' it to the authorities. Once it is approved, developers often dismiss the team and utilise local firms to design and build something of a poorer quality and much less expensive.

Overall, the difference between architects' and urban designers' work is the same in all countries: one is in charge of the 'object' for a specific client and on a site; the other prepares the layout of an area with a variety of uses and users, and including buildings and the spaces around them. Urban designers tend to be part of a team which comprises professionals of various backgrounds, and they know that their work is of a collaborative nature. The French expression of 'coordinating architect' seems to best summarise the role of the urban designer.

Urban form

In Britain, urban designers reacting against modernism have returned to more traditional morphologies and typologies, and have developed a kind of quality checklist. Words like permeability, connectivity, legibility, walkability, densification and mixed use have become part of these practitioners' vocabulary. Some of these designers, trained in Britain (including contributors to this book), have been working in various countries and have taken their 'toolkit' with them. In spite of this, the results are far from uniform and the concepts listed above sometimes only partially incorporated in schemes. Connectivity and permeability have been lost in the gated projects described in many chapters such as Argentina, Egypt, Dubai, India, Morocco or South Africa. Although these schemes may aim at all the right characteristics inside the gates, they are almost by definition (and certainly by desire on the part of their clients) disconnected from their wider environments and create large impermeable enclaves. They may be legible and walkable internally, but they are rarely dense or well served by public transport.

The perimeter block with a clear separation of private and public space, and buildings that face and animate the streets, another element of the British urban design canon, is also frequently lost, particularly in new urban extensions. This may be due to different views of the division between public and private space. Garden city and modernist based typologies appear to be still dominant in many schemes, even in some that are not gated: the Spanish example in Ponferrada is resolutely modernist, and the more New Urbanist Riedeberg in Germany also has also a morphology that is not based on the traditional perimeter block. In China, the requirement to have south-facing buildings results in parallel high-rise blocks, though their bases may enclose a usable space.

Regeneration schemes in former industrial or harbour areas do appear to be more similar to the British models, with attempts to densify, revitalise, reconnect urban neighbourhoods and to introduce new amenities and open spaces. Public transport is often a core element of these projects (New Zealand, Germany, USA, Australia, France, Italy, the Netherlands), as are mixed uses and mixed tenures.

Building forms and styles seem to be the most easily transferable or even copied; the suburban house appears in a number of countries – mostly, though not only, in the gated estates. The iconic tower is also frequently used as a symbol of a place, from Malmö to Dubai and Casablanca to Yingkou, both in new districts and in regeneration schemes. Neither of these types are necessarily rooted in the place, nor do they necessarily result from what would be considered sound urban design.

Heritage and an interest in urban history also lay at the origins of urban design in Britain. This concern does have parallels in a number of countries: the regeneration schemes cited involve, almost in every case, the renovation of some historic structure and its incorporation in the project (France, Italy, New Zealand, Argentina, Brazil). Equally, however, some of the contributors to this book acknowledge that the practice of urban design in their countries often militates against a respect for heritage. Christopher Benninger is particularly critical of India's attitude towards it, but China and Egypt do not seem to be very different. It may be that an Islamic, an Indian or a Chinese model of urban design, more closely related to those historical traditions, will eventually emerge; but as long as the main projects' clients come from an international elite, this is unlikely to go beyond pure architecture style.

How urban design travels

The globalisation of ideas in architecture and urban design is not a new phenomenon. As has already been mentioned, in the 19th century the French Beaux-Arts tradition had a major impact on the North American City Beautiful movement, and on designs as far apart as Argentina and Egypt. In the 20th century, modernism and the International Style spread worldwide and similar schemes appeared in very different parts of the world. The examples of Chandigarh and Brasilia are perhaps the most celebrated, but many other less famous designs emulated other countries' ideas.

The situation is no different today, and if anything concepts travel even faster. New Urbanism, for instance, a movement that started in the US as a reaction to suburban sprawl, has been adopted by several countries (Australia, Egypt, India, Sweden). British models of urban design – in turn inspired by North Americans Jane Jacobs and Kevin Lynch – are exported to Australia, South Africa and Dubai to mention just a few cases. Ease of travel throughout Europe has meant that ideas are easily interchanged between professionals.

It is not just the ideas that travel, but also the practitioners. Throughout this book examples of work by 'foreigners' have been mentioned, and working abroad is an important part of professional life at all levels: students going abroad to get an urban design qualification, young graduates gaining experience in a different country, individual professionals being contracted abroad because of their specific expertise, or practices opening a branch in another country. Movement happens in all directions and enriches the profession: ideas spread, but are also transformed as they adapt to new contexts. Space Syntax, for example, started in London as a research team at University College London, and has now become a global consultancy exporting a specific methodology to all corners of the world.

The ways in which these movements are generated, and work in another country is established, do not necessarily follow a clear pattern, and there is no 'magic guide to working abroad', but some elements seem to recur. As urban design is not a 'registered' profession in any country no membership of such a professional body can be demanded, although, as has been mentioned in chapter after chapter, 'architect–urbanist' is the standard qualification of most urban designers. This does give a certain amount of flexibility to jobseekers. On the other hand, some countries may impose restrictions on employing foreigners and there may be tax considerations that need to be checked – as is the case, for instance, in the USA and Brazil.

Some practices have a long tradition of networking internationally, either by having members give lectures in different countries and participating in conferences and symposia, or by travelling as part of a trade mission. A chance encounter and a personal contact are in most cases the first step to collaboration, and may start with a simple exchange of ideas. The initial exchange may be limited to asking/giving expert advice on a specific issue, and in some cases it will stop there. Many of the countries surveyed have their own urban design firms and will only need or want outside help for non-ordinary schemes or those requiring specific knowledge (say, on sustainability). Brazil, for instance, has over the years developed its own urban design tradition (which originated from lecture tours by international experts) and no longer needs much input from elsewhere. South Africa, on the other hand, needs to protect its own professionals and to adapt international ideas to its specific context. In neither of these countries will there be much of a market for outsiders, though lessons may be learned from them.

Competitions or tenders are another standard way of getting to work abroad, and architects have a long tradition of participating in these processes. Large schemes or masterplans are more likely to be the subjects for which competitions are open to international participants, rather than small local schemes. However, in most cases and probably in all countries, a local partner would be required and this would apply even without a competition; as a minimum, a local firm would help with language and with the details of local regulations. This is also true in the European Union even though legally it may not be a requirement. Scanning the professional journals and websites is a useful way to find out about competitions, but, again, a local contact may provide a useful shortcut.

As we saw earlier in this chapter, in quite a few countries a split exists between the more public day-to-day kind of work and the large – mostly private – schemes. The latter, often commissioned by international firms and for a global market, are more likely to be offered to non-local firms and through competitions, although even in these cases local partners will be needed. In addition to a good knowledge of the local legislation, an understanding of customs and of whom to contact will be essential. In France, for instance, every architect, planner or urban designer knows that a visit to the local mayor is always the first step. The influence of *feng shui* in the orientation of buildings in China, and compliance with *vaastu* in India are similarly accepted as a given.

Well-established or historical contacts between countries mean that certain types of movements are most likely and easier than others: for instance, between Commonwealth countries, between France and Morocco, or between Spain and Latin America (common language is one factor). Australian practices seem to have a wider Pacific influence. However, these links are not permanently fixed and political events tend to change allegiances or interests – as is well described in the chapter on Egypt, where European models were replaced by Soviet ones and these, in turn, by American ones, which are not likely to be favoured in the future. Similarly, in Morocco a Korean group replaced a French one for the design of the Structure Plan for Marrakech.

A respectful attitude towards local culture, practices and local colleagues will help not only in obtaining jobs abroad but also in maintaining a good relationship with clients. This seems particularly important in China. At the same time, patience in dealing with local bureaucracies and a robust standing can also be necessary, as pointed out in the 'quick guides' to a few of the countries. The reasons for employing a foreign consultant must also be understood: clients may be looking for specific expertise, for image and prestige or for political leverage, or they may not have in-house resources. The agenda behind the contract may be an important element in the choice of consultant.

Finally, good reputations travel: a practice that is well known for either its designs, the high quality of its methodology or for a particular specialism will have its work published and recognised internationally. This is a good form of introduction to clients, wherever they may be. At the same time, the particular requirements of a market must be understood; for instance, experience in sustainable design will be an asset for the foreseeable future that practices will be able to exploit.

Sustainability and the future

Climate change will be one of the fundamental concerns in the future design of cities. In most developed countries, and increasingly in others, regulations are improving the sustainability of buildings and new technologies are being introduced; to a certain extent, the use of the car is being limited and water-conservation systems are being implemented. Beyond this, not enough is known about how to design more sustainable cities and little is being done. Much research and experimentation is needed, and it may lead to different layouts from the ones we know. It is likely that (environmental) engineers will once again have an important role, just as their predecessors had in the 19th century; they are already part of urban design teams and their influence will expand as technological solutions to climate change are sought. Designs rooted in topography, climate and local materials and techniques, rather than universal ideas, may become the source of inspiration. The argument between Landscape Urbanists and New Urbanists in the US, both being anti-suburb, indicates that professionals are searching for more sustainable solutions to urban development.

The relationship between the car and the city has been at the core of the debate on urban design for almost a century now. This debate is likely to continue, but at least in developed countries the private car is now seen as a problem rather than as a solution, and suburbs are not as attractive as they once were. Hence, the densification schemes described in such diverse places as the Czech Republic, the US, Australia and Germany, all connected to good public transport. In Europe, though cities may still expand, uncontrolled sprawl is no longer acceptable; the cost of commuting and the loss of countryside has reduced the attraction of distant suburbs. Even in the US, it appears that the housing crash has affected these much more than city centres.

This is not yet the case in Egypt, Dubai, India, Argentina or South Africa, where the wealthy want to live, shop and play far from the dense urban centres, and development continues to rely on the private car. Even China is increasing its facilities for the motorcar and reducing those for cycling, although, at least there, major investment in public transport is taking place at the same time. All contributors to this book are well aware of the current problems in their respective countries, and critical of the approach taken if it is environmentally unsustainable and increases social segregation. Brazil, notably, is at least experimenting with solutions better adapted to its particular situation.

Having promoted higher densities, walkable cities, urban greenery, the use of public transport and adaptation to context, urban designers are well placed to lead the search for sustainable cities, but they will have to work hard to have these ideas universally accepted. The fact that urban design is concerned with how places work and not just how they look is probably accepted in some countries, but this doesn't mean that the profession is on a firm footing. It will have to continue to prove its value, and this may be best achieved by bringing other disciplines to the table, advocating sustainability and acting as a well-informed coordinator.

As sustainability includes the three pillars of environmental, social and economic measures, urban designers will need to be concerned with all three. Practitioners in Brazil and South Africa have embraced the social aspects earlier than most, Swedish and German ones are stronger than others on environmental matters, and the French are at least grappling with all three. Learning lessons from others has always been a good way of improving practice in any profession; urban design is particularly susceptible to international influences, and hopefully this book can help practitioners to share and learn from experiences from a wide spectrum of countries.

Notes

France

1 The Ile-de-France Region has since asked for the number of dwellings to be increased to 2,000, partly to densify around railway stations but also to make the project financially viable.

Germany

1 Source: Statistical Yearbook 2010 For the Federal Republic of Germany.

2 The time before the Bologna Process commenced with the signing of the Bologna Declaration in 1999, which made academic standards across Europe more easliy comparable. As a result of the introduction of the European Higher Education Area and the definition of academic standards, the German diploma was displaced by the BA and MA qualifications.

3 BauGB 1997, Chapter 1, Scope, Definition and Principles of Land Use Planning.

4 In other literature and translations of the Federal Building Code, these Acts are usually referred to as 'Urban Regeneration Measures' (URM) and 'Urban Development Measures' (UDM). However, for clarity and ease of understanding they are referred to as Acts within this publication.

5 Federal Building Code – Chapter One, Part One, Subdivision One, Section 136 (2).

6 Today: Trojan Trojan + Partner, located in Darmstadt.

Spain

1 Observatorio de la Sostenibilidad en España, Universidad de Alcalá de Henares, Ministerios de Medio Ambiente y de Fomento (2006) Cambios de ocupación del suelo en España. Implicaciones para la sostenibilidad. Madrid: Mundi-Prensa Libros.

2 Several journals deal with the teaching of urbanism in Spain: , 'La enseñanza del urbanismo. Una perspectiva europea' Ciudades No 2, 1995; Inés Sánchez de Madariaga, 'La enseñanza del urbanismo en España', Urban, No 6, 2001; Fernando de Terán Troyano, 'Sobre la enseñanza del Urbanismo en España', Urban, No 10, 2005.

3 There are only a few of these: Carlos Martínez Caro and Juan Luis de las Rivas (1990) Arquitectura Urbana. Elementos de teoría y diseño. Madrid: Ed. Bellisco; José Antonio López Candeira (1999) Diseño urbano: teoría y práctica. Madrid, Munilla-Lería; and JM Ordeig Corsini (2004) Diseño urbano y pensamiento contemporáneo. Barcelona: Instituto Monsa. The relevant translations of urban design classics arrived slowly in Spain: G Cullen's Townscape in 1976; the GLC manual, 'Introduction to Housing layout', in 1985; F Gibberd's 1959 book, Town Design, was translated in Argentina in 1961; R Unwin's Town Planning in Practice had to wait until 1984.

4 This can be seen in the work on both public spaces and buildings by the Spain's best-known architects: Moneo in Madrid or Murcia; Navarro Baldeweg in Salamanca; Piñon and Viaplana, Miralles, and Bohigas in the centre of Barcelona; Tuñon y Mansilla in Zamora; and León; Mangado in Olite or Madrid.

5 Storm & stress, Fundación Caja de Arquitectos, 2010, is the latest catalogue of this European landscape biennial.

6 Visit bcnecologia.net for details.

7 See the journal a+t, Nos 25–28, for case studies.

8 See JL de las Rivas Sanz (2008) 'Parque de la Juventud en Ponferrada. Diseño urbano en proceso', AM No 1, pp. 150–159.

Czech Republic

1 Although urban design and urbanism have very similar meanings in the Czech context, the former is seen as having a wider scope, more akin to town planning, and the latter relates more to practical implementation. However, for the purpose of this chapter both terms are seen as interchangeable.

Brazil

1 See also del Rio and Siembieda (2010) and del Rio (2010).

2 According to the ministry of the cities at www.cidades.gov.br/index.php?option=com_content&view=article&id=350:campanha-plano-diretor&catid=92&Itemid=120.

3 Leme (1999); Pereira (2002).

4 There are numerous publications in English on the evolution of Brazilian modern architecture, although few deal with urbanism. Among them see Fraser (2000) and Andreoli and Forty (2004).

5 The word 'design' in Portuguese translates as *desenho*, the most frequently used meaning of which is the noun 'drawing', and at the time was rarely associated with a project.

6 Although from the wider 'urbanism' approach, this discussion and several case studies can be found in del Rio and Siembieda (2010).

7 The plan for Palmas was drawn up by Grupo Quatro Arquitetos Associados from Goiania. In 1989, the first governor for Tocantins personally decided to hire the group and requested that the plan be ready in less than a year – a particularly short deadline given all the surveying and environmental studies that had to be done.

8 The case of Curitiba is well covered by the international literature. See, for instance, Schwartz (2003), Irazabal (2004 and 2010) and Santos (2011).

Australia

1   www.planning.nsw.gov.au/plansforaction/pdf/north_coast_
    design_guide_complete.pdf www.planning.nsw.gov.au/
    LinkClick.aspx?fileticket=MJKJRtoUz0E%3D&tabid=69&lang
    uage=en-US
    www.dlgp.qld.gov.au/resources/boards/urban-places/
    queensland-places-charter.pdf www.dlgp.qld.gov.au/resources/
    guideline/tod/tod-guide.pdf www.subtropicaldesign.org.
    au/images/stories/pdf/Reseach%20Project/subtropical_
    handbook/subtropical_design_seq.pdf
    www.dpcd.vic.gov.au/planning/urbandesign/urban-design-
    charter-for-victoria['page not found', as of 27.03.12]
    www.dpcd.vic.gov.au/planning/urbandesign/what-
    is-urban-design www.dpcd.vic.gov.au/__data/assets/
    pdf_file/0006/33927/Activity_Centre_Design_Guidelines.pdf
    www.dpcd.vic.gov.au/planning/urbandesign/guidelines/
    guidelines-for-higher-density-residential-development-
    four-or-more-storeys www.dpcd.vic.gov.au/__data/assets/
    pdf_file/0011/41231/Safer_Design_Guidelines.pdf

2   The origin of these guidelines was a voluntary code published
    by the federal government, known as Amcord:
    www.lgpmcouncil.gov.au/publications/files/amcord.pdf

3   For further information, see www.epra.wa.gov.au/Projects/
    Claisebrook-Village

Bibliography

Great Britain

Bentley I, et al (1985) Responsive Environments: A Manual for Designers. London: Architectural Press.

Cowan, R (2005) The Dictionary of Urbanism. Tisbury, Wiltshire: Streetwise Press.

Cullen, G (1961) Townscape. London: The Architectural Press.

Department of the Environment Transport and the Regions, and the Commission for Architecture and the Built Environment (2000) By Design – Urban Design in the Planning System: Towards Better Practice. London: DETR.

English Partnerships (2000) The Urban Design Compendium. London: English Partnerships and the Housing Corporation.

Jacobs, J (1961) The Death and Life of Great American Cities. New York: Random House.

Lynch, K (1990) The Image of the City. Cambridge, MA: MIT Press.

Tibbalds, F. (1992) Making People-Friendly Towns: Improving the Public Environment in Towns and Cities. London: Longman Press.

Urban Design Group, Urban Design, quarterly publication and available at: www.udg.org.uk

Urban Task Force (1999) Towards an Urban Renaissance. London: E&FN Spon.

Italy

Aymonino, C (1975) Il significato delle città. Laterza, Rome and Bari: Laterza.

Boeri, S, Infussi, F and Ischia, U (eds) (1989) 'Progetto urbano I'. Urbanistica, 95, pp. 57–72.

Capitanucci, MV (2009) Milano. Verso l'Expo. La nuova architettura. Milan: Skira.

Cataldi, G, Maffei, GL and Vaccaro, P (2002) 'Saverio Muratori and the Italian School of Planning Typology.' Urban Morphology, vol 6, 1.

Colarossi, P and Latini, PA (eds) (2007–8) La progettazione urbana, 3 vols: 'Principi e storie, Metodi e materiali, Declinazioni e strumenti', Il Sole 24 ORE, Milan: Confindustria.

Cremaschi, M (1994) Esperienza comune e progetto urbano. Milan: Franco Angeli.

De Carlo, G (1992) Gli spiriti dell'architettura. Rome: Editori Riuniti.

De Carlo, G (1989) 'L'interesse per la città fisica.' Urbanistica, 95, pp. 15–18.

De Carlo, G (1964) Questioni di architettura e urbanistica. Urbino: Argalia.

Dente, B, Bobbio, L, Fareri, P and Morisi, M (1990) Metropoli per progetti. Attori e processi di trasformazione urbana a Firenze, Torino, Milano. Bologna: Il Mulino.

Di Biagi, P and Gabellini, P (eds) (1992) Urbanisti italiani. Rome and Bari: Laterza.

Ferrari, M (2005) Il progetto urbano in Italia: 1940–1990. Florence: Alinea.

Gabellini, P (2008) 'Un piano che ripensa Bologna e l'urbanistica.' Urbanistica, 135, pp 51–64.

Gasparrini, C (ed.) (2005) 'Città contemporanea e progetto urbano in Italia.' Urbanistica, 126, pp. 7–41.

Gasparrini, C (1999) Il progetto urbano: una frontiera ambigua tra urbanistica e architettura. Napoli: Liguori

Gravagnuolo, B (1991) La progettazione urbana in Europa 1750–1960. Rome and Bari: Laterza.

Gregotti, V (1992) 'Elementi di disegno urbano ordinati secondo i principi della modificazione critica.' Casabella, 588, pp. 2–3.

Gregotti, V (1966) Il territorio dell'architettura. Milan: Feltrinelli.

Infussi, F (2007) 'L'esplorazione di un'opportunità e l'orientamento di un processo'. Territorio, 40, pp. 35–41.

Mancuso, F (1989) 'La pratica del disegno urbano.' Urbanistica, 95, pp. 11–14.

Marinoni, G (2005) Metamorfosi del progetto urbano. Milan: Franco Angeli.

Mazza, L (1997) Trasformazioni del piano. Milan: Franco Angeli.

Morandi, C (2007) Milan. The Great Urban Transformation. Venice: Marsilio.

Morandi, C (2006) 'Riflessioni sulla didattica della progettazione alla scala urbana'. In C Morandi and S Gullino (eds) Milano. Esercizi di urban design. Milan: Clup.

Morandi, C and Pucci, P (1998) Prodotti notevoli. Ricerca sui fattori di successo dei progetti di trasformazione urbana. Milan: Franco Angeli.

Nicolin, P (2007) 'Milano Boom. Dall'etica della produzione all'estetica del consumo.' Lotus international, 131, pp. 4–9.

Palazzo, D (2008) Urban Design. Un processo per la progettazione urbana. Milan: Mondadori.

Palermo, PC (2009) I limiti del possibile. Governo del territorio e qualità dello sviluppo. Rome: Donzelli.

— (2001) Prove di innovazione. Nuove forme ed esperienze di governo del territorio in Italia. Milan: Franco Angeli.

Palermo, PC and Ponzini, D (2009) Spatial Planning and Urban Development. Critical Perspectives. Berlin, Heidelberg and New York, NY: Springer.

Portas, N (1998) 'L'emergenza del progetto urbano.' Urbanistica, 110, pp. 51–60.

Quaroni, L (1967) La Torre di Babele. Padua: Marsilio.

Rogers, EN (1959) 'Per l'autonomia della cultura.' Casabella, 244, p. 3.

Rossi, A (1966) Architettura della città. Padua: Marsilio.

Samonà, G (1959) L'urbanistica e l'avvenire delle città. Rome and Bari: Laterza.

Secchi, B (1989) Un progetto per l'urbanistica. Turin: Einaudi.

Secchi, B (1986) 'Una nuova forma di piano.' Urbanistica, 82, pp. 6–13.

Secchi, B (1984) 'Le condizioni sono cambiate.' Casabella, 498–9, pp. 8–13.

Selicato, F and Rotondo, F (2010) Progettazione urbanistica. Teorie e tecniche. Milan: McGraw-Hill

Zucchi, C (2000) 'Una città non è un albero'/ Nuovi modelli di spazio urbano. In Ciorra, P and D'Annuntiis, M (eds) Nuova architettura italiana. Il paesaggio italiano tra architettura e fotografia. Milan: Skira.

The Netherlands

Charretteteam Hoboken 2030 (2009) Gebiedsvisie Rotterdam 2030, Internationaal topmilieu met ruimte voor lichaam en geest. Rotterdam: Rotterdam Municipality.

Department of Urban Planning of Rotterdam Municipality and Maxwan Architects and Urbanists (2008) Centraal district Rotterdam, Stedenbouwkundig plan 2007. Rotterdam: Rotterdam Municipality.

Florida, Richard (2010) The Great Reset. London: HarperCollins Publishers.

Marlet, Gerard (2009) De aantrekkelijke stad. Nijmegen: VOC uitgevers.

Projectbureau Hart van Zuid and Westerlengte (2011) Ambitiedocument Hart van Zuid. Rotterdam: Rotterdam Municipality.

Rotterdam Municipality (2007) Rotterdam Urban Vision 2030. Rotterdam: Rotterdam Municipality. English translation: KA Jakimowicz.

Sassen, Saskia (2008) Stad moet niet schoon en net zijn. Het Parool.

Czech Republic

Literature in English
Books
Berger, Jiří (2006a) Czechia from the Air. Pilsen: Fraus.

Berger, Jiří (2006b) Prague from the Bird's Eye View. Prague: Soukup & David s.r.o.

Maier, Karel et al (1998) Urban Development of Prague: History and Present Issues. Prague: Czech Technical University.

Norberg-Schulz, Christian (1984) Genius Loci. Towards a Phenomenology of Architecture. New York, NY: Rizzoli

Society of Czech Architects (1995) Czech Architecture 1945–1995. Prague: Society of Czech Architects

Literature in Czech
Books
Broncová, Edita (2006) Praha 13 – Město uprostřed zeleně. Prague: MILPO MEDIA s.r.o.

Česká komora architektů (2009) Miroslav Baše. Město – Suburbie – Venkov. Prague: ČKA.

Halík, P, Kratochvíl, P and Nový, O (1996) Architektura a město. Prague: Academia.

Hnilička, Pavel (2005) Sídelní kaše. Otázky k suburbánní výstavbě rodinných domů. Brno: ERA.

Hrůza, Jiří (1989) Město Praha. Prague: Odeon.

Hrůza, Jiří (1960) Česká města. Prague: NČVU.

Hrůza, Jiří (1958) Stavba měst v Československu. Prague: Svaz architektů ČSR.

Irop (2008) Výstavba Prahy ve druhé polovině 20. století. Prague: Irop.

Maier, Karel (2004) Územní plánování. Prague: Vydavatelství ČVUT.

Articles
Oberstein, Ivo (2005) 'Jihozápadní město', Architekt, 3/2005: 29–33.

Oberstein, Ivo (2003) 'Centrální park na pražském Jihozápadním Městě.' Zahrada – Park – Krajina, 5/2003, 7–11.

'O hraně města 21. Století'. Architekt, 7/2002, 20–8.

Říha, Martin (2002) 'Mezi městem a krajinou', Architekt, 7/2002, 18–19.

'Za námi sídliště.' Architekt, 6/2001, 43–45.

'Zlatý Anděl – administrativně-obchodní centrum v Praze'. Architekt, 5/2008, 3–23.

Dubai

Ramos, Stephen J (2010) Dubai Amplified: The Engineering of a Port Geography. Farnham, Surrey: Ashgate.

Zack, Stephen (2007) 'Beyond the Spectacle', Metropolis, November 2007. Available at: www.metropolismag.com/story/20071121/beyond-the-spectacle

Egypt

Abu Lughod, J (1971) Cairo: 1001 years of the City Victorious. Princeton, NJ: Princeton University Press.

Akbar, J (1988) Crisis in the Built Environment: The Case of the Muslim City. Leiden: EJ Brill.

Bianca, S (2000) Urban Form in the Arab World: Past and Present. London: Thames and Hudson.

Dover, Kohl and Partners (2008) 'A New Traditional Community, New Giza, Egypt', charette booklet.

Hakim, B (1986) Arabic-Islamic Cities – building and planning principles. London and New York: Kegan Paul International.

Hanna, N (1984) 'Construction Work in Ottoman Cairo (1517–1798)', Supplement aux Annales Islamologiques, Cahier 4, pp. vi–71.

Nasser, N (2003) 'Cultural Continuity and Meaning of Place: An Approach to Sustaining Historic Cities of the Islamicate World', Journal of Architectural Conservation, 1, pp. 77–94.

Steinberg, F (1991) 'Architecture and Townscape in Today's Cairo, the Relevance of Tradition', Ekistics, 58, pp. 75–86.

Stewart, D (1999) 'Changing Cairo: The Political Economy of Urban Form', International Journal of Urban and Regional Research, 23, pp. 128–46.

Volait, M (2003) 'Making Cairo Modern (1870–1950): Multiple Models for a European-style Urbanism', in J Nasr and M Volait (eds) Urbanism Imported or Exported? Native aspirations and Foreign Plans. Chichester: Wiley-Academy.

Morocco

Boumaza, N (2006) Villes réelles, villes projetées. Villes maghrebines en fabrication. Paris: Maisonneuve & Larose.

Cohen, JL and Eleb, M (2004) Casablanca. Mythes et figures d'une aventure urbaine. Paris: Hazan.

Dryef, M (1994) Urbanisation et droit de l'urbanisme au Maroc. Paris: CNRS editions, Editions de la Porte.

Institut d'Aménagement et d'Urbanisme Ile de France (2010) 'Le Maroc s'ouvre au XXIe siècle', les Cahiers (special issue) No. 154.

Navez-Bouchanine, F (1996) 'La médina au Maroc: elites et habitants. Des projets pour l'esapce dans des temps différents', Annales de la recherché urbaine, No. 72, pp. 15–22.

Signoles, P et al (1999) L'urbain dans le monde arabe. Politiques, instruments et acteurs. Paris: CNRS editions.

South Africa

Dewar, D and Uytenbogaardt, RS (1991) South African Cities: A Manifesto for Change. Cape Town: Urban Problems Research Unit, University of Cape Town.

Argentina

Asher, F (2004) Los nuevos principios del urbanismo. Madrid: Alianza Editorial.

Aslan, L, Joselevich, I, Novoa, G, Saiegh y, D and Santaló, A (1992) Inventario de Patrimonio Urbano Puerto 1887–1992. Santiago de Chile: Facultad de Arquitectura – UBA.

Corporación Antiguo Puerto Madero SA (1999) 1989–1999, un modelo de gestión urbana. Buenos Aires: Corporación Antiguo Puerto Madero.

Evans, JM (2009) Sustentabilidad en arquitectura: Compilación de antecedentes de manuales de buenas prácticas ambientales para las obras de arquitectura, junto a indicadores de sustentabilidad y eficiencia energética. Buenos Aires: Consejo Profesional de Arquitectura y Urbanismo.

Novick, A (1991) Técnicos locales y extranjeros en la génesis del urbanismo argentino. Buenos Aires, 1880–1940. In Anales del Instituto de Arte Americano. Buenos Aires: FADU-UBA.

Tella, G (2009) Buenos Aires Albores de una ciudad moderna. Buenos Aires: Nobuko.

Brazil

Abers, R (1998) 'Learning Democratic Practice: Distributing Government Resources through Popular Participation in Porto Alegre, Brazil', in M Douglass and J Friedmann (eds) Cities for Citizens: Planning and the Rise of Civil Society in a Global Age. New York: John Wiley & Sons.

Andreoli, Elisabetta and Forty, Adrian (eds) (2004) Brazil's Modern Architecture. London: Phaidon.

Brakarz, José with Margarita Green and Eduardo Rojas (2002) Cities for All: Recent Experiences with Neighborhood Upgrading Programs. Washington, DC: Inter-American Development Bank.

del Rio, Vicente (1992) 'Urban Design and Conflicting City Images of Brazil', Cities, vol. IX # 4.

— (1990) Introdução ao Desenho Urbano no Processo de Planejamento. Sao Paulo: Pini.

del Rio, Vicente (ed.) (2010) 'Urban design in Brazil – Research and Practice', Urban Design International (special issue) vol. 15, # 2, summer 2010.

del Rio, Vicente; Burcher, Lise; Kesner, Brian; and Nelisher, Maurice (2002) 'A Model for Undergraduate Study in Urban Design', Unpublished paper. Baltimore, MD: Proceedings of the National Conference of the Association of Collegiate Schools of Planning.

del Rio, Vicente and Gallo, Haroldo (2000) 'The Legacy of Modern Urbanism in Brazil', DOCOMOMO International Journal, 23, pp. 23–27.

del Rio, Vicente and Santos, Ana Cristina (1988) 'A Outra Urbanidade: A Construção da Cidade Pós-Moderna e o Caso da Barra da Tijuca', in V del Rio (ed.) Arquitetura: Pesquisa & Projeto. Sao Paulo: Pro-Editores.

del Rio, Vicente and Siembieda, William (eds) (2009) Contemporary Urban Design in Brazil: Beyond Brasilia. Gainesville, FL: University Press of Florida.

Del Rio, Vicente, Levi, Daniel and Duarte, Cristiane (2011) Perceived Livability and Sense of Community: Lessons for Designers from a Favela in Rio de Janeiro. In F Wagner and R Caves (eds) Community Livability. San Francisco: Routledge.

Duarte, Cristiane and Magalhaes, Fernanda (2009) 'Upgrading Squatter Settlements into City Neighborhoods: The Favela Bairro Program, Rio de Janeiro', in V del Rio and W Siembieda (eds) Contemporary Urban Design in Brazil: Beyond Brasilia. Gainesville, FL: University Press of Florida.

Fernandes, Edesio (2001) 'New Statute Aims to Make Brazilian Cities More Inclusive', Habitat News.

Fernandes, Edesio and Valença, Marcio (2001) 'Urban Brazil', Geoforum (special issue) vol. 32 # 4.

Fraser, Valerie (2000) Building the New World: Studies in the Modern Architecture of Latin America, 1930-1960. London: Verso.

Holston, James (1989) The Modernist City: An Antropological Critique of Brasilia. Chicago: University of Chicago Press.

Irazabal, Clara (2010) 'Urban Design, Planning and the Politics of Development in Curitiba', in V del Rio and W Siembieda (eds) Contemporary Urban Design in Brazil: Beyond Brasilia. Gainesville, FL: University Press of Florida.

— (2004) City Making and Urban Governance in the Americas – Curitiba and Portland. London: Ashgate.

Leme, Maria Cristina Dias (ed.) (1999) Urbanismo no Brasil, 1895-1965. Sao Paulo: Studio Nobe/FUPAM.

Machado, Rodolfo (ed.) (2003) The Favela Bairro Project: Jorge Mario Jauregui Architects. Cambridge, MA: Harvard University Graduate School of Design.

Menegat, Rualdo (2002) 'Participatory democracy and sustainable development: integrated urban environmental management in Porto Alegre, Brazil', Environment & Urbanization, vol. 14 # 2.

Pereira, Margareth Dias (2002) 'The Time of the Capitals: Rio de Janeiro and Sao Paulo', in A Almadoz (ed) Planning Latin American Capital Cities: 1850–1950. London: Routledge.

Perlman, Janice (2010) Favela – Four Decades of Living on the Edge in Rio de Janeiro. Oxford: Oxford University Press.

— (1976) The Myth of Marginality: Urban Poverty and Politics in Rio de Janeiro. Berkeley, CA: University of California Press.

Santos, Carlos Nelson Ferreira dos (1988) A Cidade Como um Jogo de Cartas. Niterói: Universitária.

Santos, Evandro (2011) Curitiba, Brazil. Saarbrücken, Germany: LAP Lambert Academic Publishing.

Ribeiro, Luiz Cesar and Cardoso, Adauto (eds) (2003) 'Reforma Urbana e Gestão Democrática. Promessas e Desafios do Estatuto da Cidade', Rio de Janeiro.

Rodrigues, Ferdinando de Moura (1986) Desenho Urbano – Cabeca, Campo e Prancheta. Sao Paulo: Editora Projeto.

Schwartz, Hugh (2003) Urban Renewal, Municipal Revitalization: The Case of Curitiba, Brazil. Falls Church, VA: Higher Education Publications.

Trindade, Dirceu (2010) 'Challenges of New Town Design in a Frontier Region: Palmas', in V del Rio and W Siembieda (eds) Contemporary Urban Design in Brazil: Beyond Brasilia. Gainesville, FL: University Press of Florida.

Turkienicz, Benamy (1984) 'Desenho Urbano. Anais do I SEDUR – Seminario de Desenho Urbano'. Cadernos de Arquitetura 12, 13 and 14. Editora Projeto, São Paulo.

Turkienicz, Benamy and Mauricio, Malta (1986) Desenho Urbano. Anais do II – Seminario de Desenho Urbano no Brasil. Sao Paulo: PINI.

Underwood, David (1991) 'Alfred Agache, French Sociology, and Modern Urbanism in France and Brazil', Journal of the Society of Art Historians, 50 (June).

USA

American Planning Association (2006) Planning and Urban Design Standards. Hoboken, NJ: John Wiley & Sons, Inc.

Broberg, Brad (Summer 2011) On Common Ground. Washington, DC: National Association of Realtors.

Chase, J, Crawford, M and Kaliski, J (eds) (1999) Everyday Urbanism. New York: The Monacelli Press.

Chase, John (2000) Glitter Stucco & Dumpster Diving. New York, NY: Verso.

Hegeman, W and Peets, E (1998) The American Vitruvius: An Architect's Handbook of Civic Art. Princeton New York: Architectural Press.

Jacobs, J (1961) The Death and Life of Great American Cities. New York: Random House.

Kelbaugh, Douglas (2002) Repairing the American Metropolis. Seattle, WA: University of Washington Press.

Krieger, Alex (Spring/Summer 2006). 'Toward an Urbanistic Frame of Mind', Harvard Design Magazine, p. 3.

Leinberger, Christopher (2007) The Option of Urbanism: Investing in a New American Dream. Washington: Island Press.

Lynch, K (1960) The Image of the City. Cambridge, MA: The MIT Press.

Marshall, Richard (Spring/Summer 2006). 'The Elusiveness of Urban Design', Harvard Design Magazine, pp. 21–32.

Plattus, Alan (1988) The American Vitruvius: Civic Art. New York, NY: Princeton Architectural Press.

Roberts, Marion (1999) 'MAUD', Urban Design Strategies Lecture at the University of Westminster, London.

Sert, JL and CIAM (1942) Can our Cities Survive? Cambridge, MA: Harvard University Press.

Spreiregen, Paul (1965) Urban Design: The Architecture of Towns and Cities. New York, NY: McGraw-Hill.

Waldheim, Charles (2006) The Landscape Urbanism Reader. New York, NY: Princeton Architectural Press.

Watson, Donald, Plattus, Alan and Shibley, Robert (2003) Time-Saver Standards for Urban Design. New York: McGraw-Hill.

2010 Harvard and 2011 Congress for the New Urbanism debates. Available at: www.newurbannetwork.com/article/street-fight-landscape-urbanism-versus-new-urbanism-14855

Australia

Australian Bureau of Statistics website: www.abs.gov.au

Boyd, R (1960) The Australian Ugliness. Melbourne: FW Cheshire.

Claisebrook Village website: www.mra.wa.gov.au/projects/Claisebrook-Village

Freestone, R (2010) Urban Nation: Australia's Planning Heritage. Melbourne: CSIRO Publishing.

Perry, M (2010) 'Australian cities must transform for population growth', Reuters Business Spectator, 15 March 2010.

Urban Design Forum Quarterly, issue 83 (September 2008).

Urban Design Forum Quarterly, issues 89 (March 2010) to 93 (March 2011).

New Zealand

Auckland City Council (1969) Auckland's Historical Background. Auckland: Auckland City Council.

— (1995) Public Transport Beyond 2000 – the Britomart Underground Terminal and Associated Development.

— (2004) Auckland City Council City Centre District Plan: Section 14 The Britomart Precinct (now part of Auckland Council District Plan).

Bernhardt, J (ed.) (2008) A Deeper Shade of Green. Auckland: Balasoglou Books.

Haarhoff, E (2010) 'Mastering the art of urban design', Urban, September 2010, pp. 11–12.

Hamilton City Council (2006) CityScope. Available at: www.hcc.govt.nz

Kawharu, H (2001) 'Land and Identity in Tamiki: A Ngati Whatua Perspective', Hillary Lecture 2001 at the Auckland War Memorial Museum. Available at: www.aucklandmuseum.com

Ministry for the Environment (2011) Signatories to the Urban Design Protocol. Available at: www.mfe.govt.nz/issues/urban/design-protocol/signatories.html

— (2010i) Taking Stock of the Urban Design Protocol and Action Plan Monitoring, CR98.

— (2010ii) Urban Design Panels: A National Stocktake, ME1023.

— (2009i) Urban Design Stocktake of Resource Management Plans and Policies: Summary Report, ME973.

— (2009ii) Urban Design Toolkit, ME922.

— (2009iii) Rethinking our Built Environment: Toward a Sustainable Future, ME 916.

— (2008i) Review of Urban Design Case Law, ME912.

— (2008ii) Urban Design Case Studies: Local Government, ME879.

— (2008iii) A National Policy Statement on Urban Design: Background Paper, ME899.

— (2006) A Survey of Local Government Authorities Urban Design Capability.

— (2005i) New Zealand Urban Design Protocol, ME579.

— (2005ii) Urban Design Action Pack, ME 580.

— (2005iii) Urban Design Case Studies, ME581.

— (2005iv) The Value of Urban Design, ME606.

— (2005v) Urban Design Research in New Zealand, ME683.

— (2002) People, Places, Spaces: A Design Guide for Urban New Zealand, ME420.

— (1999) Proposed Approach for Indicators for Urban Amenity, Technical Paper No 54.

New Zealand Planning Institute (2009) Education Policy and Accreditation Procedures. Auckland: New Zealand Planning Institute.

North Shore City Council (2010) District Plan Section 21 Plan Change 30 (now part of Auckland Council District Plan).

Index

Rossi, Aldo 50
Rotterdam 69–75
Royal Town Planning Institute 6
Rueda, Salvador 86

Sao Paulo, Brazil 257, 260
Sassen, Saskia 76
Seaside, Florida 280
security 262 (*see also* crime prevention; gated communities)
Sennett, Richard 278
Sert, Jose Luis 279
shanty-towns *see* informal settlements
shared public space 68 (*see also* public spaces)
Sitte, Camilo 31, 327
slums *see* informal settlements
social integration 232, 266, 269, 331
social segregation 179, 257, 331 (*see also* gated communities)
socialist approaches 116–17, 198–9
Solá Morales, Manuel de 85
South Africa 178–93
Spain 80–95
squares *see* public spaces
Städtebau 31
Stadtplanung 31
stakeholder participation 25, 39, 72, 268
standards *see* design standards
streetscape 141, 276, 284
suburban development 6, 22, 121, 151, 152, 181, 299, 304–5
sustainable development 335–6 (*see also in chapters for each country*)
Sweden 96–111

terminology *see* definitions
Thamesmead 5
Thays, Carlos 241
Tibbalds, Francis 6
Tigre, Buenos Aires 250–2
town planning 4, 31, 32, 49, 88, 329
Transit-Oriented Development (TOD) 185, 281
transport and mobility 53, 58, 185, 203, 300, 336
Transportation Investment Generating Economic Recovery (TIGER) 281–2
Turkienicz, Benamy 261
Turning Torso, Malmö 108

United Kingdom 3–11
United States 274–89
Urban Design Alliance (UDAL) 7
Urban Design Group 6, iv
urban design practice 330–2 (*see also in chapters for each country*)
urban design profession 325–6, 328–9 (*see also in chapters for each country*)
urban extensions 23–7, 37–42, 123–6, 140–2, 152, 153–7, 229–32, 250–2
urban form 8, 11, 152, 332 (*see also* grids; public squares; streetscape)
'urban planners' 31, 32, 43
urban redevelopment *see* redevelopment schemes
'urban renaissance' 10
Urban Task Force 7, 10
urbanisme 15
urbanistes 17

Valle, Gino 56

Wadala Metropolitan Centre, Mumbai 229–32
Waldheim. Charles 277
water management 68, 185, 204, 300
waterfronts 85, 101, 103–8, 138, 140–2, 213–14, 317–20
Wind Comb, San Sebastian 85
World Architecture Congress (WAC) 135
World Architecture Forum 134

Yingkou Peninsula 210–12

Zevi, Bruno 49

Image credits

239	Instituto geografico militar argentino	275	Geoff Dyer of PlaceMakers LLC		
241	Historic print	279	Old illustration		
242	(top) Taullard, A, Los planos más antiguos de Buenos Aires, 1580–1880. Buenos Aires, 1940	280	Old illustration		
242	(bottom) Dirección del catastro y via pública, City of Buenos Aires, 1970	283	Art Cueto		
243	Sebastian Loew	284	MP Architects – Stefanos Polyzoides		
245	Corporación Antiguo Puerto Madero	286	Howard Blackson of PlaceMakers LLC		
246	Corporación Antiguo Puerto Madero	287	Howard Blackson of PlaceMakers LLC		
247	(top) Sebastian Loew	292	Jenny Donovan		
247	(bottom) Sebastian Loew	293	Based on a map by Alexander C. Townsend & David A. Bruce, Barbara Hardy Centre for Sustainable Urban Environments, School of Natural & Built Environments, University of South Australia, City East Campus, North Terrace, Adelaide, South Australia		
250	Nordelta Argentina				
251	Nordelta Argentina				
252	Sebastian Loew				
256	Vicente del Rio				
259	Adapted by V. del Rio from original illustration in: Prefeitura do Districto Federal; Cidade do Rio de Janeiro: Extensão – Remodelação – Embellezamento; sob a direcção geral de Alfred Agache; Paris: Foyer Bresilien, 1930	297	Image supplied courtesy of the National Capital Authority		
		298	Mark Sheppard		
		299	Lend Lease		
		301	Prepared by David Lock Associates using a NearMap PhotoMap		
260	Vicente del RIo	302	Mark Sheppard		
262	Luis Fernando Teixeira, Grupo Quatro Arquitetos Associados	303	Mark Sheppard		
		308	David Truscott		
263	Newton Paniago; used by permission	311	David Truscott		
264	Vicente del Rio	314	Waterfront Auckland		
265	Jean Pierre Janot; used by permission	315	David Truscott		
267	Jorge Mario Jauregui	316	David Truscott		
268	Illustration adapted by V. del Rio from the original courtesy of Pedro da Luz Moreira, Archi 5	317	Waterfront Auckland		
		318	David Truscott		
269	Vicente del Rio	319	(top) David Truscott		
270	Vicente del Rio	319	(bottom) Waterfront Auckland		
274	Howard Blackson	320	Architectus		
		324	Sebastian Loew		

Front cover (from top)

Chengdu Financial City Investment & Development Co., Ltd

Atkins China

Palmbout Urban Landscapes, A2studio

National Capital Authority

Old engraving

Adapted by V. del Rio from original illustration in: Prefeitura do Districto Federal; Cidade do Rio de Janeiro: Extensão – Remodelação – Embellezamento; sob a direcção geral de Alfred Agache; Paris: Foyer Bresilien, 1930

Old illustration

Stadt Frankfurt am Main, Stadtplanungsamt

Ivo Oberstein, 2006

PGOU of Ponferrada 2007

Back cover

J.L. de las Rivas 2008

Note

The editor and publisher have made every effort to contact copyright holders and will be happy to correct, in subsequent editions, any errors or omissions that are brought to their attention.